Richard Y. Farnsworth, M.D.
Utah Valley Pediatrics, L.C.
1275 N. University Ave. #18
Provo, Utah 84604-2693
(801) 373-8930

Richard Y. Farnsworth /mo

9/29/03

AF761870

Pediatric Transfusion Therapy

AABB PRESS

Other related publications from the AABB:

Informed Consent for Blood Transfusion
Edited by Christopher Stowell, MD, PhD

Pediatric Hemotherapy Data Card
Edited by Patricia Pisciotto, MD

Technical Manual, 14th edition
Edited by Mark E. Brecher, MD

Standards for Cord Blood Services, 1st edition

Transfusion Support for Patients with Sickle Cell Disease
Edited by Wendell F. Rosse, MD; Marilyn J. Telen, MD; and Russell E. Ware, MD, PhD

Pediatric Transfusion Therapy

Editors

Jay H. Herman, MD
Cardeza Foundation for Hematologic Research
Thomas Jefferson University
Philadelphia, Pennsylvania

Catherine S. Manno, MD
The Children's Hospital of Philadelphia
Philadelphia, Pennsylvania

AABB Press
Bethesda, Maryland
2002

Mention of specific products or equipment by contributors to this AABB Press publication does not represent an endorsement of such products by the AABB Press nor does it necessarily indicate a preference for those products over other similar competitive products.

Efforts are made to have publications of the AABB Press consistent in regard to acceptable practices. However, for several reasons, they may not be. First, as new developments in the practice of blood banking occur, changes may be recommended to the AABB *Standards for Blood Banks and Transfusion Services.* It is not possible, however, to revise each publication at the time such a change is adopted. Thus, it is essential that the most recent edition of the *Standards* be consulted as a reference in regard to current acceptable practices. Second, the views expressed in this publication represent the opinions of authors. The publication of this book does not constitute an endorsement by the AABB Press of any view expressed herein, and the AABB Press expressly disclaims any liability arising from any inaccuracy or misstatement.

To purchase additional copies of this book, please call our sales department at (301)215-6499 or fax orders to (301)907-6895. AABB sales representatives are available from 8:30 am to 5:00 pm, EST, Monday through Friday, for telephone access. For other book services, including chapter reprints and large quantity sales, ask for the Senior Sales Associate.

Visit the American Association of Blood Banks Web site on the Internet at www.aabb.org or e-mail our sales department at sales@aabb.org.

American Association of Blood Banks
8101 Glenbrook Road
Bethesda, Maryland 20814-2749

ISBN NO. 1-56395-162-2
Printed in the United States

Contributors

David Bigos, MD
Temple University Children's
Medical Center
Philadelphia, Pennsylvania

Linda A. Chambers, MD
American Red Cross
Arlington, Virginia

Anne F. Eder, MD, PhD
The Children's Hospital of Philadelphia
Philadelphia, Pennsylvania

Andrew K. Feng, MD
Floating Hospital for Children
Boston, Massachusetts

Christopher J. Festa, MD
Temple University Children's
Medical Center
Philadelphia, Pennsylvania

David F. Friedman, MD
The Children's Hospital of Philadelphia
Philadelphia, Pennsylvania

Michael Goodstein, MD, FAAP
York Hospital
York, Pennsylvania
Pennsylvania State University
Hershey, Pennsylvania

Jed Gorlin, MD
Memorial Blood Centers
University of Minnesota
Minneapolis, Minnesota

Stephan Grupp, MD, PhD
University of Pennsylvania
The Children's Hospital of Philadelphia
Philadelphia, Pennsylvania

Haewon C. Kim, MD
University of Pennsylvania
School of Medicine
The Children's Hospital of Philadelphia
Philadelphia, Pennsylvania

Norma B. Lerner, MD
University of Rochester School of
Medicine and Dentistry
Galisano Children's Hospital at Strong
Rochester, New York

Cathy Litty, MD
St. Christopher's Hospital for Children
Philadelphia, Pennsylvania

Naomi L.C. Luban, MD
Children's National Medical Center
George Washington University
Medical Center
Washington, District of Columbia

Catherine S. Manno, MD
University of Pennsylvania School
of Medicine
The Children's Hospital of Philadelphia
Philadelphia, Pennsylvania

Geralyn M. Meny, MD
American Red Cross
Philadelphia, Pennsylvania

David N. Moolten, MD
American Red Cross
Musser Blood Center
Philadelphia, Pennsylvania

Sandra Taddie Nance, MS, MT(ASCP)SBB
American Red Cross
Philadelphia, Pennsylvania

Patricia T. Pisciotto, MD
University of Connecticut Health Center
Farmington, Connecticut

Joseph G. Pressey, MD
The Children's Hospital of Philadelphia
Philadelphia, Pennsylvania

Susan D. Roseff, MD
Virginia Commonwealth University
School of Medicine
Virginia Commonwealth University
Health Systems
Richmond, Virginia

Kim Smith-Whitley, MD
University of Pennsylvania School of
Medicine
The Children's Hospital of Philadelphia
Philadelphia, Pennsylvania

Ronald G. Strauss, MD
University of Iowa College of Medicine
DeGowin Blood Center
University of Iowa Hospitals and Clinics
Iowa City, Iowa

David Stroncek, MD
National Institutes of Health
Bethesda, Maryland

Jessica Wang-Rodgriguez, MD
University of California, San Diego,
La Jolla, California

Table of Contents

Preface

FOUR YEARS AGO, THE AMERICAN ASSOCIATION OF BLOOD Banks approached us to develop a comprehensive text that unifies the special aspects of transfusion therapy for neonatal and pediatric patients. Although certain topics are well referenced in this area, there are few sources of information that focus exclusively on the practice of pediatric transfusion therapy.

Over the past 30 years, common practices have been developed to address issues of blood collection, administration, and storage specific to the needs of children. The changing metabolic profile and small body size of neonates and children are often overlooked by standard techniques and policies, and misapplication of certain adult principles may harm young transfusion recipients. As is true for transfusion medicine in general, controlled studies in pediatric populations that facilitate evaluation of specific practices are often lacking. Rather, there is reliance on small, uncontrolled studies of clinical transfusion practice. Many of these practices have their roots shrouded in history, and were based on concerns that were clinically relevant at the time, but which have now outlived their need for application.

For example, two decades ago, it was standard practice to insist that all newborns receive RBCs stored for no more than 7 days. This practice began when respiratory distress syndrome of the premature was rampant, and the effect of red cell 2,3-DPG depletion was of particular concern in these severely hypoxic, acidemic infants. The advent of surfactant therapy has brought dramatic changes to the respiratory support of these very small infants, and has led to the realization that 2,3-DPG levels are of little clinical relevance today. Still, the push to limit donor exposure through dedicating separate units for individual neonates has been hampered by the continued insistence on blood remaining "fresh" for every transfusion. Clinicians have felt that there must be sound blood bank reasons for fresh blood and therefore continued to order it, while blood bankers have felt that there must be clinical reasons why it was being ordered and so continued to collect, stock, and administer it.

In an effort to remedy this kind of information gap, we charged the chapter authors to keep foremost the differences of pediatric patients and to remember that the intended audience for this book cuts across many disciplines and professions, and includes anyone involved in the transfusion of children. We recognize that not all children are transfused in pediatric-oriented institutions, and that many practices in children's hospitals may not easily transfer to a transfusion service that predominantly focuses on the transfusion of adult patients. While many pediatric physicians and nurses know how they practice transfusion medicine, the principles that justify these practices are often not taught. Conversely, many technical staff may not be well versed in understanding the clinical concerns that dictate pediatric modification of transfusion polices and procedures originally developed for adults. We hope that this book will foster communication among those involved in the transfusion of children.

Some topics deserved a straightforward and didactic review, while others required a balanced assessment of the pros and cons of the more controversial aspects of pediatric transfusion therapy. The latter often involve firmly held opinions that have much theory but little data to support them. Whenever possible, the authors have included studies of pediatric and neonatal populations. However, many transfusion studies in adults can be applied to these age groups and must suffice when the proper age group studies have not been performed.

The book starts with a discussion of the fetal and neonatal immune response, which has begun to have its mechanisms elucidated. This has direct bearing on the special circumstances involving compatibility testing for neonates and children. Chapters on the indications for red cells and other components for neonates follow, as well as an overview of the immune cytopenias and the use of special components such as granulocytes.

This section is followed by exploration of more controversial areas in pediatric transfusion. Those authors were charged with presenting a balanced discussion regarding which additive solutions to use, how old blood can be, and whether to irradiate the components, along with a review of the risks of cytomegalovirus transmission and prevention methods. Donor limitation practices and the special adaptations for blood collection and transfusion in pediatrics are then addressed.

A series of clinical chapters for older children follow, beginning with the transfusion needs of pediatric patients with hemoglobin disorders, which includes a discussion of phenotype matching for sickle cell patients. The role of fresh whole blood for cardiac surgery is addressed, followed by an overview of transfusion support for pediatric surgical, intensive care, and trauma patients. Although not widely used, intraoperative blood recovery can be applied to pediatric patients and this topic seemed to fit nicely at this point.

More specialized topics follow, including chapters on transfusion therapy for the hemophilias and immune thrombocytopenic purpura. The choice between apheresis and pooled platelet concentrates is considered, as well as transfusion therapy for pediatric oncology and hematopoietic transplant patients. This leads to a chapter on peripheral blood progenitor cell collection, which is followed by one on the indications and techniques for therapeutic apheresis for children, including erythrocyte exchange. The book concludes with a discussion of adverse reactions of transfusion in pediatric patients.

Because many of the topics themselves have a degree of overlap, it was impossible to prevent redundant discussions of issues from one chapter to the next. We feel this is actually fortunate, as we anticipate that the book will be read one chapter at a time more often than all in a single sitting. We have tried to ensure that where there is overlap, there is no significant disagreement among the authors.

In order to keep the book focused on the practice of pediatric transfusion, specialized areas such as transfusion consent were not included. This particular issue has much broader scope that encompasses all of Pediatrics, involving the dynamics of autonomy and guardianship of minors. Antenatal transfusion and "bloodless medicine" are practiced at only a handful of special centers, and we felt inclusion of these would not benefit the use of this text as a practical reference.

In conclusion, we would like to thank the publication staff at the AABB for their support and patience, especially Laurie Munk and Jennifer Boyer, who have diligently worked with us over the past 2 years as this project has come to fruition. We would also like to thank those of our friends and colleagues who agreed to author the chapters. We admire their energy and perseverance in the face of the ever-growing decline in available time for educational pursuits. We thank the technical staffs in our respective blood banks where much of the difficult, exacting practice of transfusion is executed every day of the year. Finally, we would like to thank all of the children we have cared for over the past two decades who have taught us so much about the practice of pediatric transfusion therapy.

Jay H. Herman, MD
Catherine S. Manno, MD
Editors

About the Editors

Jay H. Herman, MD, is Director of Transfusion Medicine at Thomas Jefferson University in Philadelphia, where he is also a member of the Cardeza Foundation for Hematologic Research and the Division of Hematology. Prior to 2001, he held the rank of Professor in the Departments of Medicine and Pathology at Temple University School of Medicine, also in Philadelphia. There he attended on the Stem Cell Transplant Unit and was Medical Director of Stem Cell Collection and Processing, and had been Director of Transfusion Medicine from 1993 until 1999. Earlier in his career, he was Director of the Transfusion Service and the Hematology/Coagulation Laboratory at St. Christopher's Hospital for Children and Medical Director of the Penn-Jersey Regional Blood Services of the American Red Cross, both in Philadelphia.

Dr. Herman received his medical degree from Harvard Medical School and continued his medical training at Grady Memorial Hospital, University of Virginia Medical Center and Johns Hopkins Hospital. He is board certified in Pediatrics, Pediatric Hematology/Oncology, and Blood Banking. He has authored over 100 papers, chapters, and abstracts related to transfusion medicine and hematology, and is coeditor of the AABB book *Current Issues in Platelet Transfusion Therapy and Platelet Alloimmunity*.

Dr. Herman is most known for his study in the field of platelet transfusion practice, but other areas of interest include pediatric transfusion practice, platelet and granuloctye immunology, and neonatal alloimmune disorders. Dr. Herman is a member of the American Association of Blood Banks, the American Society of Hematology, the American Society of Pediatric Hematology/Oncology, the American Society for Apheresis, and the International Society for Cellular Therapy.

Catherine S. Manno, MD, is currently the Acting Chief of the Division of Hematology at The Children's Hospital of Philadelphia, and Medical Director of the Blood Bank and Transfusion Service there. She is also an Associate Professor of Pediatrics at the University of Pennsylvania School of Medicine.

Dr. Manno received her Bachelor of Arts degree in Zoology from Duke University in Durham, and her medical degree from Hahnemann Medical College in Philadelphia. She completed her residency in Pediatrics at St. Christopher's Hospital for Children in Philadelphia and a fellowship in Hematology at The Children's Hospital of Philadelphia.

In addition to membership in the AABB, Dr. Manno is a member of the American Society of Hematology, the American Society of Pediatric Hematology/Oncology, and the American Society of Gene Therapy. She has volunteered on several organizational committees, and is currently the chair of the Medical Advisory Committee of the American Red Cross Penn-Jersey Region.

Dr. Manno's areas of interest include the treatment of hemophilia and other hematologic disorders in children, and the development of gene-based therapies. She is currently serving as an investigator in clinical trials with the objectives of developing gene-based therapies for hemophilia A and B. She is a frequent lecturer and has authored or co-authored many research articles, book chapters, and reviews.

In: Herman JH, Manno CS, eds.
Pediatric Transfusion Therapy
Bethesda, MD: AABB Press, 2002

1

The Fetal/Neonatal Immune Response

JESSICA WANG-RODRIGUEZ, MD

THE DEVELOPMENT OF THE NEONATAL IMMUNE SYStem is poorly understood. The neonatal immune system appears immature in its limited ability to respond to microbial challenges, while other aspects are entirely functional at the time of birth, even in very premature infants. Clinically, newborn infants are at increased risk for a variety of viral, fungal, and bacterial infections. The study of animal models as well as human cord blood can enhance our current understanding of the developing neonatal immune system at the cellular and molecular level.

The immune system in premature infants is characterized by extremely immature T-cell, B-cell, phagocytic, and natural killer (NK) cell functions.[1] This chapter reviews the key elements of

Jessica Wang-Rodriguez, MD, Associate Clinical Professor of Pathology, University of California, San Diego, La Jolla, California

natural and acquired neonatal and fetal immunity as we currently understand them and highlights the differences between immunity in the newborn child and in the adult. In addition, many recent studies regarding the immune response after an antigenic challenge such as blood transfusion are discussed, as are the uncertainties of its long-term effect.

Neutrophils

Neutrophils (polymorphonuclear leukocytes), which possess abundant cytoplasmic granules, participate in the effector phase of specific immune responses. These cells play important roles in inflammation and natural immunity and function to eliminate microbes and dead tissues. They respond rapidly to chemotactic stimuli, and they phagocytose and destroy foreign particles, such as microbes. They can also be activated by cytokines produced primarily by macrophages and endothelial cells, and they are the major cell population in the acute inflammatory response. Neutrophils also express receptors for IgG and complement proteins; thereby, they phagocytose opsonized particles and function as effector cells of humoral immunity.[2]

In newborns, the total white blood cell (WBC) count is quite high during the first hours of life, which is probably due to demargination from the "stress" of delivery.[2] Circulating neutrophils have a half-life of 8 hours. Fetal and neonatal marrow contains expanded precursor cell populations, and the basal proliferative rate of these cells is nearly maximal.[3] The neutrophil storage pool in human neonatal marrow is considerably smaller than that in adult marrow, and, in the face of sepsis, it may be rapidly exhausted. A seriously infected neonate may rapidly consume the limited neutrophil stores, which will diminish the capacity to accelerate proliferation, leading to neutropenia.

Cytokines such as granulocyte colony-stimulating factor (G-CSF) and granulocyte-macrophage colony-stimulating factor (GM-CSF), which are responsible for neutrophilic proliferation and maturation, are severely depressed in premature neonates.[4] The levels decrease with less gestational age or lower birth weight.[5] Trials of G-CSF or GM-CSF in infants with sepsis showed a rapid neutrophilia in treated infants, but no clear evidence of survival advantage.[6,7] Further, prophylactic treatment with GM-CSF does not appear to reduce the incidence of nosocomial infections.[7]

Premature neonates are more deficient in neutrophil adherence, chemotaxis, oxidative metabolism, bacterial killing, and phagocytic activity than term neonates, who in turn have lower activity than adult neutrophils. The phagocytic ability of neutrophils to ingest *Escherichia coli* bacteria was measured among the stressed, well, maturing, and term infants. All of the preterm neutrophils (stressed, well, maturing) ingested significantly fewer bacteria than the term neutrophils.[8] The impaired phagocytic function and chemotaxis may be in part due to a decreased expression of lymphocyte function-associated antigen (LFA-1) and complement receptor 3 (CR3, Mac-1CD11b/CD18) in the premature neonates.[9]

Lymphocytes

T Cells

T lymphocytes initiate specific immunity, cell-mediated and humoral, by recognizing portions of protein antigens (peptides) bound to major histocompatibility complex (MHC) Class II molecules on the surface of antigen-presenting cells (APCs). T cells recognize antigen through the T-cell receptor (TCR), which is structurally similar to immunoglobulin[10] (Fig 1-1). The TCR is composed of an α/β or γ/δ heterodimer, each containing proximal constant and distal variable regions.[11-13] The variable region forms an antigen-binding domain, while the constant region links the TCR to the cell membrane. The antigen-recognition site is determined by variable (V), diversity (D), and joining (J) regions through DNA recombination. The germline DNA sequences encoding these polypeptide chains undergo rearrangement during T-cell development in the thymus, producing as many as 10^8 combinations of α and β chains. Additional diversity is achieved by random splicing of the V and J chains and of additional nontemplated nucleotides attached by the enzyme terminal deoxynucleotidyl transferase. The TCR associates on the cell sur-

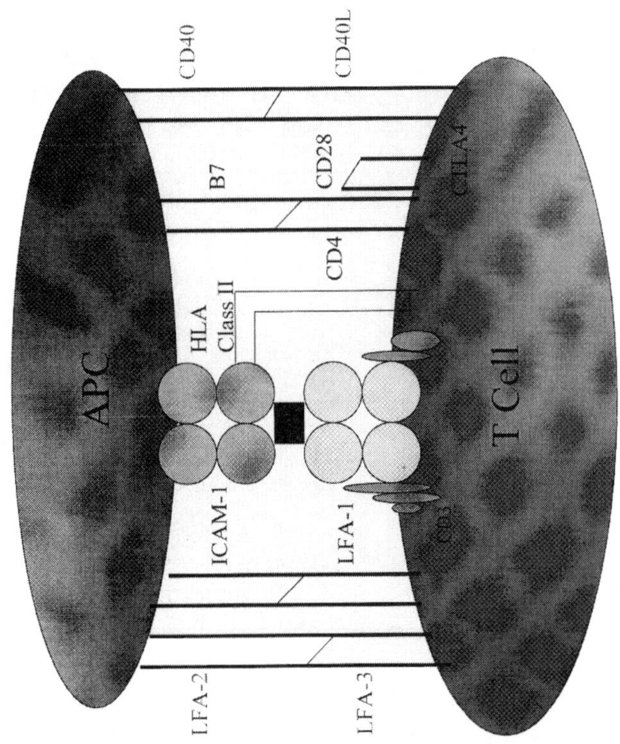

Figure 1-1. The interaction between an APC and a T cell. Various accessory molecules (CD4 or CD8) and costimulatory molecules need to be present for T-cell activation. Inhibition of the costimulatory molecules would give an anergic effect.

face with the pentameric CD3 complex, which links the TCR to other cellular components needed to mediate transduction of signals from the receptor to the cell interior.[14]

For T-cell activation to occur, the TCR in the CD3 complex has to bind a peptide fragment in the groove of the MHC molecule from an APC,[15] a phenomenon known as allorecognition. Peptides (self or non-self proteins, alloantigens, or viral proteins) are endogenously processed by the APCs and expressed in the specific HLA site.[16,17] For complete activation to occur, secondary costimulatory molecules must also be present. The best-characterized costimulatory interaction is through the receptor CD28 and CTLA4 on T cells and on B7 (CD80) on the APCs (Fig 1-1). Without the costimulatory molecules' interaction, a state of "anergy" or "tolerance" occurs.[18-22] Inactivating this pathway can potentially aid in the treatment of autoimmune disease, organ transplantation, and graft-vs-host disease (GVHD). Other proposed costimulatory pathways include the CD27/CD70,[23] the LFA-1 and intercellular adhesion molecule (ICAM-3),[24,25] the CD2/CD58,[26] and the CD5/CD72,[27] as well as the CD40-CD40L pathway that appears to costimulate CD4 but not CD8 T cells.[28]

Other cell surface receptor-ligand pairs are involved in cell adhesion, activation, and specific effector functions. LFA-1 (CD11a/18) on T cells interacts with ICAM-1 (CD54), ICAM-2, and ICAM-3 on APCs to facilitate cell adhesion. Similarly, vascular leukocyte antigen-4 (VLA-4) interacts with its ligand vascular cell adhesion molecule-1. Accessory molecules may mediate the interactions of lymphocytes with the extracellular matrix, which itself has effects on lymphocyte function, including lymphocyte activation. Some of the major molecules involved in T-cell recognition of peptide are shown schematically in Fig 1-1.

Cytokine Production

After activation, T cells are identified and divided into subsets on the basis of developmental history, cell surface markers, and cytokine production. Cytokines are small peptide molecules that transmit signals for growth and differentiation of other cells, as well as activation of other cell types to regulate and modulate the immune response against foreign antigens. On the basis of their cytokine production, the CD4+ helper cells are further divided into Th1 and Th2 cells. Th1 cells produce inflammatory cytokines such as interleukin (IL)-2, interferon-γ, and tumor necrosis factor (TNF)-β, whereas Th2 cells produce immunoregulatory cytokines such as IL-4, IL-5, IL-6, IL-9, IL-10, and IL-13. Th1 is involved in phagocyte-dependent inflammatory response against specific intracellular pathogens, whereas Th2 cells stimulate antibody production and eosinophil and mast cell differentiation, independently of phagocytic functions. T cells expressing cytokines of both patterns, designated as Th0, are intermediate forms based on the ratio of cytokines produced and the nature of the responding cells. Th3 cells are characterized as producing increased amounts of transforming growth factor (TGF)-β.[29-31] Th1 and Th2 subpopulations are responsible for a variety of immune consequences in many clinical conditions (Table 1-1).

Another pathway for T-cell activation independent of TCR has been identified. IL-12 and IL-18, produced by dendritic cells and

Table 1-1. Th1 vs Th2 Cytokine Response

TH1 Immune Response	TH2 Immune Response
IgG2a	Support of B-lymphocyte differentiation and production of IgE, A, M→G
Activation of macrophage; cellular immunity; delayed-type hypersensitivity	Inhibition of macrophage; activation of eosinophils and mast cell
Destruction of intracellular parasites, bacteria, virus	Destruction of extracellular parasites, response to allergens
Organ autoimmune disease	Hypereosinophilic syndrome
Crohn's disease	Atopic disorder
Allograft rejection	Graft tolerance
Spontaneous abortion	Normal pregnancy
Tuberculosis, leprosy	Lepromatous leprosy
Cutaneous Leishmania	Visceral Leishmania

macrophages, can upregulate CD40/CD40L in the presence of interferon (INF)-γ and -α and thereby promote the Th1 differentiation.[32] In addition, IL-12 stimulates the production of other cytokines and proinflammatory agents, such as TNF-α, GM-CSF, macrophage-CSF, IL-3, IL-8, and IL-2, from NK and T cells. IL-12 also enhances the cytolytic activity of resting and activated NK and lymphokine-activated killer cells.[33] The T-cell differentiation and cytokine production are illustrated in Figs 1-2 and 1-3.

During the neonatal T-cell development, the T precursors migrate to the thymus at 8 weeks of gestation. In the thymus, prothymocytes acquire the TCR and the CD3 complex and express both CD4 and CD8 on the cell surface. These CD4+/CD8+ thymocytes undergo a process of self-recognition and clonal deletion of autoreactive T cells. The mature T cells express either CD4 or CD8 and recognize non-self-antigens only. The complete human thymic differentiation occurs by 18 to 20 weeks of gestation. However, the diversity of TCR is limited, as a result of either immature TCR repertoire or limited exposure of antigens. The limited TCR repertoire may be partly due to nonrandom usage of TCR D and J elements and limited nucleotide additions to V-D and D-J joining sites. This leads to shorter and flatter antigen-binding sites.[34,35] The antigen-binding sites apparently increase in size and complexity with an increase in gestational age. In the study of cord blood TCRs, oligoclonal expansion of T-cell third complementarity-determining region (CDR3) was greater than that in the adult peripheral blood T cells, with the greatest expansion at 29 to 33 weeks of gestation, and a gradual decline at term.[36]

Once the immunologically naïve T cells are activated by selected, internally processed antigens, CD4 and CD8 T cells differentiate in the expression of different CD45 isoforms.[37] The cytokines produced by the activated T cells direct the cells to undergo proliferation and remain as memory T cells (CD45RA−/RO+). Secondary or memory immune responses are more vigorous against targeted antigens. Unlike adults, neonates have immature T-cell development, both qualitatively and functionally. The distribution of naïve and memory T-cell subpopulation differs in neonates and adults. Studies of umbilical cord blood shows that most of the T lymphocytes in the neonates are naïve

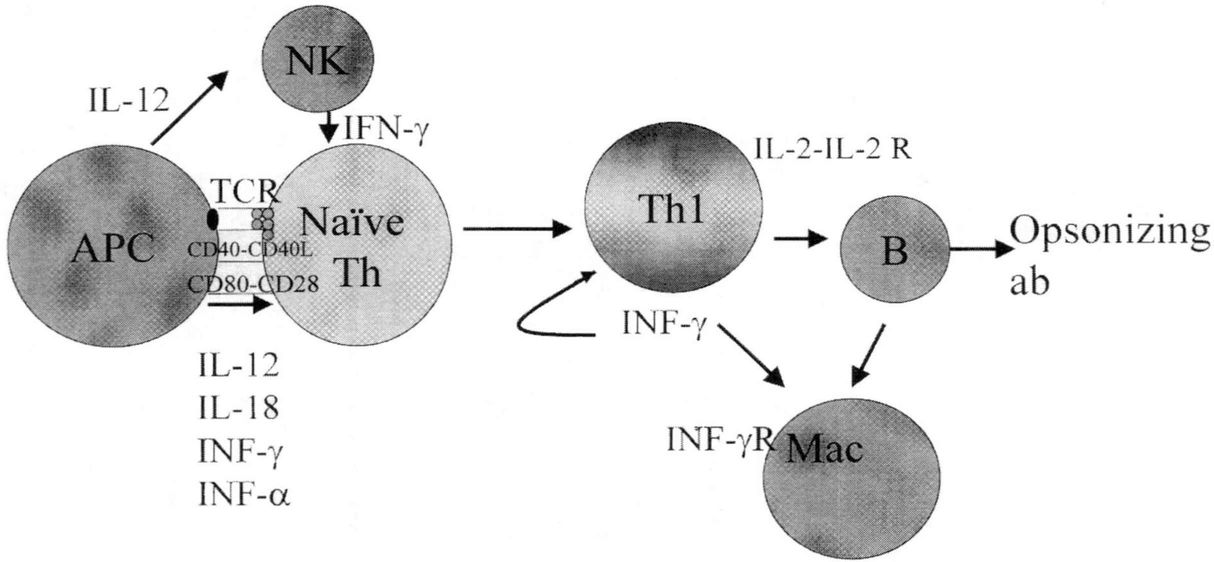

Figure 1-2. Th1 response after T-cell activation. Various cytokines are elaborated following naïve helper T-cell stimulation. IL-2 and INF-γ are secreted by Th1 cells and further activate B cells and macrophages (Mac).

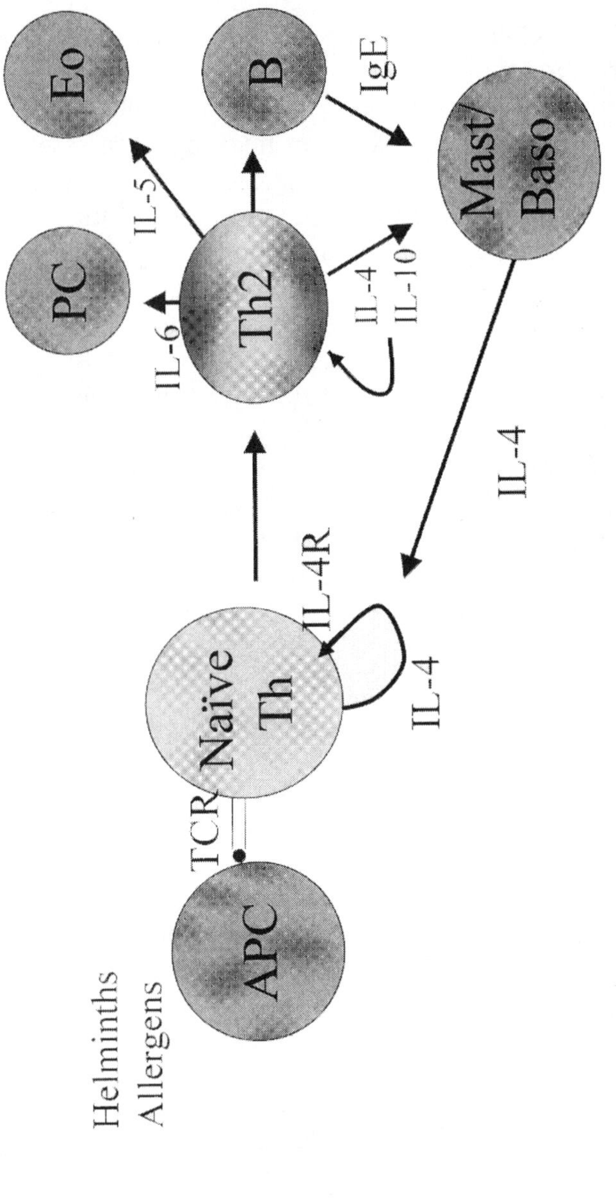

Figure 1-3. Th2 response after T-cell activation. The principal cytokine IL-4 is the initial force for Th2 differentiation, which further activates plasma cells (PC), eosinophils (Eo), B cells, and mast cells or basophils (Mast/Baso).

helper T cells (CD4+/CD45RA+/CD45RO−/CD29dim), with an absence of memory helper T cells (CD4+/CD45RO+/CD45RA−/CD29bright).[38] The CD45RA+ T cells in the cord blood are in the range of 61 to 90%, whereas adult peripheral blood T cells are 30 to 67%. The CD45RO+ cells in the cord blood are 0 to 6%, whereas adult peripheral blood T cells are 20 to 66%.[39,40]

CD45RA is the first antigen expressed by T cells during their intrathymic maturation, and it continues to be expressed by the majority of the immunologically naïve T cells in the neonate. CD45RA+/RO− T cells are involved mainly in immune suppression, either directly or via the induction of suppressor activity by CD8 cells. The CD45RA T cells are relatively unresponsive to antigenic stimulation.[41] As increased age allows increased antigenic exposure, CD45RA+ T cells co-express the lymph node homing receptor L-selectin (CD62L), lose the CD45RA, acquire CD45RO, and eventually lose CD62L.[42] CD45RA−/CD45RO+ memory cells become the predominant T cells in the circulation, and these cells are capable of recalling antigens and initiating B-cell antibody production. Umbilical cord blood T cells from term infants are capable of differentiating from naïve helper T cells to memory, adult-type, helper T cells upon mitogen stimulation ex vivo.[38] However, another report suggested a lower response rate in very low birth-weight infants than in adults.[43] The low level of CD45RA−/RO+ T cells in the neonates suggest some induction of antigen-specific T-cell memory, possibly initiated in utero.

It is unknown whether maternal influence contributes to the early selective memory T-cell formation and cytokine production. A variety of reports suggested that maternal exposure to allergens, infectious agents, food, alcohol, or steroid use may play a role.[44-47] Maternal history of atopy may boost the offspring's production of IFN-γ.[44] Monocytes derived from the cord blood of HIV-infected newborns have distinctly lower ability to produce IL-12 than those from noninfected infants.[45] Infants born of mothers who are kidney transplant recipients and who have been chronically treated with cyclosporine and methylprednisolone showed an impairment in the normal development of T, B, and NK cells, as manifested by depressed CD4 and CD8+ lymphocytes at birth, low CD25 (IL-2) receptor, and decreased

HLA-DR expression. CD57+ non-MHC-restricted cytotoxic lymphocytes also were lower than in normal newborns.[46] The long-term immune effects on these infants of the immunosuppressants of the mother are uncertain.

In a BALB/c mouse model, prenatal exposure to a certain antigen (ovalbumin) disposes neonatal mice to preferentially develop Th2 response with increased response to immunoglobulin production to immunization and higher frequencies of immediate-type skin test response. However, when the presensitized newborns are stimulated with PMA/ionomycin (Sigma, St Louis, MO), a decreased Th1 response is evident with a lower production of IFN-γ.[48]

Functionally, neonates are immature as well. CD45RA cord blood T lymphocytes secrete very little INF-γ and IL-4.[49] Term neonates are incapable of producing an adult level of IL-2 upon challenge by superantigens such as *Staphylococcus* enterotoxin B (SEB). In addition, compared with adult T cells, neonate T cells were hyporesponsive to IL-2 in the secondary response, despite an upregulation of IL-2 receptors after stimulation. The neonate T cells in the presence of SEB proliferated much less in the presence of exogenous IL-2 than did non-SEB-treated cells. Furthermore, the neonate cells do not respond to exogenous IL-4 at all,[50] probably as a result of the lack of memory T cells, as activated memory T cells generate IL-4 more efficiently than naïve T cells. Activated neonatal T cells also express less IL-2 receptor (CD25).[51] These findings suggest an inability to promote immunoglobulin synthesis by B cells, which may all contribute to neonatal susceptibility to serious infections, such as cytomegalovirus (CMV), herpes simplex, and rubella.

B Cells

In the normal stage of B-lymphocyte maturation, precursor B cells can produce heavy chains only cytoplasmically and not on the cell surfaces. There is no light chain production. Precursor B cells are capable of producing surface IgM but not IgG or IgA. Mature B cells express IgM and IgD and are capable of immunoglobulin gene rearrangement to switch classes to IgG, IgA, and IgE.

The immunoglobulin gene rearrangement is an antigen-driven process. In neonates, IgG and IgA production is impaired when the neonate B cells are stimulated with pokeweed mitogen.[1] Clinically, it is also apparent that repeated immunizations are necessary to achieve protective levels of antibody.

B cells are activated through surface cell-to-cell interaction with the activated T cells or through direct antigenic exposure. The B-cell receptor complex that contains surface IgM Igα and Igβ interacts with the antigen. Helper T lymphocytes, through interaction with the APCs, directly stimulate B lymphocytes through CD40 on the B-cell surface and a variety of cytokines (Figs 1-2 and 1-3) to produce antibodies. Once the B cells are fully differentiated, they become either plasma cells that produce a specific antibody or memory B cells.

IgM is the first antibody response formed by the B lymphocytes after antigenic exposure. These antibodies are pentamers with low affinity and nonspecificity. They can bind bacterial polysaccharides independent of T-cell activation. However, the response is not long-lived and does not produce B-cell memory. T- and B-cell activation is required for antigen-specific IgG production, which occurs late in the primary antigenic encounter. Upon secondary exposure to the same antigen, IgG can be rapidly produced by the memory B cells in high titers. IgA is synthesized primarily in the mucosa-related B lymphocytes and contributes to gut immunity. In infants, the primary source of IgA is from the IgA produced by breast milk. IgE production requires T-cell activation. Its primary role is to respond to allergic and parasitic disease. IgE in neonates is poorly studied, and its clinical role is uncertain.

B-cell immunoglobulin production is low in healthy neonates, as the majority of the circulating immunoglobulin is derived from maternal source. This low immunoglobulin production may be in part due to the immature neonatal B cells' inability to internalize, process, and present exogenous antigens to activate T cells to produce IL-2, as the processing and presenting of antigen by neonatal B cells is not adult-like until 28 days of age.[52] After acquisition of the antigen-presenting skills, IgM is required for antigen processing. However, neonatal B cells are unable to produce immunoglobulins beyond IgM until approximately 1 year of age. In addition, the interaction of the CD40 on B cells and CD40L on activated T cells is pivotal in immunoglobulin synthesis. In cord blood mononuclear cells, the CD40/CD40L interaction is ineffective, because of a lack of expression of CD40L on CD45RA/CD4+ cord blood cells, and it thereby contributes to a reduced immunoglobulin production in the neonates.[53]

IgG levels in the neonate at term are comparable to those in the adults, whereas premature infants (<32 weeks of gestational age) have extremely low IgG levels, which suggests that the majority of the transplacental passage of the IgG occurs during the last 4 to 6 weeks of gestation.[54] The low level of IgG may contribute to the premature neonate's susceptibility to infections. A recent meta-analysis did not show a reduction of septic episodes with prophylactic administration of intravenous immune globulin (IVIG), but a significant sixfold benefit in using IVIG in treating neonates with sepsis was shown.[55]

NK Cells

NK cells are a subset of large granular lymphocytes that are important in antigen-independent cytotoxicity. This MHC-independent cytolysis is important in clearing virus-infected cells prior to T-cell-mediated antigen recognition. In addition, NK cells with TCR are important in the rejection of malignant tumors and the regulation of autoimmune disease. Fc receptor (CD16) allows NK cells to recognize and directly kill antibody-coated cells. NK-cell cytolytic activities are composed of 1) recognition of and binding to a target cell, 2) lysis of the target, and 3) repetition of this lytic sequence by recycling. All three NK functions appear to be depressed in newborns, and they gradually improve with age. Cytolytic activity by NK and CD8+ cells is markedly decreased in neonates when measured by the level of killing of K562 cells,[56,57] which is clinically manifested by unusually severe viral infections such as herpes simplex virus.[58] Quantitatively, we and others have observed significantly fewer NK cells, as marked by CD3–/CD16+CD56+, in premature, very low birthweight infants than in term infants.[59-61]

The lack of functional NK cells could be due to insufficient cytokine signals such as IL-2 and INF-γ.[49,62,63] Recently, IL-12, a cytokine secreted by monocytes, macrophages, and dendritic cells, received much attention because it activates NK cytotoxicity in healthy adult cells and in HIV-infected patients with low levels of IL-12.[64] The mRNA expression of IL-12 and the level of IL-12 are lower in neonatal mononuclear cells than in adult mononuclear cells.[33] The diminished cytolytic activity by cord blood NK cells can be boosted by exogenous IL-12 in vitro.[65] Combined IL-2 and IL-12 can enhance the antibody-dependent cellular cytotoxicity as well as increase NK-cell functions quantitatively and functionally.[66]

Tolerance

Induction of tolerance can be achieved by a variety of ways: 1) stimulation of CD4+ T cells without the presence of costimulatory molecules and interaction from APCs; 2) preferential selection for the Th2 response; 3) insufficient antigenic particle presentation on an APC due to low expression; 4) inaccessibility of tissue or the cells for the APC presentation (naïve T cells do not gain access to peripheral nonlymphoid tissues, in contrast to activated/memory T cells, which can migrate into tissues); 5) induction of signal cannot change the naïve state of a T cell, therefore leaving it unrecognized; and 6) HLA similarity prevents recognition of non-self antigens.

Anergy can be induced in vivo by blocking CTL antigen (CTLA-4) or CD28, each of which binds to B7 receptor family on APCs. Embryonic tissue grafts that are devoid of hematopoietic cells can induce tolerance. Anergy is manifested by an inhibition of cytokine production and proliferation of Th1 response. For example, treating mice with soluble, hapten-conjugated proteins induced a selective inhibition of Th1 response but not of Th2 response.[67] Anergy can be overcome in some systems by the addition of accessory cells, including activated B cells, which may deliver costimulatory signals via receptors expressed on the T lymphocytes.

Response to Blood Transfusion

In adults, blood transfusion has certain immunomodulatory effects, presumably because of the presence of passenger leukocytes, as manifested by clinically observed febrile nonhemolytic reactions, GVHD, immune tolerance to allografts, and alloimmunization. Other, less clear effects include an increased incidence of postoperative wound infection and a reactivation of latent endogenous CMV.[68-75] The immune effects of blood transfusion in infants are not well studied, mainly because of the inability to collect multiple, large-volume blood samples from the infants for in vitro assays. Blood transfusion is a unique alloantigenic challenge for the neonatal immune system and is hypothesized as a T-cell-mediated response. Because of immature T-cell functions, neonatal production of red blood cell (RBC) alloantibody is rare,[76,77] and only a few case reports have appeared in the literature, including a report of HLA antibody production.[78] Furthermore, with limited donor exposure program in various transfusion centers,[79,80] repeated exposure to allogeneic WBCs from the same donor may impose a profound immunomodulatory effect.

Passenger leukocytes in RBCs may enhance the immunomodulation of blood transfusion, as reported in a prospective, randomized, double-blind study comparing the immune effect of blood transfusion of leukocyte-reduced and non-leukocyte-reduced RBCs in very low birthweight infants (birthweight <1000 g; gestational age 26±2 weeks) at various intervals for up to 2 weeks after transfusion.[61] Several observations were noted that were not previously reported in the literature. First, there was an increase in CD45RA and CD45RO cell population in both transfusion arms 5 to 7 days after transfusion, which suggests additional recruitment of CD45RA cells from the thymus and subsequent maturation into CD45RO cells.

Second, cells bearing CD3–/DR+ increased after transfusion, but the costimulatory molecule CD28 on T cells did not, which suggests that transfusion in general causes an immunosuppressive (Th2) effect, rather than immune activation. In addition, a decreased CD4:CD8 ratio was observed in infants who received either unmodified or leukocyte-reduced blood. This finding was also observed in another set of studies with larger infants.[1] The increase in HLA-DR along with upregulation of CD25 (IL-2 receptor) two days after exchange transfusion was observed previously, using unmodified whole blood.[81] However, another group did not detect any difference in CD3, CD4, CD8, or CD19 + lymphocytes or of IL-2 receptor (CD25) or HLA-DR expression 3 to 7 days after transfusion,[82] when using irradiated, washed, and partially leukocyte-reduced RBCs. Production of cytokines such as IL-2 and INF-γ was not altered by transfusion either. An additional study to include a large number of infants and a uniform method is necessary to settle the difference.

Third, the NK-cell population increased to near that in term infants approximately 2 weeks after blood transfusion, but it is uncertain whether this was due to a process of normal maturation of neonates or a specific response to blood transfusion, because the NK function was not studied. In previous studies of immunocompetent adults undergoing surgery or hemophiliac patients who receive multiple blood transfusions, NK activity in cell lysis was suppressed.[83-85] All of our findings were seen in both leukocyte-containing and leukocyte-reduced groups, which suggests that transfused blood containing cellular and humoral components in general affected the neonates' immune constitution and triggered a response that was more suppressive than stimulatory.

In addition, the kinetics of the irradiated donor leukocytes in the neonates after blood transfusion were studied. It is interesting to note that donor leukocytes are detected for no more than one day after blood transfusion. This rapid clearing of the transfused donor cells in the neonates is in contrast to the persistence of nonirradiated donor cells in adult trauma patients who received multiple transfusions.[86,87] These findings confirm the efficacy of irradiation of lymphocytes and imply that there is a neonatal functional capability to eliminate irradiated foreign cells.

Neonates may not be able to rapidly eliminate nonirradiated cells, however. A previous paper described the persistence of 1 to 10% of donor cells in infants receiving blood transfusion of maternal blood for up to 2 years after transfusion, but infants who received exchange or fetal transfusion of banked blood had a clearance of banked donor cells within 4 months. The failure to immediately eliminate allogeneic donor cells may be due to the presence of the nonirradiated cells. However, the fetus is tolerant of its mother's lymphocytes when the cells are directly infused into the peritoneal cavity.[88] There is, however, no mention of irradiation of the units, and no report of transfusion-related GVHD was mentioned. The best explanation is that HLA similarity between the mother and the fetus created a form of graft tolerance.

The potential effect in neonates of receiving coincidental, non-related, presumed HLA Class II-haploidentical blood may be further immune tolerance. This hypothesis was derived from transplant reports that the transfusion of HLA-haploidentical blood prolongs graft survival.[89] With a very small number of patients (n=2), we found that the patients who received presumed HLA Class II-haploidentical units developed necrotizing enterocolitis 2 and 3 months after the initial transfusion. One can speculate whether this is a fortuitous coincidence or is related to anergic response to microbial infection. A larger trial is necessary to confirm or refute this hypothesis.

Clinical manifestations from the possible immunosuppressive effect of blood transfusion in neonates are not well reported, because of many confounding factors such as infection and the neonate's baseline immaturity. An earlier report showed no difference in the incidence of infections in neonates at 4 months corrected age, regardless of whether they received a transfusion or not. The lymphocyte phenotypes (CD3, CD4, CD8, CD19, CD3−/CD56, CD8/CD11b+ or CD11b−, CD3+/DR+) and serum IgG concentrations were not statistically different in infants given frozen, deglycerolized, or CMV-negative, irradiated blood perinatally and in normal, nontransfused term infants.[90] The long-term effects of blood transfusion early in neonatal life are even more speculative. It is not known how these infants will react to future immunologic events such as solid organ or bone marrow transplantation, malignancy, surgery, or trauma. The early changes in immune antigenic markers after blood transfusion described so far can only begin to stimulate the imagination to sort out the risks and benefits of blood transfusion in neonates.

References

1. Burgio G, Ugazio A, Notarangelo L. Immunology of the neonate. Curr Opin Immunol 1990;2:770-7.
2. Schelonka R, Infante A. Neonatal Immunology. Semin Perinatol 1998; 22:2-14.
3. Christensen RD. Hematopoiesis in the fetus and neonate. Pediatr Res 1989;26:531-5.
4. Suen Y, Lee S, Qian J, et al. Dysregulation of lymphokine production in the neonate and its impact on neonatal cell mediated immunity. Vaccine 1998;16:1369-77.
5. Rondini G, Chirico G. Hematopoietic growth factor levels in term and preterm infants. Curr Opin Hematol 1999;6:192-7.
6. Gillan E, Christensen R, Suen Y, et al. A randomized, placebo-controlled trial of recombinant human granulocyte colony-stimulating factor administration in newborn infants with presumed sepsis: Significant induction of peripheral and bone marrow neutrophilia. Blood 1994;84: 1427-33.
7. Cairo MS, Agosti J, Ellis R, et al. A randomized, double-blind, placebo-controlled trial of prophylactic recombinant human granulocyte-macrophage colony-stimulating factor to reduce nosocomial infections in very low birth weight neonates. J Pediatr 1999;134:64-70.
8. Falconer A, Carr R, Edwards S. Impaired neutrophil phagocytosis in preterm neonates: Lack of correlation with expression of immunoglobulin or complement receptors. Biol Neonate 1995;68:264-9.
9. McEvoy L, Zakem-Cloud H, Tosi M. Total cell content of CR3 (CD11b/CD18) and LFA-1 (CD11a/CD18) in neonatal neutrophils: Relationship to gestational age. Blood 1996;87:3929-33.
10. Davis M, Bjorkman P. T-cell antigen receptor genes and T-cell recognition. Nature 1988;334:395-402.
11. Brenner M, McLean J, Dialynas D, et al. Identification of a putative second T-cell receptor. Nature 1986;322:145-9.
12. Strominger J. Developmental biology of T cell receptors. Science 1989; 244:943-50.
13. Watschinger B, Gallon L, Carpenter C, et al. Mechanisms of allorecognition. Recognition by in vivo-primed T cells of specific major histocompatibility complex polymorphisms presented as peptides by responder antigen-presenting cells. Transplantation 1994;57:572-6.

14. Fling S, Arp B, Pious D. HLA-DMA and -DMB genes are both required for MHC class II/peptide complex formation in antigen-presenting cells. Nature 1994;368:554-8.
15. Michielin O, Luescher I, Karplus M. Modeling of the TCR-MHC-peptide complex. J Molec Biol 2000;300:1205-35.
16. Heath W, Kane K, Mescher M, et al. Alloreactive T cells discriminate among a diverse set of endogenous peptides. Proc Natl Acad Sci U S A 1991;88:5101-5.
17. Dalchau R, Fangmann J, Fabre JW. Allorecognition of isolated, denatured chains of class I and class II major histocompatibility complex molecules. Evidence for an important role for indirect allorecognition in transplantation. Eur J Immunol 1992;22:669-77.
18. Linsley P, Brady W, Grosmaire L, et al. Binding of the B cell activation antigen B7 to CD28 costimulates T cell proliferation and interleukin 2 mRNA accumulation. J Exp Med 1991;173:721-30.
19. Koulova L, Clark E, Shu G, et al. The CD28 ligand B7/BB1 provides costimulatory signal for alloactivation of CD4+T cells. J Exp Med 1991; 173:759-62.
20. Gimmi C, Freeman G, Gribben JG, et al. B-cell surface antigen B7 provides a costimulatory signal that induces T cells to proliferate and secrete interleukin 2. Proc Natl Acad Sci U S A 1991;88:6576-9.
21. Gimmi C, Freeman G, Gribben JG, et al. Human T-cell clonal anergy is induced by antigen presentation in the absence of B7 costimulation. Proc Natl Acad Sci U S A 1993;90:6586-90.
22. Greenfield E, Nguyen D, Kuchroo V. CD28/B7 costimulation: A review. Crit Rev Immunol 1998;18:389-418.
23. Hintzen R, Jong RD, Lens SMA, et al. CD27: Marker and mediator of T-cell activation? Immunol Today 1994;15:307-11.
24. Hernandez-Caselles T, Rubio G, Campanero MR, et al. ICAM-3, the third LFA-1 counterreceptor, is a co-stimulatory molecule for both resting and activated T lymphocytes. Eur J Immunol 1993;23:2799-806.
25. Campanero M, Pozo MD, Arroyo AG, et al. ICAM-3 interacts with LFA-1 and regulates the LFA-1/ICAM-1 cell adhesion pathway. J Cell Biol 1993;123:1007-16.
26. Brown M, Cantrell D, Brattsand G, et al. The CD2 antigen associates with the T-cell antigen receptor CD3 antigen complex on the surface of human T lymphocytes. Nature 1989;339:551-3.
27. Beyers A, Spruyt L, Williams A. Molecular associations between the T-lymphocyte antigen receptor complex and the surface antigens CD2, CD4, or CD8 and CD5. Proc Natl Acad Sci U S A 1992;89:2945-9.
28. Cayabyab M, Phillips J, Lanier L. CD40 preferentially costimulates activation of CD4+ T lymphocytes. J Immunol 1994;152:1523-31.
29. Romagnani S. T-cell subsets (Th1 versus Th2). Ann Allergy Asthma Immunol 2000;85:9-21.

30. Abbas A, Murphy K, Sher A. Functional diversity of helper T lymphocytes. Nature 1996;383:787-93.
31. Romagnani S. Human Th1 and Th2: Doubt no more. Immunol Today 1991;12:256-7.
32. Armant M, Armitage R, Boiani N, et al. Functional CD40 ligand expression on T lymphocytes in the absence of T cell receptor engagement: Involvement in interleukin-2-induced interleukin-12 and interferon-gamma production. Eur J Immunol 1996;26:1430-4.
33. Lee S, Suen Y, Chang L, et al. Decreased interleukin-12 (IL-12) from activated cord versus adult peripheral blood mononuclear cells and upregulation of interferon-γ, natural killer, and lymphokine-activated killer activity by IL-12 in cord blood mononuclear cells. Blood 1996;88:945-54.
34. Schroeder H, Mortari F, Shiokawa S, et al. Developmental regulation of the human antibody repertoire. Ann N Y Acad Sci 1995;764:242-60.
35. Kormori T, Okata A, Stewart V, et al. Lack of N regions in antigen receptor variable region genes of TdT-deficient lymphocytes. Science 1993;261:1171-5.
36. Schelonka R, Raaphorst F, Infante D, et al. T cell receptor repertoire diversity and clonal expansion in human neonates. Pediatr Res 1998;43:396-402.
37. Clement L. Isoforms of the CD45 common leukocyte antigen family: Markers for human T-cell differentiation. J Clin Immunol 1992;12:1-10.
38. Neubert R, Delgado I, Webb J, et al. Assessing lymphocyte functions in neonates for revealing abnormal prenatal development of the immune system. Teratog Carcinog Mutagen 2000;20:171-93.
39. Morimoto C, Letvin N, Distaso J, et al. The isolation and characterization of the human suppressor inducer T cell subset. J Immunol 1985;134:1508-15.
40. Morimoto C, Letvin N, Boyd AW, et al. The isolation and characterization of the human helper inducer T cell subset. J Immunol 1985;134:3762-9.
41. Hayward A, Groothuis J. Development of T cells with memory phenotype in infancy. Adv Exp Med Biol 1991;310:71-6.
42. Picker L, Treer J, Ferguson-Darnell B, et al. Control of lymphocyte recirculation in man. 1. Differential regulation of the peripheral lymph node homing receptor L-selectin on T cells during the virgin to memory cell transition. J Immunol 1993;150:1105-21.
43. Bussel J, Cunningham-Rundles S, LaGamma E, Shellabarger M. Analysis of lymphocyte proliferative response subpopulations in very low birth weight infants and during the first eight weeks of life. Pediatr Res 1988;23:457-62.
44. Prescott S, Holt P, Jenmalm M, Bjorksten B. Effects of maternal allergen-specific IgG in cord blood on early postnatal development of allergen-specific T-cell immunity. Allergy 2000;55:470-5.
45. Chougnet C, Kovacs A, Baker R, et al. Influence of human immunodeficiency virus-infected maternal environment on development of infant interleukin-12 production. J Infect Dis 2000;181:1590-7.

46. DiPaolo S, Schena A, Morrone L, et al. Immunologic evaluation during the first year of life of infants born to cyclosporine-treated female kidney transplant recipients: Analysis of lymphocyte subpopulations and immunoglobulin serum levels. Transplantation 2000;69:2049-54.
47. Wolcott R, Jennings S, Chervenak R. In utero exposure to ethanol affects postnatal development of T- and B-lymphocytes, but not natural killer cells. Alcoholism Clin Exp Res 1995;19:170-6.
48. Herz U, Ahrens B, Scheffold A, et al. Impact of in utero Th2 immunity on T cell deviation and sebsequent immediate-type hypersensitivity in the neonate. Eur J Immunol 2000;20:714-18.
49. Lewis DB, Yu CC, Meyer J, et al. Cellular and molecular mechanisms for reduced interleukin-4 and interferon-γ production by neonatal T-cells. J Clin Invest 1991;87:194-202.
50. Macardle P, Wheatland L, Zola H. Analysis of the cord blood T lymphocyte response to superantigen. Human Immunol 1999;60:127-39.
51. Hassan J, Reen D. Cord blood CD4+ CD45RA+ T cells achieve a lower magnitude of activation when compared with their adult counterparts. Immunology 1997;90:397-401.
52. Morris J, Hoyer J, Pierce S. Antigen presentation for T cell-interleukin-2 secretion is a late acquisition of neonatal B cells. Eur J Immunol 1992;22:2923-8.
53. Brugnoni D, Airo P, Graf D, et al. Ineffective expression of CD40 ligand on cord blood T cells may contribute to poor immunoglobulin production in the newborn. Eur J Immunol 1994;24:1919-24.
54. Landor M. Maternal-fetal transfer of immunoglobulins. Ann Immunol 1995;74:279-83.
55. Jenson H, Pollock B. The role of intravenous immunoglobulin for the prevention and treatment of neonatal sepsis. Semin Perinatol 1998;22: 50-63.
56. Yabuhara A, Kawai H, Komiyama A. Development of natural killer cytotoxicity during childhood: Marked increases in number of natural killer cells with adequate cytotoxic abilities during infancy to early childhood. Pediatr Res 1990;28:316-22.
57. Merrill JD, Sigaroudinia M, Kohl S. Characterization of natural killer and antibody-dependent cellular cytotoxicity of preterm infants against human immunodeficiency virus-infected cells. Pediatr Res 1996;40:498-503.
58. Landers DV, Smith JP, Walker CK, et al. Human fetal antibody-dependent cellular cytotoxicity to herpes simplex virus-infected cells. Pediatr Res 1994;35:289-92.
59. Keever C. Characterization of cord blood lymphocyte subpopulations. J Hematother 1993;2:203-6.
60. Mills K, Gross T, Varney M, et al. Immunologic phenotype and function in human bone marrow, blood stem cells, and umbilical cord blood. Bone Marrow Transplant 1996;18:53-61.

61. Wang-Rodriguez J, Fry E, Fiebig E, et al. Immune response to blood transfusion in very-low-birthweight infants. Transfusion 2000;40:25-34.
62. Milosevits J, Pocsik E, Schimdt B, et al. Immunotypic and functional characteristics of haemopoietic cells from human cord blood. Scand J Immunol 1995;42:493-500.
63. Chehimi J, Valiante NM, D'Andrea A, et al. Enhancing effect of natural killer cell stimulatory factor (NKSF/interleukin-12) on cell-mediated cytotoxicity against tumor-derived and virus-infected cells. J Immunol 1993;23:1825-30.
64. Lau AS, Sigaroudinia M, Yeung MC, Kohl S. Interleukin-12 induces interferon-γ expression and natural killer cytotoxicity in cord blood mononuclear cells. Pediatr Res 1995;39:150-5.
65. Suen SLY, Chang L. Decreased interleukin-12 (IL-12) from activated cord versus adult peripheral blood mononuclear cells and up regulation of interferon-gamma, natural killer, and lymphokine-activated killer activity by IL-12 in cord blood mononuclear cells. Blood 1996;88:945-54.
66. Nguyen Q, Roberts R, Ank B, et al. Enhancement of antibody-dependent cellular cytotoxicity of neonatal cells by interleukin-2 (IL-2) and IL-12. Clin Diagn Lab Immunol 1998;5:98-104.
67. Burstein H, Shea C, Abbas A. Aqueous antigens induce in vivo tolerance selectively in IL-2 and IFN-gamma-producing cells. J Immunol 1992;148: 3687-91.
68. Blumberg N, Triulzi D, Heal J. Transfusion-induced immunomodulation and its clinical consequences. Transfus Med Rev 1990;4:24-35.
69. Fernandez L, MacSween M, You C, Gorelick M. Immunologic changes after blood transfusion in patients undergoing vascular surgery. Am J Surg 1992;163:263-9.
70. Jensen LS, Andersen A, Christiansen P, et al. Postoperative infection and natural killer cell function following blood transfusion in patients undergoing elective colorectal surgery. Br J Surg 1992;79:513-16.
71. McRae J, Lampe H, Banerjee D. Blood transfusions and phenotypic immune profile in head and neck cancer patients undergoing surgical resection. J Otolaryngol 1991;20:310-14.
72. Lang P, Bierling P, Buisson C, et al. Influence of posttransplantation blood transfusion on kidney allograft survival: A one-center, double-blind, prospective, randomized study comparing cryopreserved and fresh red blood cell concentrates. Transplant Proc 1993;25:616-18.
73. Triulzi D, Vanek K, Ryan D, Blumberg N. A clinical immunologic study of blood transfusion and postoperative bacterial infection in spinal surgery. Transfusion 1992;32:517-24.
74. Ziv Y, Shohat B, Gelerenter I, Wolloch Y. The influence of perioperative transfusions on the immunological profile of patients with colorectal adenocarcinoma. Panminerva Med 1992;34:4-12.
75. Klein H. Wolf in wolf's clothing. Is it time to raise the bounty on the passenger leukocytes? Blood 1992;80:1865-8.

76. Ludvigsen C, Swanson J, Thompson T, McCullough J. The failure of neonates to form red blood cell alloantibodies in response to multiple transfusions. Am J Clin Pathol 1987;87:250-1.
77. Floss AM, Strauss R, Goeken N, Knox L. Multiple transfusions fail to provoke antibodies against blood cell antigens in human infants. Transfusion 1985;26:419-22.
78. Russell AB, Rivers R, Darvey N. The development of anti-HLA antibodies in multiply transfused preterm infants. Arch Dis Child 1993;68:49-51.
79. Strauss R. Red blood cell transfusion practices in the neonate. Perinatal Hematol 1995;22:641-55.
80. Wang-Rodriguez J, Mannino F, Liu E, Lane T. A novel strategy to limit blood donor exposure and blood waste in multiply transfused premature infants. Transfusion 1996;36:64-70.
81. Romano M, El Marsafy A, Marseglia G, et al. Increased percentage of activated Ia+ T lymphocytes in peripheral blood of neonates following exchange blood transfusion. Clin Immunol Immunopathol 1987;43:301-7.
82. DePalma L, Duncan B, Chan M, Luban N. The neonatal immune response to washed and irradiated red cells: Lack of evidence of lymphocyte activation. Transfusion 1991;31:737-42.
83. Jensen L, Andersen A, Christiansen P, et al. Postoperative infection and natural killer function following blood transfusion in patients undergoing elective colorectal surgery. Br J Surg 1992;79:513-16.
84. Mathiesen O, Lund L, Brodthagen U, et al. The effect of previous blood transfusion on lymphocyte subsets and natural killer cell function in patients with colorectal cancer. Vox Sang 1994;67:36-41.
85. Kaplan J, Sarnaik S, Gitlin J, Lusher J. Diminished helper/suppressor lymphocyte ratios and natural killer activity in recipients of repeated blood transfusions. Blood 1984;64:308-10.
86. Lee T, Donegan E, Slichter S, Busch M. Transient increase in circulating donor leukocytes after allogeneic transfusions in immunocompetent recipients compatible with donor cell proliferation. Blood 1995;85:1207-14.
87. Lee TH, Paglieroni T, Ohto H, et al. Longterm multi-lineage chimerism of donor leukocytes in transfused trauma patients. Blood 1996;88(Suppl 1):265a.
88. Hutchinson D, Turner J, Schlesinger E. Persistence of donor cells in neonates after fetal and exchange transfusion. Am J Obstet Gynecol 1971;109:281-4.
89. Bayle F, Masson D, Zaoui P, et al. Beneficial effect of one HLA haplo- or semi-identical transfusion versus three untyped blood units on alloimmunization and acute rejection episodes in first renal allograft recipients. Transplantation 1995;59:719-23.
90. Kutvirt S, Armon M, Simon T, Lewis S. Lymphocyte phenotypes and infection incidence in transfused preterm neonates. Transfus Med 1996;6:329-36.

In: Herman JH, Manno CS, eds.
Pediatric Transfusion Therapy
Bethesda, MD: AABB Press, 2002

2

Compatibility Issues in Neonatal and Pediatric Transfusion

SANDRA TADDIE NANCE, MS, MT(ASCP)SBB, AND
GERALYN M. MENY, MD

AS IN OTHER AREAS OF transfusion medicine, compatibility testing for neonatal and pediatric patients shares similarities with testing for adult recipients. However, as one might expect, there are several unique issues that must be considered in the transfusion of neonatal and pediatric patients. One issue is that of samples for testing—the balance between obtaining enough blood to perform the testing and avoiding excessive blood loss. An-

---

Sandra Taddie Nance, MS, MT(ASCP)SBB, Director, Technical Services, Penn-Jersey Region, and Director, National Reference Laboratory for Blood Group Serology, American Red Cross; and Geralyn M. Meny, MD, Medical Director, American Red Cross, Penn-Jersey Region, Philadelphia, Pennsylvania

other issue is the source of blood for testing—the advantages and disadvantages of umbilical cord, capillary, or venous blood. Additional issues concern the necessary modifications to testing methods. This chapter highlights these unique issues and concerns.

Neonatal Compatibility Testing

Initial pretransfusion testing required by AABB *Standards for Blood Banks and Transfusion Services*[1] includes determination of ABO group and Rh type. Repeat ABO grouping and Rh typing may be omitted during the remainder of the neonate's hospital admission.

The test for unexpected antibodies may be performed on a sample from either the neonate or the mother.[1] Alloimmunization following red cell transfusion to a neonate is an unlikely event. Ludvigsen et al[2] did not detect antibody production during the first 3 months after birth in 90 neonates who received a mean of 14.1 transfusions from an average of 8.9 donors. In another report, 53 infants failed to produce unexpected clinically significant red cell alloantibodies after receiving 683 red cell transfusions from 503 different donors during the first 4 months of life.[3] Thus, if the initial antibody screen is negative, repeat testing for unexpected antibodies may be omitted during the remainder of the neonate's hospital admission, provided group O red cells are transfused. If a non-group-O neonate needs to receive non-group-O red cells that are incompatible with the maternal ABO group, the neonate's serum or plasma should be tested for anti-A or anti-B at the antiglobulin phase and compatible blood should be issued. If the initial antibody screen detects clinically significant unexpected red cell antibodies, the neonate should receive either units lacking the corresponding antigen(s) or units compatible by antiglobulin crossmatch. If there is difficulty obtaining components, testing of current and future neonate samples for unexpected antibodies should be performed to determine if maternal antibody continues to be present in the neonate. This will determine the antigen type of units that are required for transfusion.

Samples for Testing

Umbilical Cord Blood

A sample of umbilical cord blood should be collected from every newborn at the time of birth. The sample may be stored for 1 week in the blood bank and used in tests to evaluate infants at risk for hemolytic disease of the newborn (HDN).

ABO (and D) testing of newborns is determined through red cell testing.[4(p505)] Umbilical cord serum ABO antibodies are frequently of maternal origin. Newborns who received intrauterine transfusions often type as D-negative because of D-negative blood transfusion in utero and may give discrepant ABO typing results. A positive direct antiglobulin test (DAT) may identify newborns with HDN. The transfusion service may confirm results using an additional blood sample from the newborn, such as a heelstick sample. The strength of the DAT does not indicate the severity of the hemolysis; however, reactions are usually weakly positive in ABO HDN and strongly positive in Rh HDN. Antibody may be eluted from the red cells and the specificity can be determined. This eluate may be used for compatibility testing if a maternal sample is unavailable. It is important to use the infant's serum in parallel tests to ensure that maternal antibodies to antigens not present on the infant's cells are detected.

Capillary or Venous Blood

Capillary blood[5] may be used for compatibility testing for neonates and infants. A poorly collected capillary sample can result in hemolysis, as well as contamination by tissue fluid. Figure 2-1 denotes the correct area of the heel to use for heelsticks. Multiple heelsticks to the same area of the heel should be avoided to prevent injury and infection. Calcified cutaneous nodules secondary to heelsticks have been reported, primarily in high-risk, preterm infants. However, there have been rare reports of this development in normal healthy infants.[6] Venipuncture may be a less painful and more effective means of obtaining a blood specimen in neonates, particularly in full-term neonates.[7,8]

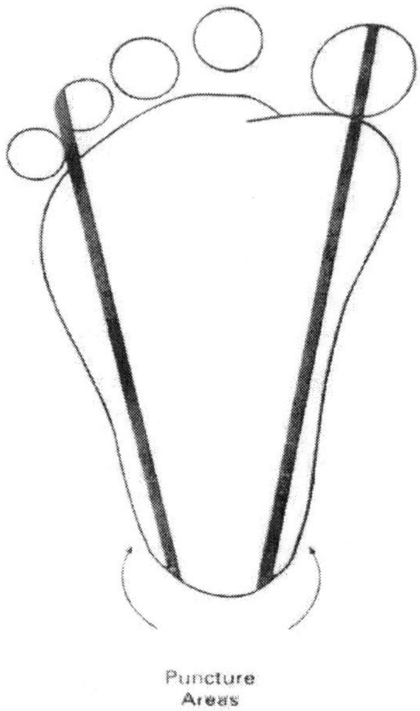

Figure 2-1. Proper heelstick locations for neonates and infants (used with permission from Jones[5]).

The ability to obtain an adequate sample size may present a problem. The amount of blood collected can be calculated as a percentage of the patient's blood volume, provided the child's weight is known (Table 2-1).[5] Mean blood volume removed for blood sampling ranges from 0.8 to 3.1 mL/kg per day for premature infants requiring intensive care during their initial weeks of life. This may result in a loss of greater than 1% of the total circulating blood volume per day to blood sampling.[9,10] A recent study by Lin et al[11] noted that the mean volume of blood drawn exceeded that requested by the hospital laboratory by 19% per test. This iatrogenic blood loss in these infants must then be frequently treated by transfusion. Clinical factors associated with greater phlebotomy overdraw included 1) blood collection in containers without fill lines (including syringes), 2) low birthweight infants, and 3) critically ill infants cared for in the neonatal intensive care unit.[11]

Table 2-1. Calculating the Amount of Blood Collected

Age	Blood Volume
Premature	115 mL/kg
Newborn	80-110 mL/kg
Infants and children	75-110 mL/kg

Hematocrit values also change as the patient ages. A newborn's hematocrit is approximately 60%, while the hematocrit decreases to approximately 35% in a 8-week-old neonate.[3] Hence, the size of the specimen collected must be adjusted if serum or plasma are needed for compatibility testing.

Maternal Blood

It is recommended that some serologic studies be performed on maternal blood when HDN is suspected: ABO, Rh (including weak D), test for fetomaternal hemorrhage (if mother is D negative and infant is D positive), and identification of antibody, if present. All clinically significant red cell alloantibodies must be considered when multiple antibodies are present in the mother's and infant's serum and transfusion is required by the newborn. In most cases, maternal serum or plasma should be used in compatibility testing in exchange transfusion.[4(p506)] Red cells selected for transfusion should be compatible with mother's ABO group and any other clinically significant antibodies. If the maternal antibodies are such that rare blood is required, it may be useful to test the infant's serum periodically to determine if the antibodies are still present. If they are not detected, further transfusions need not be of rare blood.

Patient Identification

Recipient identification systems[12] are an important part of any protocol designed to enhance transfusion safety. The transfusion recipient is frequently identified by information imprinted on a wristband. This information may be their name and hospital number, or it may consist of preprinted alphanumeric codes that are part of a dedicated transfusion system. Difficulties in using wristbands as a means of patient identification were described by the College of American Pathologists.[13] The mean total error rate in 712 hospitals was 2.2%. Errors noted were: absent wristband (49.5%); patients wearing more than one wristband containing different information (18.3%); wristbands with incomplete data (17.5%); wristbands with illegible data (5.7%); and patients with wrong wristbands (0.5%). Suggestions for improvement included: have wristbands placed by admission personnel; have phlebotomists check wristbands; and designate the ankle as the alternate site for band placement. Other systems developed have included the use of computers and bedside bar code scanners[14] or the incorporation of a mechanical barrier[15] that "forces" the transfusionist to identify the recipient before gaining access to the unit.

Although adaptable for use in the pediatric population, the above systems appear to have been designed with adult recipient rather than pediatric recipient identification in mind. Identification of the pediatric patient in the literature focuses on techniques (eg, footprinting,[16] DNA analysis[17]) for preventing infant abduction or "baby switching" rather than ensuring transfusion of the correct unit of blood.

Methods of Testing

Methods for sample testing for compatibility are the same as for adults with some modifications. This section discusses ABO/Rh typing, direct antiglobulin testing, antibody detection, and crossmatching methods.

ABO/Rh Typing

For transfusion purposes, an initial pretransfusion sample must be tested to determine ABO and D type.[1] The red cell typing is the same as for adults—anti-A, anti-B, and anti-D (control as required). For the serum type, it should be recognized that the antibodies that are present are derived from the mother. If a serum type is performed, it will reflect the IgG antibodies present in the mother's serum. For that reason, only cell typing is used to determine the blood group of the neonate. According to AABB *Standards* ABO/D typing may be omitted for the remainder of the neonate's hospital admission.[1]

Interfering substances can be a problem. Because sample collection varies, it may be necessary to wash the red cells prior to testing to obtain a valid type. Substances such as Wharton's jelly or contamination with maternal sample may result in invalid or confusing results. If there is any question about the results, a new specimen should be obtained.

There may be the appearance of two populations of cells when the ABO/Rh tests are interpreted. There are a few reasons this may occur.

- **Intrauterine Transfusion.** If the neonate has received transfusion as a fetus, generally group O D-negative blood would have been used. Therefore, if the infant was any other ABO type, ABO test results would appear to be mixed-field, indicating that two (or more) populations of red cells are present.
- **Maternal-Fetal Bleeding.** If there were a large enough maternal hemorrhage into the infant's circulation, then testing of the neonate's blood could indicate that two blood types are present.
- **Chimera.** Although rare, it is possible that there are two populations of cells being produced and are circulating in the neonate. This may be a transient or permanent condition and may result in what is known as a chimera, where two populations of cells co-exist.

In circumstances where there is a strongly positive DAT, the results of the D typing may be in question, so the use of Rh control sera or suitable control as recommended by the manufacturer is advised.

Direct Antiglobulin Testing

In most hospital settings, there is no routine DAT testing on every sample. Rather, umbilical cord samples are reserved for testing, if the clinical situation warrants it. When a DAT is ordered, there is usually a suspicion that there may be immune cell destruction in the neonate. The DAT should be performed with washed red cells from the neonate and tested with polyspecific antihuman globulin or with monospecific anti-IgG *and* anti-C3.

If the DAT is positive, the mother is known to be group O, and eluate studies are indicated, A_1 and B cells should be included in testing of the neonate's eluate. If the mother's red cell antibody status is positive and the antibody identification is known, it may be of little value to perform an eluate of the neonate's blood (or cord blood) as no new information may be gained.

In the performance of the DAT, it is important always to include a control of 6% albumin (or suitable solution) to detect spontaneous agglutination of the red cells (ie, the cells agglutinate in the absence of antiglobulin sera). If this control is positive, the DAT is invalid and further testing by the transfusion service laboratory or an immunohematology reference laboratory may be indicated.

Antibody Detection

If initial screening of the neonate's sample for red cell antibodies is negative, repeat testing may be omitted for the rest of the neonate's admission. If the initial screen is positive and the mother's sample has not been tested, it is prudent to obtain the mother's sample for antibody studies. Not only is the mother's sample a larger volume, but the antibody may be more strongly reactive.

If the mother's sample is not available, then identification of the antibody in the neonate's serum should be performed. Because the volume of the sample may be small, conservation of the serum is very important. It may be useful to obtain the cord sample for this and for elution studies, if they are indicated.

One of the newer techniques, the gel test, is an excellent way to conserve serum yet be able to perform antibody identification using established techniques.[18] Other microtechniques, such as capillary technique, have proven to be very useful in identifying antibodies when only a small volume of sample is available.[19]

If the initial antibody screen demonstrates clinically significant antibodies, then units that are negative for the corresponding antigen must be made available. AABB *Standards* requires that units shall be compatible by the antiglobulin crossmatch until the antibody is no longer demonstrated in the neonate's sample.[1] This can be very valuable if the neonate's serum contains multiple antibodies or an antibody to a high-prevalence antibody of maternal origin. If there is a long hospitalization, it is possible that the antibody may decrease in reactivity (as quantity of antibody decreases) and may not be detected by a crossmatch, thus allowing transfusion of routinely available units.

If the mother is known to have multiple red cell antibodies or an antibody to a high-prevalence antigen before delivery, there are some preparatory steps that can be taken. First, if the mother is a suitable donor for her child, autologous or directed donation can be initiated. This blood can be stored in aliquots and frozen so that small amounts can be deglycerolized for use by the infant. If the mother is not a suitable donor or time does not permit sufficient blood to be obtained, the siblings of the mother can be tested for compatibility (especially if the antibody is to a high-prevalence antigen). If the sibling route is not available or productive, the American Rare Donor Program (ARDP) may be accessed through an ARDP member. In dire situations when compatible blood is not available, consideration should be given to use of incompatible blood. Clinical and laboratory observation will dictate further need for transfusion.

Crossmatching

In rare circumstances, the maternal serum may contain antibody to an antigen of low-prevalence present on the father's red cells and inherited by the infant. Such an infant is at risk for HDN. In these cases, a crossmatch between the mother's serum and father's red cells (if ABO compatible) is valuable. It may also be of value to test the infant's eluate with the father's red cells if the mother's serum is ABO incompatible with the father. If the paternal red cells are ABO incompatible, it may be necessary to refer the parent's samples to an immunohematology reference laboratory for identification studies. Provision of blood for this situation is easy, because almost all units will be compatible with the mother's serum. Full (antiglobulin phase) crossmatches will be needed until the antibody is no longer detected. If a non-group-O neonate is to receive non-group-O red cells that are incompatible with maternal ABO, then the neonate's sample must be tested for anti-A or anti-B. This testing must be performed at the antiglobulin phase, because the maternal antibody that crosses the placenta will be IgG in nature. If there is anti-A or anti-B detected in the antiglobulin phase, then group O red cells should be used.

Blood Group Antigens

Table 2-2 details what is known about the development of antigens after birth.[20] Antigens in some systems (such as Rh, Kell, and Kidd) are known to be fully developed at birth. Some are known to be of weak strength (eg, ABO, Lutheran, P), and others are very weak or not detected on cord cells (eg, Lewis, Vel, Yt^a).

Therefore, it is easy to understand why some very potent antibodies present in the maternal serum do not cause HDN. Caution is advised if transfusion is needed when there is a maternal antibody such as those in Table 2-2 that are known to be potentially clinically significant, but ineffective at causing HDN (eg, anti-Vel). Because adult cells will be selected for transfusion to the neonate, the maternal antibody will quite readily react with the transfused adult cells and may potentially lead to cell destruction in the neonate. Because some of the antigens listed in Table 2-2 are weak or not developed at birth, the neonate's red cells should not be assessed for presence of those antigens on the cells. A few rare cases of auto- or alloantibody reactivity have been reported; this may be further diminished with the advent of universal leukocyte reduction.[21]

The relative strength of the i antigen has been used to differentiate transient erythroblastopenia of childhood from rare congenital hypoplastic anemias, especially Diamond-Blackfan syndrome in children.[22] It has been suggested that the strength of the i antigen is increased in Diamond-Blackfan anemia. Because i antigens decline in strength as the child ages, it is important to

Table 2-2. Antigen Strength on Umbilical Cord Red Cells

Normal Adult Expression	Weaker than Adult Expression	Very Weak or Absent
Rh	**ABO**	*Vel*
Kell	**P**	*Yt*[a]
Kidd	*Hy*	*AnWj*
Duffy	**Lutheran**	*Ch1*
MNS	*Xg*[a]	*Rg1*
Colton	*Gy*[a]	**Lewis**
Diego	*Jo*[a]	**I**
Do[a]	**H**	*Sd*[a]
Do[b]	**Knops**	
Scianna	**Indian**	
Yt[b]		
Landsteiner-Wiener		
Kx		
Gerbich		
Cromer		
Cost		
Er		
GLOB		

Bold = blood group systems; italic = blood group antigens; no emphasis = blood group collection

test an age-matched control (as close as possible to the age of the affected child) in parallel with the affected child's sample. If the i antigen strength is dramatically increased above that of the age-matched control, then this provides a piece of evidence for Diamond-Blackfan syndrome as a cause of the anemia vs transient erythroblastopenia of childhood.

Acknowledgment

The authors thank Margaret C. Manigly for expert assistance in manuscript preparation.

References

1. Gorlin JB, ed. Standards for blood banks and transfusion services, 21st ed. Bethesda, MD: American Association of Blood Banks, 2002:48.
2. Ludvigsen C, Swanson NK, Thompson TR, McCullough J. The failure of neonates to form red cell alloantibodies in response to multiple transfusions. Am J Clin Pathol 1987;87:250-1.
3. Floss AM, Strauss RG, Goeken N, Knox L. Multiple transfusions fail to provoke antibodies against blood cell antigens in human infants. Transfusion 1986;26:419-22.
4. Brecher ME, ed. Technical manual, 14th ed. Bethesda, MD: American Association of Blood Banks, 2002.
5. Jones PM. Pediatric laboratory medicine. In: McKenna RW, Keffer JH, eds. The handbook of clinical pathology, 2nd ed. Chicago, IL: American Society of Clinical Pathologists, 2000:527-32.
6. Williamson D, Holt PJ. Calcified cutaneous nodules on the heels of children: A complication of heel sticks as a neonate. Pediatr Dermatol 2001;18:138-40.
7. Shah V, Ohlsson A. Venipuncture versus heel lance for blood sampling in term neonates. Cochrane Database System Review 2000;(2):CD001452.
8. Larsson BA, Tannfeldt G, Lagercrantz H, Olsson GL. Venipuncture is more effective and less painful than heel lancing for blood tests in neonates. Pediatrics 1998:101;882-6.
9. Strauss RG. Neonatal anemia: Pathophysiology and treatment. In: Wilson SM, Levitt JS, Strauss RG, eds. Improving transfusion practice for pediatric patients. Arlington, VA: American Association of Blood Banks, 1991:1-17.
10. Nexo E, Christensen NC, Olesen H. Volume of blood removed for analytical purposes during hospitalization of low-birth weight infants. Clin Chem 1981;27:759-61.
11. Lin JC, Strauss RC, Kulhavy JC, et al. Phlebotomy overdraw in the neonatal intensive care nursery. Pediatrics 2000;106:E19.
12. Wenz B, Mercuriali F, AuBuchon JP. Practical methods to improve transfusion safety by using novel blood unit and patient identification systems. Am J Clin Pathol 1997;107(Suppl 1):S12-S16.
13. Renner SW, Howanitz PJ, Bachner P. Wristband identification error reporting in 712 hospitals. Arch Pathol Lab Med 1993;117:573-7.
14. Jensen NJ, Crosson JT. An automated system for bedside verification of the match between patient identification and blood unit identification. Transfusion 1996;36:216-21.
15. AuBuchon JP, Littenberg B. A cost effectiveness analysis of the use of a mechanical barrier system to reduce the risk of mistransfusion. Transfusion 1996;36:222-6.
16. Butz AM, Oski FA, Repke J, Rosenstein BJ. Newborn identification. Compliance with AAP guidelines for perinatal care. Clin Pediatr 1993;32:111-3.

17. DePancorbo MM, Rodriguez-Larcon J, Castro A, et al. Newborn genetic identification: A protocol using microsatellite DNA as an alternative to footprinting. Clin Chim Acta 1997;263:33-42.
18. Lapierre Y, Rigal D, Adam J, et al. The gel test: A new way to detect red cell antigen-antibody reactions. Transfusion 1990;30:109-13.
19. Chown B. A rapid, simple and economical method for Rh agglutination. Am J Clin Pathol 1944;14:114-15.
20. Vengelen-Tyler V. The serologic investigation of hemolytic disease of the newborn caused by antibodies other than anti-D. In: Garratty G, ed. Hemolytic disease of the newborn. Arlington, VA: American Association of Blood Banks, 1984:145-72.
21. DePalma L. Review: Red cell alloantibody formation in the neonate and infant: Considerations for current immunohematologic practice. Immunohematology 1992;8:33-7.
22. Cooper AG, Hoffbrand AV, Worlledge SM. Increased agglutininability by anti-i of red cells in sideroblastic and megaloblastic anemia. Br J Haematol 1968;15:381.

In: Herman JH, Manno CS, eds.
Pediatric Transfusion Therapy
Bethesda, MD: AABB Press, 2002

3

Neonatal Red Cell Transfusion

MICHAEL GOODSTEIN, MD, FAAP

OXYGEN DELIVERY TO THE tissues is crucial to the survival of the neonate. Arterial saturation, cardiac output, and hemoglobin are the most powerful determinants of oxygen delivery to the tissues. Increasing red cell mass and hemoglobin concentration quickly and effectively increases tissue oxygenation in the sick neonate.

Premature infants tend to be transfused liberally for multiple reasons: severe respiratory disease resulting in poor oxygenation, poor weight gain, apnea, tachycardia, patent ductus arteriosus, infection, and iatrogenic losses. Whatever the indica-

Michael Goodstein, MD, FAAP, Staff Neonatologist, Division of Newborn Medicine, York Hospital, York, Pennsylvania, and Clinical Assistant Professor of Pediatrics, College of Medicine, Pennsylvania State University, Hershey, Pennsylvania

tion, *the decision to transfuse is a clinical one.* Guidelines have been established and have been modified over the years, but there is little evidence-based medicine in the literature. This chapter reviews the clinical situations for which red cell transfusion is considered, explores alternative strategies to transfusion, and discusses the rationale behind the decision-making process.

Causes of Anemia

The normal hemoglobin concentration (obtained from the umbilical cord) in the full-term infant at birth ranges from 14 to 20 g/dL with a mean of 17 g/dL.[1] The hemoglobin concentration increases rapidly during the last weeks of gestation; thus, premature infants demonstrate lower hemoglobin concentrations at birth. Causes of anemia in the neonate can be categorized as: red cell aplasia (either congenital or acquired), acute hemorrhage, perinatal blood loss, hemolysis (including iso- or alloimmune disease, red cell enzyme defects, red cell membrane defects, and hemoglobinopathies), and physiologic anemia of prematurity. Some of these problems cannot be diagnosed in the newborn period and most will not require early transfusion.

Red Cell Aplasias

Congenital anemias are the result of erythrocyte underproduction and include: congenital hypoplastic anemia (CHA) or Diamond-Blackfan syndrome, Fanconi syndrome, Shwachman syndrome, osteopetrosis (Albers-Schonberg disease), anemias of endocrine insufficiency, and other rare conditions. CHA is characterized by decreased erythroid precursors in the marrow, peripheral reticulocytopenia, macrocytosis, elevated levels of hemoglobin F, and expressions of the "i" antigen on the surface of the erythrocytes. Fanconi syndrome is an autosomal recessive syndrome characterized by a pancytopenia resulting from a defect in replication of progenitor and stem cells in each cell line. Shwachman syndrome is an autosomal recessive disorder characterized by short stature, neutropenia, and pancreatic insufficiency, which results in diarrhea.

Transient erythroblastopenia of childhood usually occurs between 6 months and 4 years of age, often following a viral infection. There is a gradual onset of a severe anemia without reticulocytosis. The disorder differs from CHA in that the mean cell volume and hemoglobin F level are normal and the "i" antigen is absent. Only supportive care is necessary and remission is usually complete. Maternally acquired viral or protozoal infections can result in a severe hemolytic anemia that may manifest prenatally as hydrops fetalis. Cytomegalovirus, rubella, toxoplasmosis, herpes simplex virus, coxsackie B, and parvovirus B19 have all been associated with hypoplasia of erythroid precursors. At birth these infants may present with a mixed hyperbilirubinemia and a hemolytic anemia with hepatosplenomegaly secondary to extramedullary hematopoiesis.

Nutritional anemias are rare in the neonate. Iron, ferritin, and folate levels are higher in the newborn than in the adult. Infants with malabsorption or intestinal resections (gastric or terminal ileum) are at risk for vitamin B12 deficiency.

Acute Hemorrhage

Prenatal and Perinatal Hemorrhage

The placenta is a focal point for fetal blood loss. Despite the fusion of fetal membranes with the uterine mucosa, the fetal and maternal blood circulations are always separated by the placental barrier. Prenatal blood losses may occur transplacentally by fetomaternal transfusion, abruptio placentae, placenta previa, vasa previa, velamentous cord insertion, or twin-to-twin transfusion. (For a summary of pre- and perinatal hemorrhage, see Table 3-1.)

Fetomaternal Hemorrhage. Given the 4- to 5-micron diffusion distance between the maternal and fetal circulations,[2] it is not surprising that fetal erythrocytes can be detected by standard methods in the maternal blood stream in approximately 50% of pregnancies.[1] Fetomaternal hemorrhage severe enough to produce anemia in the newborn is estimated to occur in 1% of pregnancies. In most cases the bleeding occurs slowly over a prolonged period and the degree of anemia can vary widely. There is

Table 3-1. Prenatal and Perinatal Hemorrhage

Condition	Key to Diagnosis	Presentation of Infant	Therapy
Fetomaternal hemorrhage (acute)	Kleihauer-Betke acid elution test	Hypovolemia/shock	Normal saline or 5% albumin 10 to 20 mL/kg over 30 minutes; RBCs if anemia is severe or symptoms persist
Fetomaternal hemorrhage (chronic)	Kleihauer-Betke acid elution test	Anemia with increase in reticulocytes, no hemolysis	Observation
Abruptio placentae	Maternal vaginal bleeding, uterine tenderness and rigidity	Hypovolemia or acidosis, pallor, hypotension	Rapid resuscitation, respiratory support, correct acidosis, restore intravascular volume (normal saline, 5% albumin, RBCs)
Placenta previa	Painless maternal vaginal bleeding, confirm by ultrasound	Usually asymptomatic, but with sudden hemorrhage can have severe hypovolemia	Fluid resuscitation as needed
Vasa previa	Sudden maternal vaginal bleeding, rapid fetal deterioration	Hypovolemia/shock, extreme pallor	Rapid volume resuscitation

Velamentous cord insertion	Sudden maternal vaginal bleeding with rupture of membranes, rapid fetal deterioration	Hypovolemia/shock, extreme pallor	Rapid volume resuscitation
Twin-to-twin transfusion (donor)	Discordant fetal growth restriction with oligohydramnios	Tachycardia, pallor	Asymptomatic: iron supplement Symptomatic: RBCs Severe symptoms: partial exchange transfusion
Damage to umbilical cord or placenta	Unattended delivery, abnormally short cord, cesarean section with anterior placenta	Ranges from asymptomatic to shock	Fluid resuscitation as needed
Umbilical cord compression (not a true hemorrhage; rather blood is trapped in placenta)	Deep variable decelerations	Ranges from asymptomatic to hypovolemia	Fluid resuscitation as needed

no evidence of hemolytic disease and the anemia is associated with an elevated reticulocyte count and increased nucleated red cells. Diagnosis is confirmed by the Kleihauer-Betke acid-elution test.

Therapy depends on the volume and acuteness of the blood loss. In acute blood loss with hypovolemia, rapid volume replacement is critical. As blood is usually not immediately available, normal saline or 5% albumin should be infused, 10 to 20 mL/kg over 30 minutes. Generally, red cell transfusions are not necessary unless there is severe anemia or persistence of symptoms. If the blood loss is chronic and the anemia mild, then no immediate therapy is necessary. If the infant is anemic and symptomatic (tachycardia, tachypnea), then a small-volume transfusion of red cells may be required. Infants with signs of heart failure and/or hydrops may not tolerate a simple transfusion, and instead, should receive a partial exchange transfusion. In cases of significant chronic blood loss, infants will require long-term iron supplementation.

Abruptio Placentae. Abruptio placentae refers to the premature separation of the normally positioned placenta from the uterine wall. Abruption occurs in approximately 1% of all pregnancies and the incidence is increased when there is maternal hypertension or cocaine abuse. In severe cases, fetal distress or death may occur. Fetal hypoxemia from loss of placental surface area for gas exchange may be exacerbated by fetal blood loss. The hemoglobin concentration at birth may not reflect the full extent of the blood loss. Once reequilibration of the intravascular volume is complete after 6 to 12 hours, the true magnitude of the anemia will be apparent. Therapy is geared toward the rapid resuscitation of the infant.

Placenta Previa. In placenta previa, the placenta lies low in the uterus and usually overlies the cervical os to varying degrees. Placenta previa occurs in approximately 1 in 250 births[3] and is characterized by the sudden onset of painless vaginal bleeding. Fetal blood loss can be identified in as many as 50% of all cases of placenta previa.[3] The majority of patients are delivered by cesarean section. In most cases, the infant will not require therapy.

Vasa Previa. Vasa previa occurs when the umbilical vessels traverse the lower uterine segment in advance of the presenting fetal part. If the vessels sit near the cervical os, they may tear during cervical dilation or upon rupture of membranes. Fetal exsanguination may occur if the infant is not delivered rapidly. Rapid volume resuscitation is essential.

Velamentous Cord Insertion. Velamentous cord insertion describes an umbilical cord that is attached to the membranes (chorion and amnion) rather than the placenta. The umbilical vessels leave the cord, unprotected by Wharton's jelly, and run between the amnion and chorion before reaching the placenta. Rupture of membranes can result in laceration of vessels and rapid fetal blood loss. This is especially true when associated with vasa previa. Again, rapid delivery is necessary to prevent fetal exsanguination.

Twin-to-Twin Transfusion. Twin-to-twin transfusion or twin transfusion syndrome occurs only in identical twins. Approximately 70% of identical twins share a placenta, but have separate amniotic sacs. Arteriovenous anastomoses allow the twin on the arterial side to infuse blood into the circulation of the other twin. The donor twin demonstrates oligohydramnios and restricted growth. Progression can lead to high output heart failure or hydrops fetalis. Tachycardia and pallor may be present at birth. Mild or severe anemia can be exacerbated by iron deficiency. Accelerated red cell production as a compensatory mechanism is exhibited by reticulocytosis and increased nucleated red cells.

The recipient twin may be significantly larger and display polyhydramnios. At birth this infant appears ruddy or plethoric, and may have hypertension, heart failure, or pulmonary edema. Polycythemia may result in hyperviscosity from the increased red cell mass. These infants are predisposed to venous thrombosis or hemorrhage, including intracranial hemorrhage (ICH). Hypoglycemia and hyperbilirubinemia may also occur.

After delivery, the donor twin may require red cell transfusion if there is symptomatic anemia. In severe cases, a partial volume exchange transfusion is preferable to prevent circulatory overload. The hematocrit should rise rapidly as red cell production has already been maximized and the ongoing losses are eliminated by delivery. The recipient twin should be treated with a partial exchange transfusion if symptomatic from polycythemia (central hematocrit greater than 65%) or asymptomatic with a central hematocrit of greater than 70%.

Other Causes. Other causes of obstetric hemorrhage are related to damage to the umbilical cord or placenta. Rupture of a normal cord may occur during a precipitous, usually unattended delivery. An abnormally short cord or one entangled with the infant may tear during a routine delivery. During cesarean delivery, incision through an anterior placenta may result in significant hemorrhage. Although not a hemorrhage, the fetus can lose significant blood volume due to cord compression, where the umbilical arteries remain patent with blood flowing away from the infant, while the umbilical vein is occluded, resulting in blood being trapped in the placenta.

Postnatal Hemorrhage

Postnatal hemorrhage in the healthy term infant is most often the result of birth trauma. Hemorrhage is more likely in infants with congenital or acquired defects in hemostasis. The bleeding may be obvious or occult and blood loss may be gradual or rapid. (For a summary of postnatal hemorrhage, see Table 3-2.)

Scalp. Hemorrhage into the subperiosteal space or cephalohematoma results in a gradual hemorrhage that often results in hyperbilirubinemia, but rarely requires transfusion. However, hemorrhage in the space between the scalp and skull bones, known as subgaleal hemorrhage, can result in significant blood loss (see Fig 3-1). This potential space can hold up to 50% of the infant's blood volume and there is no way to effectively tamponade the bleeding. Management involves repeated measurements of head circumference and hematocrit. Volume replacement may be clinically indicated.

Intracranial Hemorrhage. Intracranial hemorrhage may occur as the result of birth trauma. In the term infant, the most common type is subarachnoid hemorrhage. The bleeding is usually minor and rarely of clinical significance. In the premature

Table 3-2. Postnatal Hemorrhage

Condition	Key to Diagnosis	Presentation of Infant	Therapy
Caput seccedaneum	Superficial bruising crossing suture lines	Stable with boggy scalp	None required
Caphalohematoma	Subperiosteal bleeding does **not** cross suture lines	Stable with firm swelling sharply demarcated by suture line	Rarely requires transfusion, monitor for jaundice, do **not** drain
Subgaleal hemorrhage	Fluctuant mass crossing suture lines and/or fontanelle	Scalp swelling, pallor, hypotonia; may progress to hypovolemic shock	Rapid restoration of blood volume
Subarachnoid hemorrhage	Lumbar puncture reveals increased red cells in cerebrospinal fluid; CT scan	Usually asymptomatic, but may present with seizures at 24 to 48 hours of life	Observation
Subdural hemorrhage	CT scan: supratentorial lesions MRI scan: infratentorial lesions	Variable from asymptomatic to severe, rapidly progressing neurologic symptoms and death	Supportive care; red cell transfusion as clinically indicated; possible surgical evacuation

(continued)

Table 3-2. Postnatal Hemorrhage (continued)

Condition	Key to Diagnosis	Presentation of Infant	Therapy
Epidural hemorrhage	Emergency CT scan reveals typical convex, lens-shaped lesion	Signs of increased intracranial pressure with bulging anterior fontanelle in first hours of life	Evacuation of lesion, usually surgically
Intraventricular hemorrhage	Preterm infants ≤34 weeks of gestation; cranial ultrasound	Ranges from asymptomatic to sudden deterioration with hypotension, coma, seizures	Maintain ventilation and perfusion; volume resuscitation as needed
Pulmonary hemorrhage	Red, frothy drainage from endotracheal tube or mouth; diffuse infiltrates on chest x-ray	Sudden deterioration with pallor, shock, cyanosis, and bradycardia	Assisted ventilation, tamponade with PEEP; volume replacement, red cell transfusion
Adrenal hemorrhage	Flank mass; abdominal ultrasound with cystic, calcified lesion in adrenal gland	Asymptomatic to findings of fever, tachypnea, yellow pallor, flank mass with skin discoloration	Red cells as needed; treat adrenal insufficiency with intravenous fluids, corticosteroids; ? surgery

Hepatic rupture	Right upper quadrant mass; abdominal ultrasound with echogenic intrahepatic hemorrhage	Initially asymptomatic, then nonspecific signs, then circulatory collapse with rigid abdomen	Rapid resuscitation with red cells; correct coagulation defects; laparotomy
Splenic rupture	Left upper quadrant mass; paracentesis with free blood in abdomen	Shock and symptoms of hemoperitoneum (abdomen distended, rigid, bluish discoloration)	Rapid resuscitation with red cells; correct coagulation defects; laparotomy
Renal hemorrhage	Gross hematuria; abdominal ultrasound with renal mass, hematoma	Ascites and flank mass; shock and symptoms of hemoperitoneum	Red cell transfusion as needed; correct coagulation defects; consider laparotomy
Necrotizing enterocolitis	Bloody stools; pneumatosis intestinalis on abdominal x-ray	Abdominal distention, peritonitis, sepsis, hypovolemic shock	Rapid resuscitation with volume and red cells; antibiotics; abdominal decompression; possible laparotomy
Stress ulcer	Bloody or coffee ground secretions in orogastric tube	Seriously ill from underlying illness	Antacids

(continued)

Table 3-2. Postnatal Hemorrhage (continued)

Condition	Key to Diagnosis	Presentation of Infant	Therapy
Hemorrhagic disease of the newborn: early	Bleeding <24 hours associated with maternal anticoagulants or anticonvulsants	Serious bleeding, may include intracranial hemorrhage	Vitamin K (slow IV infusion K_1); consider FFP with serious bleeding and red cells as needed; emergency purified Factor IX
Hemorrhagic disease of the newborn: classic	Bleeding at 1 to 7 days in infant who has not received vitamin K prophylaxis	Cutaneous or gastrointestinal hemorrhage, bleeding after circumcision	Vitamin K (slow IV infusion K_1); consider FFP with serious bleeding and red cells as needed; emergency purified Factor IX
Thrombocytopenia	CBC with decreased platelet count	Petechiae, bruising; may be asymptomatic unless there is spontaneous hemorrhage	Transfusion with appropriate platelets based on platelet count and degree of prematurity

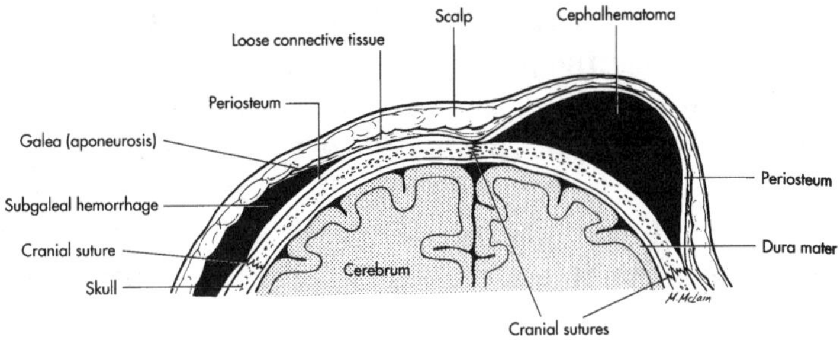

Figure 3-1. Subgaleal hemorrhage *(SGH)* and cephalohematoma.

infant, intraventricular hemorrhage in the first days of life is a fairly common complication. The hemorrhage originates from a fragile vascular network in the subependymal germinal matrix. Hemorrhage may be minor or severe, filling the ventricles with blood. The most severe intracranial hemorrhage extends into the parenchyma and may be the result of venous infarction in the periventricular white matter.[4] The infant usually presents with a sudden deterioration and will require red cell transfusion.

Pulmonary Hemorrhage. Pulmonary hemorrhage most commonly occurs in premature infants during the acute phase of hyaline membrane disease. An acute rise in pulmonary capillary pressure may be seen with such predisposing factors as hypoxia, hypervolemia, or congestive heart failure.[5] Studies suggest that often the hemorrhage represents hemorrhagic pulmonary edema due to left-sided heart failure.[6] There is speculation that after surfactant administration, improvement in lung compliance allows for increased left-to-right shunting through the ductus arteriosus, increased pulmonary capillary pressure, and intra-alveolar hemorrhagic edema. In some cases there is true hemorrhage rather than hemorrhagic pulmonary edema. Bleeding may also be associated with trauma related to suctioning of the upper airway. The infant usually presents with a sudden deterioration requiring increased ventilatory support (especially PEEP to tamponade the hemorrhage) and transfusion.

Intra-abdominal Hemorrhage. Intra-abdominal bleeding, although rare, may occur in the liver, spleen, kidneys, or adrenal glands. Such hemorrhages may be associated with traumatic delivery, breech extraction, prematurity, abnormalities of hemostasis, and conditions that predispose to distension of the abdominal organs (erythroblastosis fetalis, congenital heart block, congenital viral syndromes).[3] Severely ill neonates may develop gastric or duodenal stress ulcers. Intestinal hemorrhage may occur with intestinal ischemia, colitis (necrotizing enterocolitis in the premature infant), allergy, infection, perforation, hemangioma, or telangiectasia.

Other Causes. Bleeding may complicate several procedures performed on the ill neonate. Laryngoscopy, umbilical vessel catheterization, orogastric tube placement, thoracostomy, bladder catheterization, and surgery can all result in postnatal blood loss.

Bleeding may be the result of congenital or acquired defects of hemostasis—either decreased production or increased destruction. Congenital defects include classic hemophilia (Factor VIII deficiency), Christmas disease (Factor IX deficiency), and von Willebrand disease. Other factor deficiencies include Factor XIII (fibrin stabilizing factor) and congenital afibrinogenemia. Thrombocytopenia may be congenital or acquired. Sepsis can cause disseminated intravascular coagulation (DIC) with consumption of clotting factors, resulting in hemorrhage.

In hemorrhagic disease of the newborn, the neonate is relatively deficient in vitamin K, which is essential in the clotting cascade. Without appropriate supplementation, serious hemorrhage may occur, especially if the infant was exposed to anticonvulsant agents before birth. Rarely, vascular malformations and soft tumors can lead to neonatal hemorrhage.

Hemolytic Anemias

Decreased red cell lifespan and anemia in the newborn may be caused by numerous disorders, such as isoimmune disorders, red cell membrane defects, red cell enzyme defects, hemoglobinopathies, and infections. Except in the case of infection, the infant is typically well-appearing with jaundice secondary to the newborn liver's inability to metabolize the increased hemoglobin load from the hemolytic process. Rapid cell turnover results in anemia and stimulates a reticulocytosis. These conditions generally do not require small-volume transfusions; however, severe hemolysis may necessitate a double-volume exchange transfusion to prevent kernicterus. Rare causes of immune hemolytic anemia include medications, collagen-vascular disease, immunodeficiency syndromes, and idiopathic hemolytic anemia.

Isoimmune Causes

Isoimmune hemolytic anemia is the result of maternal IgG antibodies crossing the placenta into the fetal circulation and reacting with the infant's cells, which leads to immune-mediated destruction of the cells. Before the introduction of Rh Immune Globulin (RhIG), Rh hemolytic disease of the newborn (HDN) or erythroblastosis fetalis due to anti-D was the most common cause of severe isoimmune hemolytic disease in the newborn. Exposure of an Rh-negative mother to as little as 0.1 mL of Rh-positive fetal blood can result in sensitization, with Rh antibody formation.[7] Because the initial exposure results in a relatively weak primary immune response that consists of IgM antibodies, which do not cross the placenta, the first fetus is spared from a significant antibody exposure. However, in subsequent pregnancies, the anamnestic response causes greater antibody production with IgG, which crosses the placenta, often resulting in an aggressive hemolytic anemia that may progress to hydrops fetalis (erythroblastosis fetalis). Several other red cell antigens can cause significant hemolytic reactions including: the minor Rh antigens, Kell, Duffy, Diego, Kidd, and MNSs.

ABO incompatibility is now the most common cause of HDN. This disorder differs from Rh HDN in that sensitization is not required. Due to similar antigens in bacteria or food, there is natural production of anti-A and anti-B in the maternal circulation prior to pregnancy. In group O mothers, these antibodies tend to be IgG and cross the placenta, interacting with the fetal red cells.

The disease tends to be less severe than Rh HDN with the spectrum of illness ranging from asymptomatic to the rare need for exchange transfusion. The decrease in severity may be due to multiple factors including dilution of the antibody throughout many tissues that carry the antigen and decreased surface expression of the A and B antigens on the fetal cells, resulting in fewer sites for reaction.[8,9]

Red Cell Membrane Defects

Deformability of the red cell membrane is critical to erythrocyte survival in the capillary circulation. Hereditary defects in the red cell membrane may present in the newborn period with hemolytic anemia. One of the most common disorders is hereditary spherocytosis, characterized by small, spherical erythrocytes on peripheral smear.[10] Multiple gene defects have been reported that result in abnormal erythrocyte membrane proteins. Membrane instability leads to membrane loss and decreased deformability. These red cells are sequestered in the splenic microcirculation and destroyed.

Other erythrocyte membrane defects include hereditary elliptocytosis, hereditary pyropoikilocytosis, and hereditary stomatocytosis. In hereditary elliptocytosis the peripheral blood smear reveals characteristic oval, cigar-shaped red blood cells. Most infants are asymptomatic. Hereditary pyropoikilocytosis is a rare cause of neonatal anemia due to protein defects resulting in decreased erythrocyte stability. The peripheral smear is notable for bizarre-shaped red cells with fragmentation and budding. Hereditary stomatocytosis is a defect of sodium and potassium transport across the red cell membrane. Excess cations increase the erythrocyte water concentration resulting in large, osmotically fragile cells.[10]

Red Cell Enzyme Defects

Although the erythrocyte lacks a nucleus, DNA, RNA, polyribosomes, and mitochondria, it has a full complement of enzymes, cofactors, and proteins to maintain adequate energy stores, reducing substances, and 2,3-diphosphoglycerate (2,3-DPG) levels. Energy is supplied by anaerobic glycolysis via the Embden-Meyerhof pathway, by oxidative glycolysis through the hexose monophosphate pathway, and through nucleotide salvage pathways.[10] Enzymatic defects in these pathways may result in varying degrees of hemolytic anemia in the newborn that may be referred to as hereditary nonspherocytic hemolytic anemias. A complete list of these defects is beyond the scope of this chapter. The most common of these defects is glucose-6-phosphate dehydrogenase (G6PD) deficiency. G6PD is the first and rate-limiting step in the hexose monophosphate pathway, which is critical in preventing oxidant injury to the red cell. The disorder can range from a mild decrease in enzyme activity manifested only after oxidative stress (90% of patients), to a severe decrease in enzyme activity with chronic moderate to severe anemia.

The most common defect in the glycolytic (Embden-Meyerhof) pathway is pyruvate kinase deficiency. Reduced adenosine triphosphate levels lead to altered cellular water content, resulting in rigid cells with decreased lifespan.[11] Other erythrocyte enzymes associated with hemolysis include: hexokinase, glucose phosphate isomerase, phosphofructokinase, phosphoglycerate kinase, pyrimidine 5´-nucleotidase, elevated adenosine deaminase levels, and enzymes involving glutathione metabolism.

Hemoglobinopathies

Defects in hemoglobin synthesis can result in hemolytic anemia in the neonate. However, disorders affecting β-globin chain synthesis (β-thalassemia, sickle cell disease) generally do not present until 4 to 6 months of age because of the presence of fetal hemoglobin. In α-thalassemia, defects in one to four of the α-globin genes results in decreased production of α-globin chains. The four clinical syndromes correlate with increasing numbers of affected genes. Although there is significant heterogeneity in the spectrum of illness, the syndromes include: silent carrier, α-thalassemia trait, Hb H disease, and hydrops fetalis where α-globin chains are completely absent. The clinical syndrome is due to a combination of inadequate hemoglobin production and unbalanced accumulation of globin subunits, which leads to hemolysis.[12] Many other mutations have been identified that yield unstable hemoglobins. Again, the majority of these involve the β-globulin chain; however, in some instances hemolytic anemia and jaundice may be seen in the newborn. Precipitated hemoglobin may be identified by staining for Heinz bodies, but this test is of little value in the neonatal period because they may be seen in normal erythrocytes at term.

Infections

Both congenital and neonatal infection can result in significant hemolytic anemia. Congenital viral infections due to cytomegalovirus (CMV), toxoplasmosis, and rubella may present with hemolytic anemia, jaundice, and hepatosplenomegaly. Other congenital infections associated with hemolytic anemia include syphilis and parvovirus B19. The latter attacks erythroid progenitor cells, which can result in severe anemia and hydrops. Neonatal sepsis can be the result of bacterial infection by such agents as group B streptococcus and gram-negative organisms (*Escherichia coli*, *Klebsiella*) or viral organisms such as herpes, influenza, and enteroviruses. Sepsis can result in hemolysis, DIC, and hemorrhage. Other infections that may present with anemia in the newborn include malaria and human immunodeficiency virus.

Anemia of Prematurity

Both term and premature infants demonstrate a gradual decline in hemoglobin concentration during the first 2 to 3 months after birth. Multiple physiologic factors result in this normal decrease in red cell mass. The transition to extrauterine life results in a dramatic increase in systemic oxygen delivery, which greatly exceeds the metabolic demands of the healthy, term newborn. Erythropoietin production becomes quiescent and erythropoiesis is suppressed. The rapid growth of the infant demands an equally rapid expansion of blood volume, resulting in a progressive decline in hemoglobin concentration to 11 g/dL on average, rarely less than 9 g/dL.

Despite the decrease in hemoglobin, neonates maintain adequate tissue oxygenation through improved oxygen off-loading. This is a result of a combination of increasing levels of adult hemoglobin and 2,3-DPG, which shifts the oxygen-hemoglobin equilibrium curve and decreases oxygen affinity for hemoglobin. However, the decline in the infant's central venous oxygen tension correlates with the stimulus to increase production of erythropoietin.[13] By 10 to 12 weeks, serum erythropoietin concentrations reach adult levels and there is an active resumption of erythropoiesis.[14] Hemoglobin concentrations gradually increase to a mean of 12.5 g/dL after 6 months and remain stable throughout the first year. In term infants, these changes are well-tolerated. Therapy with iron or other hematinic agents has no effect on this normal progression.

Premature infants also experience a decrease in hemoglobin concentration after birth; however, compared to the term infant, the decrease occurs earlier, is more profound, and resolves more slowly. Many very low birthweight infants are profoundly ill at birth and require frequent blood sampling for management of complications. Such infants may have phlebotomy losses of 1 to 4 mL/kg daily, resulting in the rapid development of anemia and a need for frequent transfusions.[15]

In stable preterm infants without transfusion, those who are more premature will develop correspondingly lower hemoglobin levels. Infants with birthweights of 1.0 to 1.5 kg have a mean hemoglobin level of approximately 8 g/dL, while infants weighing less than 1 kg at birth have a mean of approximately 7 g/dL.[16,17] This anemia is normocytic and normochromic and does not respond to iron, folate, vitamin E, or other nutrients. As in the term infant, factors involved in this anemia of prematurity include decreased fetal erythrocyte survival and hemodilution secondary to expansion of the plasma volume from rapid growth. The late anemia is also accentuated by increased phlebotomy. However, a major reason behind the premature infant's lower nadir is a diminished capacity to increase plasma erythropoietin levels in the face of anemia. In many extremely preterm infants, this anemia is associated with clinical signs and symptoms that may be attributed to anemic hypoxia and may respond to red cell transfusion.

Hydrops Fetalis

Hydrops fetalis is a condition defined by the pathologic accumulation of excess body water in the fetus, resulting in fluid collections in the serous cavities or edema in the soft tissues. The hydropic fetus may have pleural and pericardial effusions, ascites, generalized edema, placental edema, and polyhydramnios. Hydrops is associated with or a complication of a wide variety of disorders. Prior to the wide availability of RhIG, HDN due to anti-D was responsible for 80% of the cases of hydrops fetalis. Other red cell antigens can cause hydrops. (For details on immune causes of hydrops, see earlier discussion on hemolytic anemias.)

Nonimmune causes of hydrops fetalis are now the most common and the incidence is estimated at 1 in 1500 to 1 in 4000 deliveries. Causes of nonimmune hydrops fetalis can be categorized as high output cardiac failure, vascular obstructions, lymphatic obstructions, fetal anemia, congenital infection, genetic disorders, metabolic diseases, and idiopathic sources.[18]

Although the conditions that produce hydrops fetalis are quite varied, they produce a series of common pathways that result in accumulation of fluid. Intrauterine heart failure is responsible for the largest proportion of cases of hydrops fetalis.[19] Limited compliance of the fetal ventricles results in right-sided cardiac failure, venous hypertension, and accumulation of vascular and extravascular fluid.

Any condition producing liver congestion will increase portal pressure, which in turn may lead to the development of ascites. Liver damage or renal loss of protein causes hypoproteinemia, resulting in decreased oncotic pressure and accumulation of fluid. Congenital infections may cause myocarditis, liver damage, hemolytic anemias, and protein leakage. Severe fetal anemia may result in high-output cardiac failure or compromise liver function by transforming it into a hematopoietic organ, promoting liver congestion, portal hypertension, and decreased protein production. Lymphatic diseases interfere with fluid reabsorption from tissues, resulting in subcutaneous edema and pleural effusions.

The overall prognosis for nonimmune hydrops is poor with a perinatal mortality rate of 50% under the best of circumstances.[20] One reason for these numbers is that many cases are associated with underlying lethal disorders. Another reason for the dismal outcomes is that the mean gestational age at diagnosis is 24 to 25 weeks with delivery at 29 to 32 weeks.[21] The best outcomes occur in cases where the underlying cause is correctable.

Fetomaternal hemorrhage is a potentially correctable cause of nonimmune hydrops through the use of intrauterine transfusions. Infection with parvovirus B19 results in marrow suppression and red cell aplasia from destruction of erythroid precursors. Again, intrauterine transfusion may be corrective. Fetal arrhythmias, in particular supraventricular tachycardia, may be controlled with maternal medication. However, once hydrops develops, it rarely resolves spontaneously in utero, and may worsen quickly.

Management goals include: 1) identifying lethal conditions to prevent maternal morbidity from futile therapy, 2) identifying conditions that may be corrected in utero and applying appropriate therapy, and 3) identifying conditions that may be corrected by delivery. The premature infant with hydrops fetalis is extremely challenging to manage and the mortality rates range from 50% to 95%.[18] A team approach including obstetrician, perinatologist, and neonatologist is crucial. Delivery and stabilization should occur at a tertiary care facility. Ventilation may be complicated by pleural effusions or pulmonary hypoplasia. Perfusion may be compromised by pericardial effusion, poor pump function, or severe anemia. Infants may require paracentesis, thoracentesis, or paracardiocentesis in the immediate postnatal period. These procedures may result in sudden fluid shifts and volume replacement may be critical. Replacement with 5% albumin may improve oncotic pressure and red cell transfusions will be beneficial in cases of severe anemia. In cases where there is risk of intravascular volume overload and congestive heart failure, partial exchange (red cells exchanged for whole blood removed) transfusion may be appropriate.[22] The volume of exchange is calculated as follows[22]:

$$\text{Infant's blood volume} \times \frac{\text{Desired Hct} - \text{observed Hct}}{\text{RBC Unit Hct} - \text{observed Hct}}$$

In conclusion, nonimmune hydrops fetalis remains a frustrating disorder with a poor prognosis. A rigorous and aggressive approach to prenatal diagnosis is critical to positively affect the minority of cases that may be salvageable. A multidisciplinary approach is essential to promote a positive outcome for the viable fetus.

Exchange Transfusions

Generally, an exchange transfusion involves the replacement of most or all of the infant's blood with compatible donor red cells and plasma. The technique was first described by Wallerstein in 1946 for the treatment of infants with erythroblastosis fetalis who did not respond to multiple red cell transfusions.[23] Multiple studies have demonstrated the utility of the double-volume exchange transfusion in the infant with erythroblastosis. However, the only randomized, controlled trial was performed by Mollison and Walker in 1952.[24] Exchange transfusion initiated in the first 9 hours of life resulted in a significant reduction in mortality compared to simple transfusion (13% vs 37%).[24] Furthermore, kernicterus was rarely seen in infants receiving an exchange transfusion, especially term infants.

Exchange transfusion has been accepted as a standard mode of therapy to prevent kernicterus. However, because the data are limited and dated, extrapolation to current problems is necessary.

Indications for Exchange Transfusion

The primary indication for exchange transfusion is to reduce unconjugated bilirubin levels to prevent kernicterus in those infants who have failed other therapies such as phototherapy, heme oxygenase inhibitors, phenobarbital, or intravenous immune globulin. Before the widespread availability of RhIG, Rh HDN was the most common condition requiring exchange transfusion. Today, ABO HDN is the most common indication. (There are several nonimmune-mediated causes of hyperbilirubinemia; however, a discussion is beyond the scope of this chapter.)

In most instances, the fetus is either blood group A or B, and the mother is group O. Placental transfer of maternal IgG antibody results in coating of fetal cells, which are then destroyed. The resulting hemolysis can lead to a more rapid production of bilirubin than the immature neonatal liver can process. Elevated levels of unconjugated bilirubin can exceed the binding capacity of albumin, leading to an increase in free serum bilirubin. Free bilirubin can cross the blood-brain barrier, staining critical structures, creating neurotoxicity and consequently, kernicterus. Although there is almost always maternal transfer of antibody, most infants remain asymptomatic, and those that do have clinical manifestations usually display mild disease. Many other antigens can potentially result in severe hemolytic disease, including Kell, Duffy, and Kidd.

Numerous benefits result from a double-volume exchange transfusion in hemolytic disease. Bilirubin is removed from the circulation and tissues, lessening the possibility of kernicterus. Antibody-coated erythrocytes, which are likely to have decreased survival, are removed from the circulation. Preventing the hemolysis of such cells limits further increase in bilirubin levels. Free maternal antibody in the circulation is removed, preventing attachment to and subsequent hemolysis of the infant's newly produced red cells. The blood returned to the infant is devoid of the offending antigen and antibody, so there is no hemolysis and the cells will have a normal lifespan.

In infants who were anemic before the procedure, a normal hematocrit can be reestablished without causing heart failure. There is the theoretic benefit of replacing fetal hemoglobin with hemoglobin A, providing improved oxygen-carrying capacity and oxygen off-loading at the tissue level. Finally, the plasma component will provide additional free albumin, which can bind bilirubin.

Timing of Exchange Transfusion

Optimal timing for intervention with an exchange transfusion in the treatment of hyperbilirubinemia is controversial. Multiple factors are involved in the decision to exchange, including: evidence of hemolysis, degree of anemia, the rate of rise of the bilirubin level, gestational age, and other clinical conditions that may alter brain susceptibility to bilirubin entry and toxicity, such as acidosis, hypoalbuminemia, or asphyxia. Current guidelines are largely based on extrapolation and clinical observation.

Procedures performed in the first 9 to 12 hours of life are considered early transfusions, and are based on cord blood hemoglobin and serum bilirubin, as well as the early rate of rise of the bilirubin. Older recommendations for early exchange transfusion have included a cord hemoglobin of less than 13 to 15 g/dL and a cord serum bilirubin level greater than 3 to 7 mg/dL.[25] These criteria have been modified over time due to conflicting data and changes in therapy, including phototherapy, intravenous immunoglobulin, and prenatal transfusion. Graphs that plot bilirubin levels over time to provide a "zone of obligatory exchange transfusion" are available for both term and preterm infants; however, they do not account for newer therapies. A reasonable guideline would be to consider early exchange in the neonate with severe anemia (hemoglobin <10 g/dL) or a rate of bilirubin rise >0.5 mg/dL/hour while under optimal phototherapy.[26]

Late exchange transfusions are those performed after 9 to 12 hours, when bilirubin levels are rising toward critical levels associated with kernicterus despite maximal therapy (see Table 3-3). Indications for late exchange transfusion are controversial and differ depending on multiple clinical factors. Traditionally, exchange transfusion has been used to prevent the total bilirubin level from exceeding 20 mg/dL. This value was based on data from studies in the early 1950s that demonstrated an association between increasing bilirubin levels and the risk of kernicterus. In these studies, the risk of kernicterus was as high as 50%

Table 3-3. Guidelines for Late (after 9-12 hours) Exchange Transfusion*

Infant Birthweight	Bilirubin Level
<1000 g	10 mg/dL
1000 - 1249 g	10 - 13 mg/dL
1250 - 1499 g	12 - 15 mg/dL
1500 - 1999 g	15 - 17 mg/dL
2000 - 2500 g	17 - 19 mg/dL
2500 g at 25 - 48 hours	20 - 25 mg/dL
2500 g at 48+ hours	25 - 30 mg/dL

*Values may vary based on age, birthweight, clinical condition of the patient, and the severity of hemolysis. See text for early exchange transfusion.
Modified from Peterec.[25]

in infants with bilirubin levels greater than 30 mg/dL, but was minimal in those infants whose levels remained below 18 mg/dL.[27,28] For the stable term infant with hemolytic disease, 20 mg/dL remains the standard. The American Academy of Pediatrics has developed evidence- and consensus-based guidelines for the healthy term infant with nonhemolytic hyperbilirubinemia.[29]

Methods of Exchange Transfusion

There are two techniques for exchange transfusions. Wallerstein[23] originally described the isovolumetric method, where blood is simultaneously withdrawn and replaced. This technique requires two sites of vascular access (usually the umbilical artery and vein) and two individuals to perform the procedure. As each aliquot of blood is removed, an equal amount is simultaneously infused into the second site, avoiding sudden changes in arterial pressure.

The other method is the discontinuous technique developed by Diamond et al.[30] This technique consists of removal and then replacement of small aliquots of blood through a single catheter.

Both methods are performed with the serial exchange of small aliquots of blood; however, this is of increased importance in the discontinuous method because the sudden removal of blood from the infant can result in altered hemodynamic stability, especially in the premature infant who is at risk for altered cerebral blood flow and intracranial hemorrhage.

A maximum of 5 mL/kg or 5% of the infant's blood volume is replaced over 2 to 4 minutes during each cycle of the exchange. The total volume exchanged is twice the infant's blood volume (85 mL/kg × 2 for the term infant, up to 100 mL/kg × 2 for the very low birthweight infant). There is no benefit to exceeding two blood volumes. Similarly, there is little lost if the volume is slightly less than twice the infant's blood volume. Practically, the actual volume used should be approximated to the nearest full RBC unit to minimize donor exposures.

The procedure takes 1 to 2 hours to perform. The procedure should not be performed too quickly, because there will be insufficient time for extraction of bilirubin from the tissues as reequilibration occurs between serum and tissue bilirubin. The procedure should not be performed too slowly, because the efficiency of the exchange is maximal initially and diminishes exponentially as the procedure continues.[31]

A single-volume exchange transfusion will remove 70% to 75% of the newborn's erythrocytes, whereas a double-volume exchange transfusion will remove approximately 90% of the fetal cells. Bilirubin levels decrease only by about 50% due to tissue reequilibration and once complete, bilirubin levels may rebound to 60% of the pre-exchange levels.[32] Levels may rebound to higher levels in cases of aggressive hemolytic disease (Rh, Kell), requiring additional exchange transfusions.

Components Used in Exchange Transfusion

Several combinations of blood components have been used for exchange transfusions. However, there are no controlled trials to evaluate superiority of any one method. Most commonly, red cells preserved less than 5 to 7 days in CPDA-1 are used, although the use of cells preserved in additive solutions has been increasing. Alternatively, frozen deglycerolized red cells may be used.

FFP is usually added to the red cells to provide plasma proteins, coagulation factors, and albumin. Supernatant preservative solution should be removed from the RBC unit to allow for the appropriate addition of the FFP to reconstitute the unit to a hematocrit of 40% to 45%. The volumes are calculated as given below.

Total volume (in mL) = infant's weight in kg × 85* mL/kg × 2

Absolute volume of RBCs required (in mL) =
Total volume × 0.45 (the desired hematocrit)

Actual volume of RBCs required (in mL) =
Absolute volume/hematocrit of unit after any manipulation

Necessary volume of FFP = Total volume required –
actual volume of RBCs required

*(85 to 100 mL/kg, depending on estimated blood volume)

The blood should be kept well-mixed throughout the procedure to maintain the same hematocrit through multiple exchange cycles. Remaining partial RBC units and FFP should be kept in the blood bank refrigerator until expiration (24 hours) in case a second exchange transfusion is required. This can avoid additional donor exposures.

Other Constituents

There is controversy as to the use of other constituents prior to or during exchange transfusion. Some clinicians will administer additional albumin to the infant to increase intravascular binding of unconjugated bilirubin. By increasing bilirubin binding capacity, the equilibrium with tissue bilirubin is shifted to allow increased diffusion into the vascular space and thus greater quantities of bilirubin to be eliminated during the exchange transfusion. In one nonrandomized study of 75 infants mostly with Rh disease, bilirubin removal was increased by 26%.[33] It is unclear whether this practice is of any benefit in infants with normal albumin levels. Furthermore, this therapy may worsen intravascular volume overload in those infants who are already in congestive heart failure or severely anemic.

Some clinicians use supplemental calcium gluconate during an exchange transfusion. The use of citrated blood may result in calcium chelation and a fall in ionized calcium. It is unclear whether such supplementation is necessary or beneficial. One study compared two groups of full-term infants undergoing exchange transfusion. One group received calcium supplementation with 100 mg calcium gluconate after each 100 mL of the procedure. There were no differences between the two groups in post-exchange ionized calcium levels.[31] If not given prophylactically, the calcium can be administered if clinical signs are present, such as irritability, tetany, or cardiac rhythm disturbance, or if measured ionized calcium levels are low.

No consensus exists concerning the temperature of the blood at the time of transfusion. Some recommend warming the blood to a maximum of 37 C, because of reports of a decrease (0.7 to 2.5 C) in rectal temperature when the blood is at room temperature.[31] There is also concern that cool blood rapidly infused could cause cardiac arrhythmia. Blood should be warmed carefully, to avoid significant hemolysis. Gentle warming in a controlled waterbath is an acceptable method. In-line blood warmers are available. Some clinicians allow the blood to warm slightly under the infant's radiant warmer. The use of non-FDA-approved microwave devices or hot towels wrapped around the tubing is not acceptable.

Complications

The infant should be monitored closely throughout the procedure, including continuous cardiopulmonary monitoring and pulse-oximetry. Feedings should be discontinued prior to the procedure and remain suspended until 12 to 24 hours after completion. Blood work should be obtained before and after the exchange transfusion including: complete blood count, electrolytes, glucose, calcium, indirect bilirubin, and blood gas (if respiratory compromise is present). Additional testing during the procedure may include blood gases, blood sugars, and ionized calcium. Medication levels may be altered by the exchange transfusion. Drug levels may need to be monitored and dosing adjusted accordingly.

In addition to all the potential complications involving blood transfusions, one must give consideration to several serious metabolic, catheter-related, and procedure-related issues. Metabolic complications include hypoglycemia, hyperkalemia, hypocalcemia, metabolic acidosis, and metabolic alkalosis. The alterations in calcium and potassium can lead to arrhythmias and cardiac arrest. Catheters can also cause arrhythmias as well as vessel perforation, emboli, thrombosis, renovascular hypertension, peripheral ischemia and necrosis, necrotizing enterocolitis, and infection. Procedure-related complications include thrombocytopenia, leukopenia, systemic blood pressure fluctuations, intracranial pressure fluctuations with possible intracranial hemorrhage, accidental hemorrhage, loss of intravascular catheters, hypothermia, and hemolysis.

The National Institute of Child Health and Human Development (NICHD) phototherapy study demonstrated a rate of 6.7% for adverse clinical problems and a mortality rate of 0.5%.[34] Jackson et al[35] found a severe complication rate of 4% and a mortality rate of 2% in a review of two hospitals' experience with exchange transfusions between 1981 and 1995. *Exchange transfusion is a procedure that is not to be undertaken lightly and should only be performed in an appropriate neonatal intensive care setting by experienced personnel.*

Erythropoietin

Erythropoietin (EPO) is the principal growth factor that regulates erythropoiesis by inhibiting programmed cell death (apoptosis) and stimulating immature erythroid progenitor cell proliferation and differentiation into normoblasts.[14,36] During fetal life the liver is the primary source of EPO, while in the adult it is the kidney.[37] In the fetus and neonate, renal EPO production begins to increase at 30 weeks' gestation; at term, approximately

75% of EPO is still hepatic. The switch is not thought to be complete until several months of age.[14] Hepatic production of EPO in response to hypoxic stress is only 10% of that produced by renal cells under similar stimulation and EPO requires a longer induction period in the liver.[14] As a result, the premature infant is likely to have a diminished response to the decreasing hemoglobin concentration seen in the first months of life.

Studies have suggested that EPO is metabolized three to four times more per kg in the preterm and term infant than in adults.[15] Studies have also found that compared to adults, neonates have increased plasma volume of distribution, shorter fractional elimination, and shorter mean residence times for EPO.[38] However, in-vitro studies have demonstrated that erythroid progenitor cells in the preterm infant are highly responsive to EPO.[39] This finding suggests that an inadequate EPO level—not marrow unresponsiveness—is the major cause of the anemia of prematurity. Furthermore, there are apparently normal concentrations of other erythropoietic growth factors that are responsible for erythrocyte production.[40]

With the development of recombinant human erythropoietin (rHuEPO), there have been more than 20 controlled trials since 1990 that have evaluated its use for the treatment and prevention of anemia of prematurity (see Table 3-4). Studies have varied in patient population, used a variety of doses and schedules, and have demonstrated mixed results, thus precluding the development of a consensus for treatment. The earliest pilot studies used adult doses of rHuEPO, and found little or no effect in the preterm infant. However, once the differences in EPO pharmacokinetics in the neonate were understood, higher doses per kilogram of body weight consistently demonstrated stimulation of erythropoiesis and moderation of neonatal anemia, without any short-term safety issues. The true objective for the use of rHuEPO, though, is not simply to increase the hematocrit, but to reduce the need for transfusion therapy. Unfortunately, many of the older studies involved infants who were relatively mature and stable. The vast majority of these infants would not require red cell transfusions using current standard care, bringing into question the efficacy of rHuEPO.

Table 3-4. Major Trials of rHuEPO for Anemia of Prematurity

Study and Size	Birth-weight (grams)	Gesta-tional Age (week)	Enrollment Criteria	rHuEPO Dose (IU/kg/dose)	Trans-fusion Criteria*	Results† (EPO followed by control)	p Value	Comment
Maier et al[41] (n = 241)	750-1499	<34	Day of life 3-42 stable respiratory status	250 SC 3 times/week +iron	Liberal	0-2 weeks: no change in transfusion needs or success rates >2 weeks: mean no. of transfusions 0.9 vs 1.3 Success rate‡ 27.5% vs 4.1%	NS 0.013 0.008	Liberal transfusion criteria resulted in more single transfusions in control group
Meyer et al[42] (n = 80)	900-1500	28-32	Age: 2-8 weeks Hct ≤0.35 stable respiratory status	200 SC 3 times/week +iron, vitamin E	Strict	Total no. of transfusions: 7 vs 21 % infants transfused; 15 vs 42.5	0.002 0.013	Improved erythropoiesis in **mature** preterm infants
Shannon et al[43] (n = 157)	≤1250	<31	Day of life 7-42 stable respiratory status Hct < 0.40	100 SC 5 times/week +iron, vitamin E	Strict	Mean no. of transfusions/infant: 1.1 vs 1.5 Volume transfused/infant: 16.5 vs 23.9 No transfusions: 43% vs 31%	0.046 0.023 0.18	Highlights importance of strict transfusion guidelines

(continued)

Table 3-4. Major Trials of rHuEPO for Anemia of Prematurity (continued)

Study and Size	Birth-weight (grams)	Gestational Age (week)	Enrollment Criteria	rHuEPO Dose (IU/kg/dose)	Transfusion Criteria*	Results[†] (EPO followed by control)	p Value	Comment
Al-Kharfy et al[44] (n = 55)	<1250	AGA mean 26	Age 10-17 days Hct <0.45 >75% risk BPD	200 SC 3 times/ week + iron, vitamin E, folate	Strict	Mean no. of transfusions/infant: 3.5 vs 5.7 No transfusion after day 28: 14 vs 3	0.0001 0.003	Decreased transfusion needs, but infants averaged 2 transfusions before entry
Donato et al[45] (n = 114)	<1250	<32	0-72 hours	250 IV 5 times/ week[§] + iron, folate	Strict	Mean no. of transfusions/infant: 1.8 vs 1.8 Mean no. of transfusions/infant to day of life 14: 0.8 vs 0.9	NS NS	Transfusion needs outweigh increase in reticulocyte counts

Ohls et al[46] protocol 1 (n = 172)	401-1000	≤32	24-96 hours and likely to survive >72 hours	400 IV or SC 3 times/week + iron, vitamin E	Strict	Infants transfused: 84% vs 87% Mean no. of transfusion/infant: 4.3 vs 5.2 Volume transfused/infant: 80 vs 95	0.56 0.09 0.16	rHuEPO stimulates erythropoiesis in very low birthweight infants, but does not reduce transfusion requirements or donor exposures (both protocols)
Ohls et al[46] protocol 2 (n = 118)	1001-1250	≤32	24-96 hours and likely to survive >72 hours	400 IV or SC 3 times/week + iron, vitamin E	Strict	Infants transfused: 37% vs 46% Mean no. of transfusions/infant: 1.0 vs 1.1 Volume transfused/infant: 39 vs 35	0.25 0.42 0.89	

*See section transfusion guidelines for definition of strict transfusion criteria
†Volume transfused is in mL.
‡Success rate defined by no need for transfusion and maintenance of a venous hematocrit ≥32%.
§Experimental infants treated for 2 weeks. All infants received rHuEPO 250 IU SC 3 times/week for 6 weeks.

rHuEPO = recombinant human erythropoietin; SC = subcutaneous; IV = intravenous; AGA = appropriate for gestational age; BPD = bronchopulmonary dysplasia; NS = not significant

Three large randomized, controlled trials evaluating the subcutaneous administration of rHuEPO to a total of 478 preterm infants have been published.[41-43] The first multicenter trial by Maier et al for the European Multicentre Erythropoietin Study Group demonstrated that rHuEPO stimulates erythropoiesis and ameliorates anemia of prematurity. However, the results are limited by the liberal transfusion criteria, which resulted in more control infants receiving a single transfusion that otherwise would have been avoided. Furthermore, liberal transfusion practices unrealistically exaggerate the potential benefit of rHuEPO by suppressing endogenous erythropoiesis and creating transfusion dependency. The study by Meyer et al confirms the findings of the European trial; however, again the population studied was at a relatively low risk of requiring a transfusion. Over half the control infants did not require transfusion, suggesting that many infants would receive unnecessary therapy if rHuEPO were administered routinely to this population. In the US multicenter study,[43] rHuEPO provided a consistent and significant boost to erythropoiesis in the preterm infant. Still, there was only a modest impact on total red cell transfusion.

More recent studies in extremely premature infants have demonstrated a decrease in the number and volume of transfusions administered to rHuEPO recipients. However, these infants continue to require multiple transfusions.[44-46] Although there is a clear enhancement of erythropoiesis and some reduction in transfusion needs, the significant phlebotomy losses, the severity of illness, and the lag time to response all prevent rHuEPO from having a dramatic impact.

These study results leave the clinician with a dilemma. The infants who demonstrate the best response to rHuEPO are the larger, more mature, clinically stable infants who are at the lowest risk for transfusion. The critically ill, extremely low birthweight infant with the greatest transfusion needs will not respond well enough to rHuEPO to eliminate the need for transfusion. Through the use of dedicated units and sterile connection devices, neonates can receive multiple transfusions from a single unit of blood for 35 to 42 days, depending on the storage medium.[47-50] With this strategy, even the smallest and sickest premature infants can generally be managed with only one or two donor exposures for the entire hospitalization. The question then becomes whether it is justifiable to expose the infant to a course of therapy that decreases the number of transfusions, but most likely has little or no impact on donor exposure.

Clinicians remain at odds over the routine use of rHuEPO in the neonate. Utility may depend on whether the facility is using strict transfusion guidelines and dedicated RBC units. Some researchers feel that although rHuEPO has been fairly extensively studied, there are still many unanswered questions regarding efficacy, patient population, dosing, cost, and long-term outcomes and effects.[51]

Other experts feel that although rHuEPO has not been approved by the FDA specifically for use in the neonate, that when combined with rigorous transfusion criteria and efforts to minimize phlebotomy losses, it is useful for reducing erythrocyte transfusions. One such group of researchers has proposed using rHuEPO in two situations: reducing transfusions in the first days of life in the ill, extremely low birthweight infant with significant phlebotomy losses, and reducing or eliminating late transfusions in the stable very low birthweight infant with anemia of prematurity.[52] They recommend a 2-week course of therapy followed by a reevaluation of the need for additional therapy. Widness and Strauss[15] feel that inadequate data exist to support the use of rHuEPO in the ill, extremely low birthweight infant and that in infants with birthweights greater than 1.3 kg, the unlikelihood of transfusion precludes its use.

However, they agree that therapy may be reasonable in the infant with a birthweight between 0.8 and 1.3 kg with the understanding and consent of the parents that it is a therapy without universal acceptance and uncertain long-term effects. They recommend continuing therapy until either red cell transfusions are no longer required or the infant is 8 to 12 weeks of age.

Because there is still a lack of clinical evidence to establish definitive guidelines for the use of rHuEPO, the individual facility should decide whether to use it to treat anemia of prematurity. If rHuEPO is used, guidelines to allow for a rational and consistent approach to rHuEPO therapy in the neonate should be developed based on available data. Such guidelines should not be rigid protocols, nor should they replace clinical judgment. Finally, given the controversial nature of the therapy, it is prudent to involve families in the decision-making process.

Transfusion Trigger

Infants with anemia of prematurity are often transfused if they have symptoms that are attributed to anemia. When hemoglobin levels begin to fall, the infant responds with compensatory mechanisms to either increase oxygen delivery or reduce consumption. If the oxygen demands exceed the compensatory response, then symptoms of anemic hypoxia will develop. Adaptive mechanisms in the infant include increasing cardiac output, mostly by increasing heart rate, increasing respiratory effort to improve oxygenation or to decrease pCO_2 to compensate for metabolic acidosis, decreasing oxygen consumption by decreasing activity, or increasing erythropoiesis to increase erythrocyte production.[53] Symptoms that may be indicative of inadequate tissue oxygenation include: periodic breathing or apnea and bradycardia, tachycardia, poor weight gain, and lactic acidosis due to anaerobic metabolism. Numerous studies have been undertaken to better understand the effects of anemia in the premature infant and the response to transfusion (Table 3-5).

In apnea of prematurity the infant's ventilatory response to carbon dioxide is diminished by hypoxia.[55] The rationale for red cell transfusion in these patients is that an increase in red cell mass will improve oxygen delivery to the central nervous system, which in turn makes the infant less sensitive to respiratory depression and apnea. Increasing heart rate is a compensatory mechanism for the anemic infant to improve oxygen delivery through increasing cardiac output. Investigators have hypothesized that increasing red cell mass through red cell transfusion would result in a decrease in heart rate and cardiac output.[56-63] Some clinicians feel that poor weight gain, especially when associated with decreased activity, is an indication for transfusion of

Table 3-5. Studies Examining Small-Volume Red Cell Transfusions in Preterm Infants[54]

Study	Patient Characteristics	Study Size and Characteristics	Hb or Hct Pre- and Posttransfusion	Results
Blank, 1984	• BW <1.5 kh • GA 27-32 week • Entered study at birth	• Randomized to keep Hb > 10 g/dL (group A, n = 26) or transfusion according to clinical indication (group B, n = 30)	• Discharge Hb (g/dL): Group A = 11.8, Group B = 9.1 (p <0.001)	• No significant differences between groups in weight gain or the incidence or severity of apnea
Stockman, 1984	• BW <1.5 kg • PNA 33-34 day • Weight gain < expected mean for BW and GA	• Observational, uncontrolled • n = 13	• Hb 8.5⟶11.4 g/dL	• Weight gain (g/kg/day): 20⟶28—change most marked in infants with pretransfusion Hb <7.5 g/dL
Joshi, 1987	• Stable infants • GA 30 week (26-36) • PNA 47 day (18-105)	• Observational, uncontrolled • n = 30	• Hct 0.27⟶0.36 (p <0.001)	• HR (beats/min): 157⟶148 (p = 0.001) • Periodic breathing (min/100 min): 6⟶1 (p = 0.01) • No. of apneic episodes 5-10 seconds/100 minutes: 9⟶5 (p = 0.05) • No. of apneic episodes 11-20 seconds/100 minutes: 0-1.1⟶0-0.4 (p = 0.05)

(continued)

Table 3-5. Studies Examining Small-Volume Red Cell Transfusions in Preterm Infants[54] (continued)

Study	Patient Characteristics	Study Size and Characteristics	Hb or Hct Pre- and Posttransfusion	Results
Alverson, 1988	• Infants with BPD (9 requiring mechanical ventilation) • GA 27 week (25-30) • BW 0.9 kg (0.7-1.1) • PNA 5 week (3-7)	• Observational, uncontrolled • n = 10	• Hb 11.2→14.8 g/dL ($p < 0.001$)	• VO_2 (mL O_2/min/kg): 10.4→9.4 ($p = 0.02$) • O_2 utilization: 0.31→0.24 ($p < 0.01$) • Hb level not a predictor for a ↓ in O_2 utilization
Ross, 1989	• GA < 32 week • PNA 1-3 month	• If candidate for transfusion (Hct ≤0.29 and BPD or symptomatic apnea/BC) randomized to receive (T, n = 18) or not to receive a transfusion (NT, n = 8)	• T: pretransfusion Hb 8.7 g/dL (post- not stated) • NT: Hb 9.7 g/dL	• Weight gain (g/kg/day): T 13.5→17.4: NT = 18.2→9.8 ($p < 0.07$) • Apnea (not further defined): according to authors, significantly improved in transfused group • Lactate levels (μmol/g blood): T 1.6→0.9 (N <0.9); NT-no change
Demaio, 1989	• Stable infants • GA 31 week (26-35) • PNA 34 day (12-75)	• Observational, uncontrolled • n = 23	• Hct 0.31→0.42 ($p < 0.001$)	• Periodic breathing (% sleep time): 4.9→1.5 ($p = 0.025$) • Apnea density (% sleep time): 6.5→3.1 ($p = 0.01$)

Keyes, 1989	• GA 29 week (25-37) • PNA > 7 day	• Observational, uncontrolled • n = 11	• Hct 0.31→0.38 ($p < 0.05$)	• No. of apneic episodes >15 seconds/24 hours: 0.3→0.3 (NS) • HR (beats/min: 154→151 (NS)
Hudson, 1990	• Stable and ill infants (10 infants on ventilators) • GA 24-34 week • PNA 25 d (2-90)	• Observational, uncontrolled • n = 24	• Hb 12.0→17.7 g/dL	• Red cell volume (mL/kg): 27→45 • CO (mL/kg/min): 286→251 • Most marked fall in CO in infants with pretransfusion red cell volume <25 mL/kg
Sasidharan, 1990	• Stable infants • GA 29.3 ± 2.4 week • PNA 42 ± 22 day	• Observational, uncontrolled • n = 10 • Transfusion guidelines defined	• Hct 0.28→0.38 ($p < 0.01$)	• Study of pulmonary mechanics • Compliance decreased in all infants; other measurements showed no significant changes
Sasidharan, 1992	• Stable infants • GA 29 week (27-32) • PNA 41 day (22-61)	• Observational, uncontrolled • n = 14	• Hct 0.27→0.36 ($p < 0.0001$)	• HR (beats/min): 160→154 ($p = 0.0001$) • Periodic breathing (% total time): 10.1→5.6 ($p = 0.01$)

(continued)

Table 3-5. Studies Examining Small-Volume Red Cell Transfusions in Preterm Infants[54] (continued)

Study	Patient Characteristics	Study Size and Characteristics	Hb or Hct Pre- and Posttransfusion	Results
Bifano, 1992	• Infants with 6-second apnea density ≥5% • GA 29-30 week • PNA 38-46 day	• Randomized to receive RBC transfusion (T = 14) or 5% albumin (NT = 12)	• Hb (g/dL): T 8.3⟶11.3 (p <0.001) NT 8.5⟶7.9 (p <0.001)	• HR (beats/minutes): T 157⟶151 (p = 0.01) NT-no change • No significant differences pre versus posttransfusion in either group for cardiac output, periodic breathing, or no. of apneic episodes >10 seconds/100 minutes • Oxygen consumption (mL/kg/minutes): T 7.3⟶6.5 (p = 0.01) NT 7.5⟶7.9 (NS) • 6-second apnea density: T 8.6⟶4.5 (p = 0.01); NT 9.0⟶4.7 (p = 0.01)

Izraeli, 1993	• Stable infants • GA 30-31 week • PNA 33-40 day	• Observational, uncontrolled • n = 37	• Hct 0.27→0.38	• HR (beats/minutes): 155→150 (p = 0.01) • No significant changes in weight gain • Infants with elevated lactate levels pretransfusion (n = 17) had significant decrease in lactate levels
Myer, 1993	• GA ≤33 week • Entered study at birth	• Randomized to keep Hct >0.35 (T, n = 9) or to no transfusion (NT, n = 10) • 14 other infants, initially randomized, removed from study because of physician decision to transfuse	• Hb (g/dL): T = 11.5→14.3 (p <0.0001); NT = 12.0→11.1	• Weight gain (g/kg/day): T = 18→27; NT = 21→25 • Apnea (not further defined): similar in both groups

(continued)

Table 3-5. Studies Examining Small-Volume Red Cell Transfusions in Preterm Infants[54] (continued)

Study	Patient Characteristics	Study Size and Characteristics	Hb or Hct Pre- and Posttransfusion	Results
Lachance, 1994	• Stable infants • GA 28 week (26-30) • PNA 35 day (33-37)	• Observational, uncontrolled • n = 12	• Hb (g/dL): 7.5→15.0	• HR (beats/minutes) 155→146 ($p = 0.05$) • CO (mL/kg/minutes): 281→199 ($p = 0.05$)
Lachance, 1994				• 7 other indices of myocardial function-no significant changes • VO_2 (mL/kg/min): 8.4→9.0 (NS) • Weight gain (mg/kg/day): 19→16 (NS)
Nelle, 1994	• Stable infants • GA 29 week (26-34) • PNA 48 day (19-100)	• Observational, uncontrolled • n = 33	• Hct: 0.27→0.37 ($p < 0.001$)	• HR (beats/min): 161→149 ($p < 0.005$) • CO (mL/kg/min): 367→311 ($p < 0.005$) • Mean blood flow velocity (mL/seconds) -Internal carotid artery: 0.24→0.22 ($p < 0.05$) -Anterior cerebral artery: 0.26→0.20 ($p < 0.05$) -Celiac trunk: 0.34→0.30 ($p < 0.05$)

Stute, 1995	• Stable infants • GA ≤32 week • PNA 39 day	• Observational, uncontrolled • n = 25	• Hb (g/dL): 7.8→11.7 ($p < 0.001$)	• No. of apneic episodes >10 seconds/day: 2.7→0.9 ($p = 0.04$) • No. of BCs <100 beats/minute: 66→13 per day ($p = 0.004$) • No. of tachycardias >200 beats/minute: 34→25 per day ($p = 0.004$)
Moller, 1995	• Entered study at birth—removed if severe cardiorespiratory disorder • GA 32 week (27-36) • PNA 30 day (3-56)	• Observational, uncontrolled • n = 56 (19 infants transfused, 37 not transfused)	• Hb (g/dL) 12.1 in nontransfused • Hb (g/dL) 9.7→12.9 in transfused	• No significant correlation between Hb and CO or serum lactate or between serum lactate and CO or O_2 delivery

Abbreviations: BW = birthweight; GA = gestational age; PNA = postnatal age; Hct = hematocrit; HR = heart rate; BPD = bronchopulmonary dysplasia; VO_2 = oxygen consumption; BC = bradycardia; CO = cardiac output; NS = not significant; d = days; s = seconds

Note: (1) Unless indicated, RBC transfusions were given as judged necessary by the treating physician. (2) Stable infants refers to infants receiving oral feedings and not on supplemental oxygen; some were receiving methylxanthines, and some may have had periodic breathing, apnea, and/or episodes of bradycardia. (3) Where no p value is given, none was given in the study. (4) Not all parameters evaluated in all the studies are shown in this table.

Hematocrit values in this table are expressed in international units.

the neonate with anemia of prematurity. Lethargy with poor nippling results in decreased caloric intake. Tachycardia or respiratory difficulties result in increased metabolic expenditures. Inadequate systemic oxygen delivery will result in cellular dysfunction and growth failure. Finally, there are some investigators who have looked at lactic acidosis as a marker of anemic hypoxia.[58,62,64] If oxygen delivery to the tissues is inadequate, anaerobic metabolism will increase, resulting in an increase in lactic acid.

Although space constraints do not allow a complete review of all the studies on transfusion trigger in anemia of prematurity, examples will illustrate the difficulty of interpreting the data. At least eight studies have evaluated the effect of small-volume red cell transfusion on respiratory control in stable premature infants.[56-59,61,65-67] The studies are all small with varying patient populations and definitions of respiratory irregularities. Only one of the studies[59] has a control group; the others use the infant as its own control. The results are inconsistent, with five of the studies finding an improvement in measures of apnea after transfusion and the other three revealing no clinical benefit. Joshi et al[56] observed that after transfusion, infants had a decrease in the following: periodic breathing, the longest episode of periodic breathing, 5- to 10-second apnea, 11- to 20-second apnea, and bradycardic episodes.

On the other hand, Keyes et al[57] found small volume red cell transfusions had no impact on respiratory rate, apneic episodes, or bradycardic episodes. In the only study with control subjects, anemic preterm infants were assigned to receive either an erythrocyte transfusion or an isovolemic infusion of 5% albumin.[59] There was no relationship between measures of oxygen delivery and respiratory irregularities. However, both groups showed a similar decrease in 6-second apnea density after infusion, suggesting that the volume expansion, not an increase in oxygen supply from an increase in hemoglobin, was responsible for the change in respiratory pattern. Additional data are needed to determine if transfusion effects on respiratory patterns are sustained because only one of the studies examined patterns beyond 12 hours after transfusion.

It should be noted that even in those trials where there were statistically significant changes in breathing patterns related to red cell transfusion, the clinical relevance is questionable. For example, Joshi et al[56] found that the median number of 11- to 20-second apneas was 0 in both groups; however, the range before transfusion was 0 to 1.1 and decreased to 0 to 0.4 after transfusion. Similarly, Stute et al[61] observed a decrease in bradycardic episodes to less than 80 beats per minute from 3.9 to 2.4. Such results are probably not clinically significant enough to justify exposing the infant to the potential risks of transfusion.

Studies have shown that the hemoglobin or hematocrit correlate poorly with red cell mass in the neonate and it is a low red cell mass that seems to be better at identifying the infant who will respond to transfusion.[68] Red cell mass is usually determined by measurement of Cr^{51}-labeled autologous cells, a technique that is not appropriate for routine use in infants. Non-radioactive biotin-labeled autologous cells have also been used to measure red cell volume, but would be difficult to use in the clinical setting.[69] Another proposed technique involves measuring the difference between pre- and posttransfusion Hb F levels. This method is limited to early postnatal life due to increasing Hb A levels from endogenous production as well as transfusion.[70] Other physiologic criteria for determining the need for transfusion have been suggested, including available oxygen, mixed venous oxygen saturation, and oxygen delivery and consumption.[38,71] Again, these techniques are not readily accessible in routine practice and studies are lacking to demonstrate efficacy over the currently used strategies and guidelines.

Transfusion Guidelines

Currently available data from studies on neonatal anemia and response to red cell transfusion do not allow for the establishment of universal transfusion guidelines at this time. Recommendations by expert opinion have been established over the years to provide guidance to the clinician caring for at-risk newborns. Recent efforts to reduce transfusion risks have focused on safely decreasing transfusions and donor exposures. Although infants cared for today are more premature and critically ill, there has been a steady decrease in transfusion requirements. One study found a progressive decrease in both red cell transfusions and donor exposures from 1982 to 1993.[72] Transfusions per infant declined from 7.0 in 1982 to 5.0 in 1989, and to 2.3 in 1993. Similarly, donor exposures per infant decreased from 4.8 and 5.0 in 1982 and 1989 respectively, to 2.2 in 1993. This is at least in part related to the institution and maintenance of stricter transfusion criteria.

There continues to be significant variation in transfusion practices among neonatal intensive care units. In 1998, Bednarek et al[73] found transfusion volumes in low birthweight infants varied by as much as 47 mL/kg per infant during hospitalization; however, there were no differences in rates of intraventricular hemorrhage, necrotizing enterocolitis, bronchopulmonary dysplasia, 28-day weight gain, or length of stay. They concluded that transfusion and phlebotomy guidelines could result in fewer transfusions, fewer complications, and reduced cost. However, we are still lacking the clinical evidence to establish definitive red cell transfusion guidelines. Based on available data, multiple groups have proposed guidelines to allow for a rational and consistent approach to erythrocyte transfusions in the neonate. Such guidelines are not meant to be rigid protocols, nor are they intended to replace clinical judgment.

The American Association of Blood Banks, the British Committee for Standards in Haematology, and the Canadian Pediatric Society each published recommendations for neonatal red cell transfusions in the early 1990s.[74-76] They all recommend maintaining a hemoglobin of 13 g/L in neonates with severe pulmonary or cardiac disease. For infants with symptomatic anemia of prematurity, these guidelines suggest red cell transfusion for a hemoglobin varying from 8.0 to 10.5 g/L. In the US multicenter erythropoietin study,[43] the researchers developed strict and rigorously defined transfusion criteria. Similar criteria were recently presented by a consensus of neonatologists to encourage uniformity of care until definitive study results are available.[52] Table 3-6 is an integration of these sources and is designed as a

Table 3-6. Guidelines for Neonatal Red Cell Transfusion

1. Transfuse all ill infants with acute blood loss with hypotension.
2. Transfuse infants with a hematocrit of ≤35% to 40% if:
   a. On mechanical ventilation requiring either a fraction of inspired oxygen (FiO_2) of greater than 35% to 40% or a mean airway pressure of greater than 6 to 9 cm H_2O.
3. Transfuse infants with a hematocrit of ≤28% to 30% if:
   a. On mechanical ventilation requiring either a fraction of inspired oxygen of less than 35% to 40% or a mean airway pressure of less than 6 to 9 cm H_2O.
   b. Weaned off of mechanical ventilation, but still have a significant supplemental oxygen requirement (>40%).
   c. Undergoing major surgery
   d. There are any of the following signs of anemia:
      1) Significant unexplained apnea (greater than 12 to 18 spells per day or two episodes per day requiring bag and mask ventilation) despite therapeutic methylxanthine therapy.
      2) Persistent, unexplained heart rate greater than 165 to 180 beats/minute or respiratory rate greater than 80 breaths/minute lasting more than 24 to 48 hours.
      3) Unexplained poor weight gain <10 g/day over 4 to 7 days despite adequate caloric intake (100-120 kcal/kg/d).
      4) Unexplained lethargy.
4. Transfuse infants with a hematocrit <20% ± reticulocyte count ≤100,000/μL, regardless of signs of anemia.
5. Do not transfuse to replace blood removed for laboratory tests alone.

framework from which individual facilities can develop standards adapted to local populations and practices.

Transfusions generally consist of 10 to 15 mL/kg body weight of type- and Rh-compatible, filtered RBCs with no detectable cytomegalovirus or Hb S administered over 2 to 4 hours. The blood may be administered more rapidly if the infant has ongoing losses or is hemodynamically unstable. The cells are irradiated when there is concern about immune deficiency, prior intrauterine transfusion, or the possibility of organ transplantation. Directed donor blood can be used at parental request, as available.

It should be noted that one area of concern regarding strict transfusion criteria is the possibility of limiting available oxygen to the developing brain of the preterm infant. The current research shows no clinical differences in measured outcomes between those infants liberally transfused compared to those managed under transfusion guidelines. However, no data exist for the long-term neurodevelopmental outcome of preterm infants exposed to severe anemia.

Conclusion

Our understanding of hematopoiesis in the perinatal period as well as the physiology and pathophysiology of neonatal anemia remains incomplete. The limitations of our knowledge result in significant practice variation and unclear cost/benefit ratios. Measurements of such physiologic indices as red cell mass, available oxygen, mixed venous oxygen saturation, and oxygen delivery and use, may provide more accurate transfusion trigger points, but are technically difficult and not easily applied in clinical practice.[38] Well-designed controlled trials are needed to evaluate risks and benefits of small-volume replacement transfusions in the neonate vs alternative therapies as well as the consequences of not intervening. Until such data are available, clinicians should strive to safely minimize transfusion needs and limit donor exposure. Phlebotomy should be reduced by judicious use of laboratory tests and increased use of noninvasive tests and microsampling techniques. The use of dedicated donor units equipped with multiple satellite bags or maintained by a sterile connection device through to expiration can significantly reduce donor exposures in those infants with the greatest transfusion needs. Recombinant erythropoietin may also have a role in reducing neonatal transfusion requirements, but questions remain regarding dosage, patient population, cost-effectiveness, and long-term neurodevelopmental and hematologic outcome. Other techniques to prevent neonatal anemia, such as delayed umbilical cord clamping, are also in need of further study. Only through the continued rigorous study of anemia in the term and preterm neonate will we uncover the best strategies for safe and effective treatment.

References

1. Shurin SB. The blood and hematopoietic system. In: Fanaroff AA, Martin RJ, eds. Neonatal-perinatal medicine: Diseases of the newborn and fetus, 5th ed. St. Louis, MO: Mosby-Year Book, 1992:941-89.
2. Kaufman P, Scheffen I. The placenta: Placental development. In: Polin RA, Fox WW, eds. Fetal and neonatal physiology. Philadelphia, PA: WB Saunders, 1992:47-56.
3. Molteni RA. Perinatal blood loss. Pediatr Rev 1990;12:47-57.
4. Papile L. Central nervous system disturbances: Periventricular-intraventricular hemorrhage. In: Fanaroff AA, Martin RJ, eds. Neonatal-perinatal medicine: Diseases of the newborn and fetus, 5th ed. St. Louis, MO: Mosby-Year Book, 1992:719-29.
5. Miller MJ, Martin RJ, Fanaroff AA. The respiratory system: Respiratory disorders in term and preterm infants. In: Fanaroff AA, Martin RJ, eds. Neonatal-perinatal medicine: Diseases of the newborn and fetus, 7th ed. St. Louis, MO: Mosby-Year Book, 2002:1025-49.
6. Cole VA, Normand IC, Reynolds EO, Rivers RB. Pathogenesis of hemorrhagic pulmonary edema and massive pulmonary hemorrhage in the newborn. Pediatrics 1973;51:175-87.
7. Bowman JM. Immune hemolytic disease. In: Nathan DG, Orkin SH, eds. Nathan and Oski's hematology of infancy and childhood. 5th ed. Philadelphia, PA: WB Saunders, 1998:53-78.
8. Voak D, Williams MA. An explanation of the failure of the direct antiglobulin test to detect erythrocyte sensitization in ABO hemolytic disease of the newborn and observations on pinocytosis of IgG anti-A antibodies by infant (cord) red cells. Br J Haematol 1971;20:9-23.
9. Romano EL, Hughes-Jones NC, Mollison PL. Direct antiglobulin reaction in ABO-haemolytic disease of the newborn. Br Med J 1973;1:524-6.
10. Gallagher PG. Disorders of erythrocyte metabolism and shape. In: Christensen RD, ed. Hematologic problems of the neonate. Philadelphia, PA: WB Saunders, 2000:209-37.
11. Segel GB. Diseases of the blood: Enzymatic defects. In: Behrman RE, Kliegman RM, Jenson HB, eds. Nelson textbook of pediatrics, 16th ed. Philadelphia, PA: WB Saunders, 2000:1488-11.
12. Bard H. Hemoglobin synthesis and metabolism during the neonatal period. In: Christensen RD, ed. Hematologic problems of the neonate. Philadelphia, PA: WB Saunders, 2000:365-88.

13. Stockman JA, deAlarcon PA. Hematopoiesis and granulopoiesis. In: Polin RA, Fox WW, eds. Fetal and neonatal physiology. Philadelphia, PA: WB Saunders, 1992:1327-62.
14. Dame C, Juul SE. Neonatal hematology: The switch from fetal to adult erythropoiesis. Clin Perinatol 2000;27:507-26.
15. Widness JA, Strauss RG. Recombinant erythropoietin in treatment of the premature newborn. Semin Neonatal 1998;3:163-7.
16. Dallman PR. Anemia of prematurity. Annu Rev Med 1981;32:143-60.
17. Wardrop CAJ, Holland BM, Veale KEA, et al. Non-physiologic anemia of prematurity. Arch Dis Child 1978;53:855-60.
18. Moore TR, Tipton EE. Amniotic fluid and nonimmune hydrops fetalis. In: Fanaroff AA, Martin RJ, eds. Neonatal-perinatal medicine: Diseases of the newborn and fetus, 6th ed. St. Louis, MO: Mosby-Year Book, 1997:312-26.
19. Gough JD, Keeling JW, Castle B, Iliff PJ. The obstetric management of nonimmunological hydrops. Br J Obstet Gynaecol 1986;93:226-34.
20. Allan LD, Crawford DC, Sheridan R, Chapman MG. Aetiology of non-immune hydrops: The value of echocardiography. Br J Obstet Gynaecol 1986;93:223-5.
21. Castillo RA, Devoe LD, Hadi HA, et al. Nonimmune hydrops fetalis: Clinical experience and factors related to a poor outcome. Am J Obstet Gynecol 1986;155:812-16.
22. Warkentin PI. The blood and hematopoietic system: Blood component therapy for the neonate. In: Fanaroff AA, Martin RJ, eds. Neonatal-perinatal medicine: Diseases of the newborn and fetus, 5th ed. St. Louis, MO: Mosby-Year Book, 1992:989-1018.
23. Wallerstein H. Treatment of severe erythroblastosis by simultaneous removal and replacement of the blood of the newborn infant. Science 1946;103:583.
24. Mollison PL, Walker W. Controlled trials of the treatment of haemolytic disease of the newborn. Lancet 1952;262:429.
25. Peterec SM. Perinatal hematology: Management of neonatal Rh disease. Clin Perinatol 1995;22:561-92.
26. Koenig JM. Evaluation and treatment of erythroblastosis fetalis in the neonate. In: Christensen RD, ed. Hematologic problems of the neonate. Philadelphia, PA: WB Saunders, 2000:185-207.
27. Mollison PL, Cutbush M. A method of ensuring the severity of a series of cases of hemolytic disease of the newborn. J Hematol 1951;6:777.
28. Hsia DY-Y, Allen FH, Gelis SS, et al. Erythroblastosis fetalis. VIII. Studies of serum bilirubin in relation to kernicterus. N Engl J Med 1952;247:668.
29. Provisional Committee for Quality Improvement and Subcommittee on Hyperbilirubinemia. Practice parameter: Management of hyperbilirubinemia in the healthy term newborn. Pediatrics 1994;94:558-65.
30. Diamond LK, Allen FH, Thomas WO. Erythroblastosis fetalis. VII. Treatment with exchange transfusion. N Engl J Med 1951;244:39.

31. Warkentin PI. The blood and hematopoietic system: Blood component therapy for the neonate. In: Fanaroff AA, Martin RJ, eds. Neonatal-perinatal medicine: Diseases of the newborn and fetus, 6th ed. St. Louis, MO: Mosby-Year Book, 1997:1252-87.
32. Valaes T. Bilirubin distribution and dynamics of bilirubin removal by exchange transfusion. Acta Paediatr Scand 1963;52S:149.
33. Waters WJ, Porter E. Indications for exchange transfusion based upon the role of albumin in the treatment of hemolytic disease of the newborn. Pediatrics 1964;33:749.
34. Keenan WJ, Novak KK, Sutherland JM, et al. Morbidity and mortality associated with exchange transfusion. Pediatrics 1985;75:422-6.
35. Jackson JC. Adverse events associated with exchange transfusion in healthy and ill neonates. Pediatrics 1997;99:E7.
36. Shannon K. Recombinant human erythropoietin in neonatal anemia. Clin Perinatol 1995;22:627-40.
37. Koury ST, Koury MJ. Erythropoietin production by the kidney. Semin Nephrol 1993;13:78-86.
38. Strauss RG. Blood banking and transfusion issues in perinatal medicine. In: Christensen RD, ed. Hematologic problems of the neonate. Philadelphia, PA: WB Saunders, 2000:405-25.
39. Rhondeau SM, Christensen RD, Ross MP, et al. Reponsiveness to recombinant human erythropoietin of marrow erythroid progenitors from infants with the "anemia of prematurity." J Pediatr 1988;112:935-40.
40. Ohls RK, Liechty KW, Turner MC, et al. Erythroid "burst promoting activity" in the serum of patients with anemia of prematurity. J Pediatr 1990;116:786-9.
41. Maier RF, Obladen M, Scigalla P, et al. The effect of epoetin beta (recombinant human erythropoietin) on the need for transfusion in very-low-birth-weight infants. N Engl J Med 1994;330:918-23.
42. Meyer MP, Meyer JH, Commderford A, et al. Recombinant human erythropoietin in the treatment of the anemia of prematurity: Results of a double-blinded, placebo-controlled study. Pediatrics 1994;93:918-23.
43. Shannon KM, Keith JF, Mentzer WC, et al. Recombinant erythropoietin stimulates erythropoiesis and reduces erythrocyte transfusions in very low birth weight preterm infants. Pediatrics 1995;95:1-8.
44. Al-Karfy T, Smyth JA, Wadsworth L, et al. Erythropoietin therapy in neonates at risk of having bronchopulmonary dysplasia and requiring multiple transfusions. J Pediatr 1996;129:89-96.
45. Donato HD, Vain N, Rendo P, et al. Effect of early versus late administration of human recombinant erythropoietin on transfusion requirements in premature infants: Results of a randomized, placebo-controlled, multi-center trial. Pediatrics 2000;105:1066-72.
46. Ohls RK, Ehrenkranz RA, Wright LL, et al. Effects of early erythropoietin therapy on the transfusion requirements of preterm infants below 1250

grams birth weight: A multicenter, randomized, controlled study. Pediatrics 2001;108:934-42.
47. Liu EA, Mannino FL, Lane TA. A prospective, randomized trial of the safety and efficacy of a limited donor exposure transfusion program for premature neonates. J Pediatr 1994;125:92-6.
48. Lee DA, Slagel TA, Jackson TM, Evans CS. Reducing blood donor exposures in low birth weight infants by the use of older unwashed packed red blood cells. J Pediatr 1995;126:280-6.
49. Strauss RG, Burmeister LF, Johnson K, et al. AS-1 red cells for neonatal transfusions: A randomized trial assessing donor exposure and safety. Transfusion 1996;36:783-8.
50. Goodstein MH, Herman JH, Smith JF, Rubenstein SD. Metabolic consequences in very low birth weight infants transfused with older AS-1-preserved erythrocytes. Pediatr Pathol Mol Med 1998/1999; 18:173-85.
51. Casadevall N, Nataf J, Viron B, et al. Pure red-cell aplasia and anti-erythropoietin antibodies in patients treated with recombinant erythropoietin. N Engl J Med 2002;346:469-75.
52. Calhoun DA, Christensen RD, Edstrom CS, et al. Consistent approaches to procedures and practices in neonatal hematology. Clin Perinatol 2000; 27:733-53.
53. Alverson DC. The physiologic impact of anemia in the neonate. Clin Perinatol 1995;22:609-25.
54. Hume H. Red blood cell transfusions for preterm infants: The role of evidence-based medicine. Semin Perinatol 1997;21:8-19.
55. Miller MJ, Martin RJ. Apnea of prematurity. Clin Perinatol 1992;19: 789-808.
56. Joshi A, Gerhardt T, Shandloff RN, Bancalari E. Blood transfusion effect on the respiratory pattern of preterm infants. Pediatrics 1987;80:79-84.
57. Keyes WG, Kimzey-Donohue P, Spivak JL, et al. Assessing the need for transfusion of premature infants and role of hematocrit, clinical signs, and erythropoietin level. Pediatrics 1989;84:412-17.
58. Ross MP, Christensen RD, Rothstein G, et al. A randomized trial to develop criteria for administering erythrocyte transfusions to anemic preterm infants 1 to 3 months of age. J Perinatol 1989;9:246-53.
59. Bifano EM, Smith F, Borer J. Relationship between determinants of oxygen delivery and respiratory abnormalities in preterm infants with anemia. J Pediatr 1992;120:292-6.
60. Lachance C, Chessex P, Fouron JC, et al. Myocardial, erythropoietic, and metabolic adaptations to anemia of prematurity. J Pediatr 1994;125: 278-82.
61. Stute H, Greiner B, Linerkamp O. Effect of blood transfusion on cardiorespiratory abnormalities in preterm infants. Arch Dis Child 1995;72: F194-6.

62. Izraeli S, Ben-Sira L, Harell D, et al. Lactic acid as a predictor for erythrocyte transfusion in healthy preterm infants with anemia of prematurity. J Pediatr 1993;122:629-31.
63. Alverson DC, Isken VH, Cohen RS. Effect of booster blood transfusions on oxygen utilization in infants with bronchopulmonary dysplasia. J Pediatr 1988;113:722-6.
64. Moller JC, Schwarz U, Schaible TF, et al. Do cardiac output and serum lactate levels indicate blood transfusion requirements in anemia of prematurity? Intensive Care Med 1996;22:472-6.
65. DeMaio JG, Harris MC, Deuber C, Spitzer AR. Effect of blood transfusion on apnea frequency in growing premature infants. J Pediatr 1989;114:1039-41.
66. Sasidharan P, Heimler R. Transfusion-induced changes in the breathing pattern of healthy preterm anemic infants. Pediatr Pulmonol 1992;3:170-3.
67. Blank JP, Shegren TG, Vajaria J, et al. The role of RBC transfusion in the premature infant. Am J Dis Child 1984;138:831-3.
68. Wardrop CAJ, Jone JG, Holland BM. Detection, correction, and ultimate prevention of anemias in the preterm infant. Transfus Sci 1991;12:257-70.
69. Hudson IR, Cavill IA, Cooke AD, et al. Biotin labeling of red cells in the measurement of red cell volume in preterm infants. Pediatr Res 1990;28:199-202.
70. Phillips HM, Holland BM, Ardell-Motz A, et al. Determination of red-cell mass in assessment and management of anaemia in babies needing blood transfusion. Lancet 1986;i:882-4.
71. Hume H, Bard H. Small volume red blood cell transfusions for neonatal patients. Transfus Med Rev 1995;IX:187-99.
72. Widness JA, Seward VJ, Kromer IJ, et al. Changing patterns of red blood cell transfusions in very low birth weight infants. J Pediatr 1996;129:680-7.
73. Bednarek FJ, Weisberger S, Richardson DK, et al. Variations in blood transfusions among newborn intensive care units. J Pediatr 1998;133:601-7.
74. AuBuchon JP, ed. Guidelines for blood utilization review. Bethesda, MD: American Association of Blood Banks, 2001.
75. Voak D, Cann R, Finney D, et al. Guidelines for administration of blood products: transfusion of infants and neonates. Transfus Med 1994;4:63-9.
76. Guidelines for transfusion of erythrocytes to neonates and premature infants. Can Med Assoc J 1992;147:1781-92.

In: Herman JH, Manno CS, eds.
Pediatric Transfusion Therapy
Bethesda, MD: AABB Press, 2002

4

Transfusion of Plasma and Platelets to Neonates

LINDA A. CHAMBERS, MD

THE THERAPEUTIC USE OF plasma and platelet transfusion for neonates is largely based on local norms and expert opinion, which has resulted in a wide variation in practice among institutions.[1,2] Published indications are often those for adult transfusion with the numeric targets, or "triggers," increased to build in a safety margin.[3-6] It is not possible for neonatal transfusion decisions and indications to be more strictly evidence based at this time, because very few randomized studies have been performed in this patient group. Yet, the knowledge that would result from such studies is needed; transfusion remains an invasive therapy akin to organ transplantation, with identifiable risks including

Linda A. Chambers, MD, Senior Medical Officer, Biomedical Headquarters, American Red Cross, Arlington, Virginia

the transmission of infectious disease. Such infections have the potential to result in more morbidity in neonates than in adults, as neonates have relatively high survival rates and long post-transfusion life expectancies, during which delayed complications, such as cirrhosis and hepatocellular carcinoma from hepatitis C infection, can develop.[7]

Even in the short run, aggressive transfusion support of neonates may not be innocuous. For example, the results of recent studies both support and refute an independent association of red cell transfusion with retinopathy of prematurity.[8,9] There is evidence that transfusion causes or aggravates the lesions of bronchopulmonary dysplasia.[10,11] In one randomized multi-institutional study comparing the treatment of shock in meningococcal sepsis with colloid or fresh frozen plasma (FFP), mortality was more than doubled in those treated with FFP.[12] And as in adults, transfusions to neonates can be shown to alter the number and phenotypes of circulating lymphocytes for many days, resulting in a subtle but measurable degree of immunosuppression.[13] These observations may have important implications, particularly for the treatment of neonates with sepsis.

Normal Status

Healthy newborns, even if premature, have circulating platelet levels comparable to those of adults, and platelet function is well developed, although there are some functional differences from adult platelets of both hyporesponsive and hyperresponsive natures.[14-17] It can be inferred that the relationship of platelet count to bleeding time and bleeding risk is similar in infants as in adults. If so, bleeding time should be normal when platelets are present in the peripheral blood at concentrations above about 100,000/μL, which has been confirmed in studies of neonates.[18] Platelet-mediated hemostasis should be intact at counts above about 50,000/μL, at which level the bleeding time is about twice the upper limit of the reference range.[19] Spontaneous bleeding risk should not increase until levels fall below about 10,000/μL, unless coincident fever or coagulopathy is present.[19] Platelet transfusion practices in neonates do not necessarily reflect these correlations, however. In a national hospital survey regarding neonatal transfusion practices, most hospitals reported that they transfused platelets to sick premature neonates if the platelet count was below 50,000/μL, whether or not bleeding was present or an invasive procedure was planned.[2]

Unlike platelets, the levels of several coagulation proteins—in particular, the vitamin-K-dependent procoagulant Factors II, VII, IX, and X—are predictably reduced in neonates to about 50% of levels in adults.[20-22] Standard laboratory tests of coagulation protein function, such as the activated partial thromboplastin time (aPTT) and prothrombin time (PT), are prolonged, reflecting this moderate reduction of multiple procoagulants. The levels of naturally occurring thrombin inhibitors (eg, protein C and antithrombin) and fibrinolytics (eg, plasminogen) are also reduced in rough proportion so that the coagulation balance is maintained.[20,21] Consequently, neither bleeding nor clotting ensues, though the neonate has little "buffer" if a consumptive process such as disseminated intravascular coagulation (DIC) develops. Replacement of coagulation proteins with FFP is not ordinarily considered necessary even for critically ill neonates, in the absence of a major hemostatic challenge such as surgery. Several specific conditions for which FFP may be inappropriately used, including hypovolemia and hypoalbuminemia, occur with some frequency in neonates, and surveys show that FFP is still transfused for volume or nutritional support, despite the publication of several sets of practice guidelines specifying that this should be discontinued because alternative nonblood therapies are safer and equally effective.[2,22,23]

Indications for Transfusion

For Perinatal Thrombocytopenia

Perinatal mild thrombocytopenia (<100,000/μL) occurs in less than 1% of neonates of all birthweights, and most of the time it is nonimmunologic in etiology, self-limiting, and clinically benign.[24] Newborns with platelet counts in the 50,000 to 100,000/μL range do not bleed abnormally, and platelet transfusion may not be required. More severe thrombocytopenia is rare and likely to be due to neonatal alloimmune thrombocytopenia as a result of maternal-fetal platelet serologic incompatibility.[24,25] Antibody to HPA-1a is most often implicated in these cases, and transfusion of appropriate antigen-negative compatible platelets will increase the platelet count in a rapid and sustained manner.[25] If collected from the mother, who is necessarily negative for the involved antigen, platelets should be washed or volume-reduced to minimize the amount of maternal plasma (which contains the pathogenic antibody) that is co-transfused. Components should be gamma-irradiated to prevent transfusion-related graft-vs-host disease when platelets are obtained from a biologic relative. Irradiation does not compromise platelet function, although washing or volume reduction may result in a loss of 10% or more of the starting platelet content.[26,27]

To Prevent Intracranial Hemorrhage

Intracranial hemorrhage, more specifically, periventricular and intraventricular hemorrhage, is a common complication of prematurity that also occurs, but at a lower incidence, in term newborns with serious illness.[28] The nature of the lesion predisposing to these hemorrhages is unknown, but it is thought to involve immaturity of the periventricular brain tissue and capillaries, and not the underlying reduced levels of procoagulants found in neonates.[29,30] There is evidence that the risk relates primarily to the development, or lack of development, of protective changes in the cerebral arterial flow during the third trimester, so that preterm labor becomes the critical antecedent event.[31,32] The risk of periventricular or intraventricular hemorrhage is inversely proportional to gestational age at birth, from about 2% in term infants to 50% in infants born at 24 to 30 weeks of gestation.[28,32]

Any contribution from mild thrombocytopenia, which develops in the first 3 days of life in approximately 0.5% of neonates, is questionable.[24,29] Even for the most at-risk subgroup—very low birthweight premature newborns in the first 72 hours of life—prophylactic platelet transfusions did not reduce the incidence or severity of intracranial hemorrhage in one randomized multi-institutional study.[29] Despite maintenance of the platelet count above 150,000/μL for the first 7 days of life (a level at which platelet-mediated hemostasis is clearly intact), intracranial hemorrhage developed or extended in transfused infants at a rate comparable to that in infants transfused with platelets only if their count fell below 50,000/μL.[29]

In Open Heart Surgery

Children undergoing open heart surgery with cardiopulmonary bypass develop a substantial dilutional coagulopathy because of the small intravascular volume of the patient relative to the volume of the bypass circuit, which is usually primed with Red Blood Cells lacking coagulation factors. The use of cardiopulmonary bypass also causes a degree of activation of the coagulation system, despite systemic heparinization, which may consume procoagulant proteins. At one tertiary-care pediatric hospital, approximately one-third of all FFP transfusions were given to children with congenital diseases, primarily during and after surgery for congenital heart disease.[33]

The effects of cardiopulmonary bypass on platelets are less predictable. In older children, the immediate postoperative platelet count is typically above 100,000/μL.[34] In neonates, however, the dilutional effects are exaggerated. Neonates are more likely to develop significant deficiencies of platelets in addition to procoagulant proteins, which leads to excessive bleeding in the postoperative period.[34] At one institution, platelet and/or FFP transfusions were required by a majority (61%) of infants less than 1 month of age after open heart surgery compared with 31% of older infants and young children.[35]

Clotting capacity in the postoperative period can be improved without transfusion if the platelets and coagulation proteins are reconcentrated in the patient at the conclusion of bypass. This can be accomplished by removing excess fluids from the patient-bypass circuit through a process called ultrafiltration, which has been shown to reduce both postoperative bleeding and FFP transfusion, particularly when the patient is very small and/or the bypass time is prolonged.[34,36]

During Extracorporeal Membrane Oxygenation

Extracorporeal membrane oxygenation (ECMO) can be thought of as continuous cardiopulmonary bypass, with all of the associated effects on platelet count, platelet function, procoagulant protein levels, and hemostasis. When ECMO is initiated after open heart surgery, the coagulation effects are additive and further complicated by the required systemic heparinization. In such a complicated setting, evaluation of the coagulation state and identification of appropriate transfusion requirements for FFP may not be possible with standard tests for fibrinogen, PT, and aPTT.[37] Consequently, non-red cell transfusions during ECMO are frequently given empirically to either prevent or treat excessive blood loss.[38,39] In one program, for example, FFP is automatically transfused in a dose of 10 mL/kg each 6 hours.[39]

ECMO results in a substantial reduction in platelet count within the first hour after initiation of bypass.[40] Platelet transfusion only transiently increases the platelet count, which returns to baseline within hours, and platelet function remains poor despite transfusion.[40] Nevertheless, it does not appear that bleeding risk is closely related to the poor integrity of platelet function in these patients, who also receive heparin. In one review of neonates treated with ECMO for heart failure after open heart surgery, excessive bleeding occurred in 43 of 65 patients who had platelet counts between 90,000/µL and 100,000/µL.[41] Yet platelets, like plasma, are apt to be transfused empirically to these patients, and this led to an average of 7 to 9 donor exposures at one institution where platelets were transfused to maintain the count above 80,000/µL.[38] The therapeutic benefits of such transfusions during ECMO have not been established in clinical studies.

With Exchange Transfusions

Double-volume whole-blood exchange in neonates with hemolytic disease of the newborn (HDN) predictably causes dilution of coagulation proteins from the approximately 50% baseline level to less than 10% (63% reduction with each exchange volume).[42] These levels are associated with prolongation of the

PT and aPTT and, in adults, abnormal hemostasis. Many programs anticipate the dilutional coagulation protein deficiency and, rather than transfuse plasma after exchange, use a source of coagulation proteins (FFP) to adjust the hematocrit of a unit of Red Blood Cells thereby creating a whole-blood-like component for neonatal exchange transfusion.

During massive transfusion in older children and adults, thrombocytopenia is uncommon, as the dilutional effect is offset by the release of platelets from the spleen. In fact, thrombocytopenia is not apparent until almost two total blood volumes have been exchanged with a platelet-poor component.[42,43] This observation matches the general experience in double-volume exchanges in neonates, in which thrombocytopenia is uncommon and platelet transfusion is not usually required. This assumes, of course, that the infant's starting platelet count is in the normal range. With preexisting thrombocytopenia, potentially problematic counts (<50,000/μL) may result from otherwise routine exchange transfusion.[42]

Partial exchange transfusion for polycythemia results in only slight decreases in coagulation factors compared with double-volume exchanges for HDN. Therefore, replacement of coagulation factors or platelets for partial exchange is not necessary, and crystalloid solutions can be used alone to replace the exchanged volume, with no adverse clinical effects.[44,45]

Disseminated Intravascular Coagulation

Sepsis within the first 3 days of life is uncommon, even in very low birthweight neonates, but it develops later in the hospitalization course in fully 25% of these infants, most often involving gram-positive organisms.[46,47] When accompanied by DIC (which it often is), consumption of procoagulants and platelets can lead to significant deficiencies requiring transfusion replacement.[48] Because coagulation factor levels begin at about half of adult levels, problematic coagulopathies may be more profound and may occur earlier in the disease course than they do in adults with sepsis.

DIC without sepsis can occur in neonates secondary to birth asphyxia associated with such events as placental abruption or breech delivery.[49] In these patients, consumption of procoagulants from the already lower starting levels can produce a significant coagulopathy relatively early in the clinical course, and transfusion replacement therapy may be required. Close monitoring of fibrinogen levels and coagulation testing is indicated.

Selection and Preparation of Plasma and Platelets for Neonatal Transfusion

Plasma for transfusion as a source of coagulation proteins is traditionally provided as FFP, that is, plasma from one apheresis or whole-blood donation that has been frozen within 8 hours of collection so that the function of labile coagulation factors (particularly Factors VIII and V) are preserved. FFP is potentially infectious for hepatitis C, hepatitis B, and HIV at the same rates as for other single-donor-exposure components (eg, RBCs). Before freezing, variable numbers of leukocytes, occasionally more than 5×10^6, are present in the plasma.[50] Most do not survive the freeze-thaw process intact, which leaves cellular fragments and contents to be infused to the patient. Although a small number of viable lymphocytes can be detected by sensitive methods in thawed FFP, transfusion of this component has not been shown to transmit cytomegalovirus infection or to cause transfusion-related graft-vs-host disease.[50]

Procoagulant protein levels of about 50% of normal are sufficient to ensure that this component of hemostasis is intact. In the worst case, when the patient has 0% of one or several procoagulants, FFP in a dose approximating 50% of the total plasma volume of the patient would ensure reestablishment of hemostatic levels. If the plasma volume of neonates is between 40 and 50 mL/kg, then 20 to 25 mL/kg of plasma is guaranteed to correct a coagulopathy due to factor deficiencies. Because most patients begin at low levels, but not at zero, the smaller "standard" dose of about 10 to 15 mL/kg is a reasonable and well-founded compromise to avoid volume overload.

Platelet dosing is inherently more complicated. There is no general agreement as to what constitutes a correct adult dose from which a neonatal dose could be scaled. Both whole-blood-derived and apheresis components contain variable concentrations of platelets (per mL) as well as total numbers of platelets per individual component, although on average each milliliter contains about 1.5×10^9 platelets in plasma.[51] Transfused into an infant with a 50 mL/kg plasma volume, and correcting for 30% retention in the spleen, a "standard" dose of 5 mL/kg of platelets should raise the platelet count by about 100,000/µL under ideal circumstances. Usually, however, this is not seen, either because the full amount is not received by the patient (eg, component lost in tubing) or the patient's platelet response is compromised by fever, sepsis, DIC, or another high-consumption state.

A key issue in deciding whether to use apheresis or whole-blood-derived platelets for neonatal transfusion is whether the remainder of the source component can be used in the future by the neonate or whether each platelet transfusion will necessarily be prepared from a new component and entail an additional donor exposure. When multiple platelet transfusions are required over a 1- to 3-day period, aliquotting apheresis platelets can substantially reduce the total donor exposures for neonates over the course of a hospitalization.[52] Aliquotting can be accomplished by subdividing the component into the two integral collection bags, if present, or by entering through a sterile connection device, with transfer of the platelet dose to a bag or syringe.[52]

The platelets contained in apheresis and whole-blood-derived components are comparable in terms of survival and function in the patient. There is evidence from culture surveillance programs that whole-blood-derived platelets are more likely to be bacterially contaminated and thus to have the potential to cause a septic transfusion reaction.[53,54] It is possible, however, that serial aliquotting of apheresis components may itself introduce opportunities for bacterial contamination, blurring the differences in ultimate risk to the recipient. Prestorage leukocyte reduction, if desired, is more readily available for apheresis platelets, although prestorage leukocyte-reduced whole-blood-derived platelets will be more widely manufactured in the future. From most suppliers, whole-blood-derived platelets are less expensive on a platelet content basis and less likely to be in short supply (Table 4-1).

Because one whole-blood-derived platelet concentrate is usually sufficient to provide a full dose, whole-blood-derived platelet transfusions are single-donor transfusions for neonates, rendering irrelevant many of the advantages of apheresis platelets for adult patients. Even the preparation simplicity of apheresis platelet transfusions for adult recipients (no pooling and relabeling necessary) is not an advantage for neonates; in fact, serial aliquotting of an assigned apheresis component entails more work for the transfusion service than would the use of whole-blood-derived platelets.

Concerns about the ABO type and plasma compatibility for platelet transfusions in neonates are discussed in Chapter 17. It should be appreciated that a 10 mL/kg platelet transfusion to a neonate delivers 10 mL/kg of plasma, which, if ABO-incompatible, is the equivalent of about three units of incompatible FFP for an adult. The potential for hemolysis is consequently higher than for a typical ABO plasma-incompatible apheresis platelet transfusion to an adult (350-mL component to a 70-kg recipient, approximately 5 mL/kg plasma), which leads some in-

Table 4-1. Differences Between Whole-Blood-Derived and Apheresis Platelets That May Be of Importance for Neonatal Transfusion

Issue	Preferred Preparation
Option for multiple dosing from one component	Apheresis
Bacterial contamination rate	Apheresis
Availability of prestorage leukocyte-reduced preparations	Apheresis
Transfusion service workload	Whole-blood-derived
Availability	Whole-blood-derived

stitutions to restrict platelet transfusions in neonates to ABO-identical or plasma-compatible components.

Formation of antibodies to leukocytes, including HLA antibodies, in preterm infants as a result of red cell transfusion either does not occur or is rare. Consequently, special transfusion maneuvers, including limited-donor programs or component leukocyte reduction specifically to reduce alloimmunization to platelet transfusions, may not be necessary for these patients.[55] Limited-donor programs remain beneficial, however, as a means to reduce the risk of infectious disease transmission. At the current very low rates of infection from transfusion (cumulatively, less than 1 in 100,000), any reduction in infection risk may not be observable or strictly cost-effective.[56]

Summary

In the absence of clinical trials of liberal and restrictive transfusion of plasma and platelets to neonates, there is plenty of opportunity for empiric transfusion and the use of transfusion triggers that are based in tradition only. This results in substantial variability among institutions and otherwise comparable programs in the use of non-red cell transfusion in this patient group. In general, there is agreement that platelets and plasma should be transfused to correct deficiencies in the function or amount of platelets and procoagulant proteins, respectively. What is missing is a clear understanding of the clinical situations for hospitalized, seriously ill neonates when these deficiencies do or do not affect bleeding risk, complication rate, or outcome.

References

1. Bednarek FJ, Weisberger S, Richardson DK, et al. Variations in blood transfusions among newborn intensive care units. J Pediatr 1998; 133:601-7.
2. Strauss RG, Levy GJ, Sotelo-Avila C, et al. National survey of neonatal transfusion practices: II. Blood component therapy. Pediatrics 1993;91: 530-6.
3. Norfolk DR, Ancliffe PJ, Contreras M, et al. Consensus conference on platelet transfusion. Royal College of Physicians of Edinburgh, 27-28 November 1997. Br J Haematol 1998;101:609-17.

4. Contreras M. Final statement from the consensus conference on platelet transfusion. Transfusion 1998;38:796-7.
5. AABB Pediatric Hemotherapy Committee. Guidelines for conducting pediatric transfusion audits. Bethesda, MD: American Association of Blood Banks, 1992.
6. Voak D, Cann R, Finney RD, et al. Guidelines for administration of blood products to infants and neonates. Transfus Med 1994;4:63-9.
7. O'Riordan JM, Conroy A, Nourse C, et al. Risk of hepatitis C infection in neonates transfused with blood from donors infected with hepatitis C. Transfus Med 1998;8:303-8.
8. Seiberth V, Linderkamp O. Risk factors in retinopathy of prematurity: A multivariate statistical analysis. Ophthalmologica 2000;214:131-5.
9. Brooks SE, Marcus DM, Gillis D, et al. The effect of blood transfusion protocol on retinopathy of prematurity: A prospective, randomized study. Pediatrics 1999;104:514-18.
10. Korhonen P, Tammela O, Koivisto AM, et al. Frequency and risk factors in bronchopulmonary dysplasia in a cohort of very low birthweight infants. Early Human Dev 1999;54:245-58.
11. Silvers KM, Gibson AT, Russell JM, Powers HJ. Antioxidant activity, packed cell transfusions and outcome in premature infants. Arch Dis Child Fetal Neonatal Ed 1998;78:F214-19.
12. Busund R, Straume B, Revhaug A. Fatal course in severe meningococcemia: Clinical predictors and effect of transfusion therapy. Crit Care Med 1993;21:1699-705.
13. Wang-Rodriguez J, Fry E, Fiebig E, et al. Immune response to blood transfusion in very-low-birthweight infants. Transfusion 2000;40:25-34.
14. Andrew M. The relevance of developmental hemostasis to hemorrhagic disorders in newborns. Semin Perinatol 1997;21:70-85.
15. Blanchette VS, Rand ML. Platelet disorders in newborn infants: Diagnosis and management. Semin Perinatol 1997;21:53-62.
16. Shenkman B, Linder N, Savion N, et al. Increased neonatal platelet deposition on subendothelium under flow conditions: The role of plasma von Willebrand factor. Pediatr Res 1999;45:270-5.
17. Pisciotto PT, Snyder EL. Platelet defects and their therapy. In: Luban NLC, ed. Transfusion therapy in infants and children. Baltimore, MD: Johns Hopkins University Press, 1991:52-93.
18. Andrew M, Castle V, Saigal S, et al. Clinical impact of neonatal thrombocytopenia. J Pediatr 1987;110:457-64.
19. Practice parameter for the use of fresh-frozen plasma, cryoprecipitate and platelets. JAMA 1994;271:777-81.
20. Andrew M, Paes B, Milner R, et al. Development of the human coagulation system in the full-term infant. Blood 1987;70:165-72.
21. Andrew W, Paes B, Milner R, et al. Development of the human coagulation system in the healthy premature infant. Blood 1988;72:1651-7.

22. Contreras M, Ala FA, Greaves M, et al. Guidelines for the use of fresh frozen plasma. British Committee for Standards in Haematology, Working Party of the Blood Transfusion Task Force. Transfus Med 1992;2:57-63.
23. Hume H, Blanchette V, Strauss RG, Levy GJ. A survey of Canadian neonatal blood transfusion practices. Transfus Sci 1997;18:71-80.
24. Uhrynowska M, Niznikowska-Marks M, Zupanska B. Neonatal and maternal thrombocytopenia: Incidence and immune background. Eur J Haematol 2000;64:42-6.
25. Blanchette VS, Johnson JM. The management of alloimmune neonatal thrombocytopenia. Baillieres Clin Haematol 2000;13:365-90.
26. Rock G, Adams GA, Labow RS. The effects of irradiation on platelet function. Transfusion 1988;28:451-5.
27. Read EJ, Kodis C, Carter CS, et al. Viability of platelets following storage in the irradiated state. A pair-controlled study. Transfusion 1988;28: 446-50.
28. Berger R, Bender S, Sefkow S, et al. Peri/intraventricular haemorrhage: A cranial ultrasound study on 5286 neonates. Eur J Obstet Gynecol Reprod Biol 1997;75:191-203.
29. Andrew M, Vegh P, Caco C, et al. A randomized, controlled trial of platelet transfusions in thrombocytopenic premature infants. J Pediatr 1993; 123:285-91.
30. Meek JH, Tyszczuk L, Elwell C, Wyatt JS. Low cerebral blood flow is a risk factor for severe intraventricular hemorrhage. Arch Dis Child Fetal Neonatal Ed 1999;81:F15-8.
31. Mari G, Abuhamad AZ, Keller M, et al. Is the fetal brain-sparing effect a risk factor for the development of intraventricular hemorrhage in the preterm infant? Ultrasound Obstet Gynecol 1996;8:329-32.
32. Gleissner M, Jorch G, Avenarius S. Risk factors for intraventricular hemorrhage in a birth cohort of 3721 premature infants. J Perinat Med 2000;28:104-10.
33. Zimmerman R, Handtrack D, Zingsem J, et al. A survey of blood utilization in children and adolescents in a German university hospital. Transfus Med 1998;8:185-94.
34. Friesen RH, Campbell DN, Clarke DR, Tornabene MA. Modified ultrafiltration attenuates dilutional coagulopathy in pediatric open heart operations. Ann Thorac Surg 1997;64:1787-9.
35. Petaja J, Lundstrom U, Leijala M, et al. Bleeding and use of blood products after heart operations in infants. J Thorac Cardiovasc Surg 1995; 109:524-9.
36. Bando W, Turrentine MW, Vijay P, et al. Effect of modified ultrafiltration in high-risk patients undergoing operations for congenital heart disease. Ann Thorac Surg 1998;66:821-7.
37. Zavadil DP, Stammers AH, Willett LD, et al. Hematological abnormalities in neonatal patients treated with extracorporeal membrane oxygenation. J Extra Corpor Technol 1998;30:83-90.

38. Minifee PK, Daeschner CW, Griffin P, et al. Decreasing blood donor exposure in neonates on extracorporeal membrane oxygenation. J Pediatr Surg 1990;25:38-42.
39. Klein MD, Shaheen KW, Wittlesey GC, et al. Extracorporeal membrane oxygenation for the circulatory support of children after repair of congenital heart disease. J Thorac Cardiovasc Surg 1990;100:498-505.
40. Robinson TM, Kickler RS, Walker LK, et al. Effect of extracorporeal membrane oxygenation on platelets in newborns. Crit Care Med 1993;21: 1029-34.
41. Raithel SC, Pennington G, Boegner E, et al. Extracorporeal membrane oxygenation in children after cardiac surgery. Circulation 1992;86(Suppl 2):305-10.
42. Leslie SD, Toy PTCY. Laboratory hemostatic abnormalities in massively transfused patients given red blood cells and crystalloid. Am J Clin Pathol 1991;96:770-3.
43. Cote CJ, Liu LM, Szyfelbein SK, et al. Changes in serial platelet counts following massive blood transfusion in pediatric patients. Anesthesiology 1985;62:197-201.
44. Deorari AK, Paul VK, Shreshta L, Singh M. Symptomatic neonatal polycythemia: comparison of partial exchange transfusion with saline versus plasma. Indian Pediatr 1995;32:1167-71.
45. Roithmaier A, Arlettaz R, Bauer K, et al. Randomized controlled trial of Ringer solution versus serum for partial exchange transfusion in neonatal polycythaemia. Eur J Pediatr 1995;154:53-6.
46. Stoll BJ, Gordon T, Korones SB, et al. Early-onset sepsis in very low birth weight neonates: A report from the National Institute of Child Health and Human Development Neonatal Research Network. J Pediatr 1996; 129:72-80.
47. Stoll BJ, Gordon T, Korones SB, et al. Late-onset sepsis in very low birth weight neonates: A report from the National Institute of Child Health and Human Development Neonatal Research Network. J Pediatr 1996; 129:63-71.
48. Shirahata A, Shirakawa Y, Murakami C. Diagnosis of DIC in very low birth weight infants. Semin Thromb Hemost 1998;24:467-71.
49. Suzuki S, Morishita S. Hypercoagulability and DIC in high-risk infants. Semin Thromb Hemost 1998;24:463-6.
50. Wieding JU, Katalin V, Dittman J, et al. Contamination of fresh-frozen plasma with viable white cells and proliferable stem cells. Transfusion 1994;34:185-6.
51. Chambers LA, Herman JH. Considerations in the selection of a platelet component: Apheresis versus whole blood-derived. Transfus Med Rev 1999;13:311-22.
52. Rosenberg EM, Chambers LA, Gunter JM, Good JA. A program to limit donor exposures to neonates undergoing extracorporeal membrane oxygenation. Pediatrics 1994;94:341-6.

53. Barrett BB, Anderson JW, Anderson KC. Strategies for the avoidance of bacterial contamination of blood components. Transfusion 1993;33: 228-33.
54. Alvarez EE, Rogge KJ, Tarrand J, et al. Bacterial contamination of cellular blood components. A retrospective review at a large cancer center. Ann Clin Lab Sci 1995;25:283-90.
55. Strauss RG, Cordle DG, Quijana J, Goeken NE. Comparing alloimmunization in preterm infants after transfusion of fresh unmodified versus stored leukocyte-reduced red blood cells. J Pediatr Hematol Oncol 1999;21:224-30.
56. Dodd RY. Current viral risks of blood and blood products. Ann Med 2000;32:469-74.

In: Herman JH, Manno CS, eds.
Pediatric Transfusion Therapy
Bethesda, MD: AABB Press, 2002

5

Neonatal Alloimmune Neutropenia and Alloimmune Thrombocytopenia

DAVID STRONCEK, MD

MATERNAL ALLOANTIBODIES CAN CAUSE severe anemia in a neonate whose red cells are incompatible with his or her mother's. During pregnancy, mothers can also become alloimmunized to neutrophil- or platelet-specific antigens. Maternal IgG can then cross the placenta and destroy the neonate's neutrophils or platelets. In hemolytic disease of the newborn, maternal alloimmunization usually occurs at childbirth, and, with subsequent pregnancies, neonates are at risk of intrauterine hemolysis. However, maternal alloimmunization to neutrophil or platelet antibodies can occur in utero and affect the first

David Stroncek, MD, Chief, Laboratory Services Section, Department of Transfusion Medicine, National Institutes of Health, Bethesda, Maryland

child. Most neonates experience isolated neutropenia or thrombocytopenia, but the cytopenias are self-limiting, and they resolve as the antibody is cleared. In both syndromes, the alloimmunized mothers produce and carry the antibodies, but the antibodies do not react with the mother's blood cells or tissues, and they have normal neutrophil and platelet counts. There are many similarities in the pathophysiology and diagnosis of alloimmune neonatal neutropenia and alloimmune neonatal thrombocytopenia, but there are also many important differences in the clinical consequences, the need for prenatal diagnosis, and treatment.

Neonatal Alloimmune Neutropenia

Neutrophil Antigens Implicated in Neonatal Alloimmune Neutropenia

Antibodies implicated in neonatal alloimmune neutropenia most often react with antigens in the NA or human neutrophil antigen-1 (HNA-1) system and NB or HNA-2 system.[1,2] Occasionally the alloantibodies react with SH antigen,[3] 5b antigen,[2] and antigens common to all Fc-γ receptor IIIb (FcγRIIIb) molecules.[4,5]

NA and Related Antigens

The neutrophil-specific NA antigen system is made up of two alleles, *NA1* and *NA2*. The antigens are also known as HNA-1a and HNA-1b (Table 5-1). Among Whites, the *NA1* gene frequency is 0.30 to 0.37 and the *NA2* gene frequency is 0.63 to 0.70.[6-9] The *NA1* and *NA2* gene frequencies vary widely among racial groups. In Japanese and Chinese populations, the *NA1* gene frequency is 0.60 to 0.66 and the *NA2* gene frequency is 0.30 to 0.33.[7-9]

The NA antigens are expressed on neutrophils but not on other blood cells. NA1 and NA2 antigens are located on FcγRIIIb (CD16).[10-12] FcγRIIIb is expressed on all segmented neutrophils, on about half of neutrophilic metamyelocytes, and on about 10% of neutrophilic myelocytes.[13] Soluble FcγRIIIb is present in

Table 5-1. Neutrophil Antigens Implicated in Neonatal Alloimmune Neutropenia

Nomenclature				Antigen Location	
Classic		ISBT			
System	Antigen	System	Antigen	Glycoprotein	CD Number
NA	NA1	HNA-1	HNA-1a	FcγRIIIb	CD16
NA	NA2	HNA-1	HNA-1b	FcγRIIIb	CD16
SH	SH	HNA-1	HNA-1c	FcγRIIIb	CD16
NB	NB1	HNA-2	HNA-2a	58-64 kDa	CD177
5	5b	HNA-3	HNA-3a	70-95 kDa	Not known

HNA = Human neutrophil antigen; ISBT = International Society of Blood Transfusion; NA = Neutrophil antigen.

plasma, and plasma FcγRIIIb has the same NA polymorphisms found on neutrophils.[14]

FcγRIIIb is a 50- to 80-kDa glycoprotein (GP) with 233 amino acids and N-linked carbohydrate side chains; it is glycosylphosphatidylinositol (GPI)-anchored.[10-12] *FcγRIIIB* encodes FcγRIIIb and its two major antigens. The NA1 form of the *FcγRIIIB* (*NA1-FcγRIIIB*) differs from the NA2 form of the *FcγRIIIB* *(NA2-FcγRIIIB)* by only five nucleotide bases in the coding region, at positions 141, 147, 227, 277, and 349.[10-12] Four of the nucleotide changes result in changes in amino acid sequences between the NA1 and NA2 forms of the GP. The fifth polymorphism at 147 is silent. The glycosylation pattern of the antigen differs between the two antigens because of two nucleotide changes at bases 227 and 277, which create two additional N-linked glycosylation sites.[10-12] NA2-FcγRIIIb is 65 to 80 kDa and has six N-linked glycosylation sites, while NA1-FcγRIIIb has four glycosylation sites and is only 50 to 65 kDa. *NA1-FcγRIIIB* and *NA2-FcγRIIIB* can be distinguished by using polymerase chain reaction (PCR) and sequence-specific primers or PCR and restriction enzymes.[15,16]

Neutrophils from approximately 1 of 1000 Whites phenotype as NA-null.[17] These neutrophils do not express NA1, NA2, or FcγRIIIb. The NA-null phenotype is caused by the deletion of *FcγRIIIB*. Women whose neutrophils have the NA-null phenotype are healthy, but during pregnancy they sometimes produce antibodies to FcγRIIIb. These antibodies are not specific for NA1 or NA2 but instead react with an FcγRIIIb epitope common to neutrophils from all donors. The NA-null phenotype is inherited in an autosomal recessive manner, and the offspring of women with NA-null neutrophils can experience alloimmune neonatal neutropenia.[4,5]

Antibodies to an additional FcγRIIIb polymorphism, SH, can also cause neonatal alloimmune neutropenia. SH is expressed on neutrophils in 4% to 5% of Whites and 25% to 38% of African Americans.[3,8] The molecular basis for SH has been shown to be a C→A substitution in *FcγRIIIB* at nucleotide 266 that results in an alanine→aspartate substitution at amino acid 78. The SH antigen has been found to be expressed only on NA2-positive granulocytes. The SH genotype can be identified by using PCR and restriction enzymes.[3]

NB Antigens

The NB or HNA-2 neutrophil antigen system is made up of the well-defined NB1 antigen and the poorly defined NB2 antigen. NB1, which has been implicated in neonatal alloimmune neutropenia, is expressed on neutrophils by approximately 97% of Whites, 95% of African Americans, and 89% of Japanese.[6,18] NB1 is expressed on neutrophils, but not on basophils, eosinophils, monocytes, lymphocytes, platelets, or red cells.[13] In the marrow, NB1 is expressed on neutrophilic metamyelocytes, myelocytes, and myeloblasts.[13] NB1 antigen is unique in that not all neutrophils from NB1-positive people express the antigen; it is expressed on subpopulations of neutrophils, the mean size of which is 56% to 64% of the total.[18]

NB1 antigen is located on a 58- to 64-kDa GP.[19,20] The NB1 GP is located on neutrophil plasma membranes and secondary granules, is GPI-anchored, and has N-linked carbohydrate side chains. CD177 monoclonal antibodies are reactive with the 58- to 64-kDa NB1 GP. Kissel and colleagues[21] reported the results of sequencing the *NB1* gene and found that *NB1* is a member of the *Ly-6* gene family. Other members of this family include urokinase-type plasminogen activator receptor, reactive inhibitor of lysis receptor (CD59), and polycythemia rubra vera gene 1. Methods to determine the *NB1* genotype have yet to be developed.

NB1 has been reported to have an allele, *NB2*, but the product of this gene cannot be reliably identified with alloantisera, and no monoclonal antibody specific for NB2 has been identified. Rabbit polyclonal antibodies that react with NB1 GP do not react with any glycoprotein on NB1-negative neutrophils in flow cytometry, immunoblotting, or immunoprecipitation assays.[19,22] Neutrophils from NB1-negative persons appear to lack the 58- to 64-kDa NB1 GP, or the NB1 GP on their neutrophils is markedly different from the NB1 GP on neutrophils from NB1-positive persons.

5b Antigen

Antigens in the 5 system are expressed by neutrophils, lymphocytes, platelets, and endothelial, kidney, spleen, and placental cells. The 5 system has two alleles, *5a* and *5b*. Antibodies to 5a are not readily available, and this antigen is not well characterized, but antibodies specific for 5b have been used to partially characterize this antigen. Among Whites, the gene frequency of 5b is 0.66, and it is located on a 70- to 95-kDa neutrophil antigen.[2] Antibodies to 5b have been implicated in alloimmune neonatal neutropenia.[2]

Neutrophil Antibodies in Neonatal Alloimmune Neutropenia

The reported incidence of alloimmunization to granulocyte antibodies during pregnancies has varied markedly, from 0.17% to 2%.[6] However, the reported incidence of alloimmune neonatal neutropenia is less, 2 or fewer per 1000 births.[6] Bux and colleagues[1] tested postpartum sera in 1016 mothers and found neutrophil-specific antibodies in 11. One of the 11 contained anti-NB1, one anti-NA1, and two anti-NA2, but none of the 11 infants became neutropenic. It is not clear why all granulocyte antibodies do not cause neutropenia. However, mothers with affected children generally have high-titer antibodies, and it may be that the titer of granulocyte antibody in most pregnant women is not high enough to cause neutropenia.

Antibodies to granulocyte-specific antigens, most commonly NA1, NA2, and NB1, have been reported to cause neonatal alloimmune neutropenia (Table 5-2).[1,2] Antibodies to SH and 5b rarely cause alloimmune neonatal neutropenia.[2,3] In addition, antibodies to FcγRIIIb (CD16) have been produced in several mothers who lack NA antigens, and these antibodies have resulted in neonatal alloimmune neutropenia.[4,5] In some cases, the alloantibodies do not show specificity to the described granulocyte antigens, and, in others, only antibodies to HLA antigens can be detected. However, HLA antibodies are not thought to cause alloimmune neutropenia. In some mothers, no neutrophil antibody can be detected.

Table 5-2. Specificities of Antibodies in Alloimmune Neonatal Neutropenia

Antigen	Bux et al[1] (n = 18)	De Hass et al[2] (n = 48)
NA1	28%	10%
NA2	22%	8%
FcγRIIIb	0%	8%
NB1	11%	2%
5b	0%	2%
Unknown	0%	15%
HLA Class I	11%	54%
Negative	28%	38%

Clinical Presentation

Before birth, fetuses are in a sterile environment, and therefore newborns with alloimmune neutropenia are usually asymptomatic. Because neutrophil counts are not routinely performed at birth, some neonates with alloimmune neutropenia likely are never diagnosed. Most often the neutropenia is detected in the first week of life, when the neonate becomes febrile or develops an infection and a neutrophil count is done. In some cases, no circulating neutrophils are present, but typically the counts are 100 to 200/μL. In general, the neutrophil counts in affected neonates fall during the first few days of life. Some neonates have normal neutrophil counts the first day of life, but they become neutropenic on their second day.[1] White blood cell (WBC) count, platelet count, and hemoglobin are usually normal, and eosinophilia or monocytosis may be present. If a marrow biopsy is performed, it often shows normal numbers of erythroid progenitors and megakaryocytes with hyperplasia of the myeloid progenitors. Segmented neutrophils and band forms of neutrophils are often present in the marrow,[2] but sometimes neutrophil metamyelocytes and band forms are absent, and the maturation of myeloid cells may appear to be arrested.[23]

The clinical course is quite variable. An occasional infant is asymptomatic,[23] but almost all affected children have an infection. The most common infections are umbilicus infections, skin infections, abscesses, and respiratory tract infections. Less commonly, infants experience otitis media, urinary tract infections, and gastroenteritis. Serious infections such as sepsis, pneumonia, and meningitis can occur. The affected neonates are often infected with gram-negative bacteria or *Staphylococcus aureus*.[1,2,23,24] These infections usually are effectively treated by prompt administration of broad-spectrum antibiotics, but fatalities have been reported in 5% of cases.[6,23] The duration of the neutropenia may be as short as a few days or as long as 28 weeks.[1,2] In their study of 18 infants, Bux and colleagues[1] found the mean duration of neutropenia was 11 weeks. In other smaller studies, the neutropenia lasted from 3 to 7 weeks.[23,24]

The differential diagnosis of neutropenia in neonates includes congenital neutropenias, aplastic anemia, leukemia, and overwhelming sepsis. Some patients with aplastic anemia or acute leukemia will become neutropenic before other manifestations of these diseases become evident. Marrow biopsies can be useful in the diagnosis of acute leukemia and severe aplastic anemia, but it may be difficult to distinguish biopsies from patients with neonatal alloimmune neutropenia from biopsies from patients with congenital neutropenia or sepsis.

Diagnosis

The best way to diagnose neonatal alloimmune neutropenia is to test for granulocyte antibodies and to determine neutrophil antigen phenotypes of neonates and their parents. Leukocyte antibodies reactive with an antigen expressed by neutrophils from the child are present in the serum of the mother and child. In an evaluation of a child with neonatal alloimmune neutropenia, blood should be obtained from the child and both parents, if possible. Samples from the mother and neonate should be tested for leukocyte antibodies, and granulocytes from the father and the neonate should be crossmatched with the mother's and neonate's serum. In many but not all mothers, antibodies to one of the well-defined granulocyte antigens can be detected.

The mother's, father's, and, if possible, the neonate's neutrophils should be phenotyped. Unfortunately, if the child is neutropenic, it is impossible to phenotype the granulocytes, but the lymphocytes can be used for genotyping for NA1, NA2, and SH antigens.[3,15] Methods to determine the genotype of other neutrophil antigens are not yet available.

Prenatal Diagnosis

Because in utero infections are not a concern, there is no need to diagnose neonatal alloimmune neutropenia before birth. There is a high incidence of recurrent alloimmune neutropenia in subsequent pregnancies, and the neutropenia appears to be worse with each affected pregnancy.[24,25] Mothers with an affected child should not be discouraged from having additional children, but neonates with affected siblings should be assessed for alloimmune neonatal neutropenia immediately after birth.

Treatment

If a child is found to have neonatal alloimmune neutropenia during a routine medical evaluation or during the evaluation of an unrelated medical problem, no immediate treatment may be required. Prompt and aggressive antibiotic treatment of children with fevers or other signs of infections is indicated. Neonates with an infection and those suspected of having an infection should be treated with intravenous antibiotics effective against both gram-negative bacteria and gram-positive bacteria, including *S. aureus*.

Intravenous immunoglobulin (IVIG) has a limited role in the treatment of neonatal alloimmune neutropenia. Bux and colleagues[1] found that an IVIG dose of 0.4 to 1.0 g/kg daily for 4 to 5 days increases neutrophil counts to near normal levels in half of the treated infants, but the effects of IVIG lasted only for a few days to a few weeks. Others found that, in two neonates, IVIG doses of 1 mg/kg daily for 2 days or 0.4 mg/kg daily for 5 days were not effective.[24]

The use of granulocyte colony-stimulating factor (G-CSF) to treat alloimmune neutropenia has also had mixed results. One study found that the administration of G-CSF elevates the granulocyte count in some but not all neonates.[2] However, Gilmore and colleagues[26] found that two neonates, one with neutropenia due to anti-NA1 and one to anti-NA2, were effectively treated with G-CSF. Neutrophil counts rose to normal levels after 2 and 4 days of treatment. One patient became neutropenic again 11 days after the G-CSF treatments were stopped, but the other neonate's counts remained normal.

Granulocyte transfusions have rarely been used to treat alloimmune neutropenia. They have been effective in at least one case,[24] but they are very difficult to give to neonates with alloimmune neutropenia. Because granulocyte concentrate transfusions in patients with leukocyte antibodies can cause severe pulmonary reactions,[27] the transfused granulocytes must lack the antigen to which the mother's antibody is directed. Even when the antibody is specific to a well-defined neutrophil antigen, blood donors are rarely, if ever, phenotyped for neutrophil antigens. The affected neonate's mother has antigen-negative granulocytes, but it is not practical for her to be a donor, as granulocyte transfusions must be given daily, and it is difficult to wash the granulocytes to remove the maternal antibody. In one case where granulocyte transfusions were felt to be effective, the granulocytes were collected by apheresis from donors with NA1-negative cells.[24] The granulocytes were volume reduced and irradiated before transfusion. In this case, only three granulocyte concentrates were given. Granulocyte concentrate donors for neonates should also be cytomegalovirus (CMV) seronegative.

Neonatal Alloimmune Thrombocytopenia

Platelet Antigens

Several platelet-specific alloantigen systems have been implicated in neonatal alloimmune thrombocytopenia (Table 5-3).[28] The antigens have been described under several different names, but the most frequently used nomenclature is that proposed by

Table 5-3. Platelet Antigens Implicated in Neonatal Alloimmune Thrombocytopenia

Nomenclature			
ISBT		Classic	
System	Antigen	System	Antigen
HPA-1	HPA-1a	Zw, Pl^{A}	Zw^{a}, Pl^{A1}
	HPA-1b		Zw^{b}, Pl^{A2}
HPA-2	HPA-2a	Ko, Sib	Ko^{b}
	HPA-2b		Ko^{a}, Sib^{a}
HPA-3	HPA-3a	Bak, Lek	Bak^{a}, Lek^{a}
	HPA-3b		Bak^{b}
HPA-4	HPA-4a	Pen, Yuk	Pen^{a}, Yuk^{b}
	HPA-4b		Pen^{b}, Yuk^{a}
HPA-5	HPA-5a	Br, Hc, Zav	Br^{b}, Zav^{b}
	HPA-5b		Br^{a}, Zav^{a}, Hc^{a}
HPA-6	HPA-6a	Ca, Tu	Ca^{b}, Tu^{b}
	HPA-6b		Ca^{a}, Tu^{a}
HPA-7	HPA-7a	Mo	Mo^{b}
	HPA-7b		Mo^{a}
HPA-8	HPA-8a	Sr	Sr^{b}
	HPA-8b		Sr^{a}
HPA-9	HPA-9a	Max	Max(a+)
	HPA-9b		Max(a–)

*International Society of Blood Transfusion. Adapted from Davis.[28]

the International Working Party on Platelet Serology of the International Society of Blood Transfusion and International Society of Hematology. The platelet-specific antigens are called HPA for human platelet antigen. The systems are numbered in chronological order by the date of description. All HPA systems described to date are biallelic; the high-incidence allele is designated by the letter a and the low-incidence allele by the letter b.

HPAs are located on specific platelet membrane GPs or GP complexes (Table 5-4). HPA-1, HPA-4, HPA-6, HPA-7, and HPA-8 are located on GPIIIA; HPA-2 on GPIb; HPA-3 and HPA-9 on GPIIb; and HPA-5 on GPIa. The difference between the two alleles in each system is due to single nucleotide polymorphisms that result in single amino acid substitutions in the GP carrying each antigen system[29] (Table 5-4). Molecular methods have been developed to distinguish the alleles of each of these genes. These methods use genomic DNA and PCR so genotyping can be performed with small numbers of lymphocytes. Several methods have been used to distinguish the alleles, including sequence-specific probes and restriction enzymes.

Table 5-4. Molecular Basis of Platelet Antigens

System	Antigen	Glycoprotein	Polymorphic Amino Acid
HPA-1	HPA-1a	GPIIIa	Leu_{33}*
	HPA-1b		Pro_{33}
HPA-2	HPA-2a	GPIb	Thr_{145}
	HPA-2b		Met_{145}
HPA-3	HPA-3a	GPIIb	Ile_{843}
	HPA-3b		Ser_{843}
HPA-4	HPA-4a	GPIIIa	Arg_{143}*
	HPA-4b		Gln_{143}
HPA-5	HPA-5a	GPIa	Glu_{505}
	HPA-5b		Lys_{505}
HPA-6	HPA-6a	GPIIIa	Arg_{489}*
	HPA-6b		Gln_{489}
HPA-7	HPA-7a	GPIIIa	Pro_{407}*
	HPA-7b		Ala_{407}
HPA-8	HPA-8a	GPIIIa	Arg_{636}*
	HPA-8b		Cys_{636}
HPA-9	HPA-9a	GPIIb	Val_{837}
	HPA-9b		Met_{837}

*HPA-1a, HPA-4a, HPA-6a, HPA-7a, and HPA-8a are the same molecule: GPIIIa Leu_{33}, Arg_{143}, Pro_{407}, Arg_{489}, Arg_{636}. HPA-1b, HPA-4b, HPA-6b, HPA-7b, and HPA-8b differ from this molecule by a single amino acid. Adapted from Valentin and Peter.[29]

Platelet Antibodies in Alloimmune Thrombocytopenia

Among Whites, the antibodies implicated in neonatal alloimmune thrombocytopenia are most often specific for HPA-1a and HPA-5b.[30,31] In Whites with clinically well-defined neonatal alloimmune thrombocytopenia, the antibodies are specific for HPA-1a in 73% to 88% of cases, HPA-5b in 6% to 19%, HPA-3a in 0% to 2%, and HPA-1b in 0% to 2%.[30,31] Asians with neonatal alloimmune thrombocytopenia most often have antibodies specific for HPA-4 antigens. Antibodies specific to HPA-2 and HPA-3 antigens have rarely been implicated in neonatal alloimmune thrombocytopenia.[32] Fetuses with neonatal alloimmune thrombocytopenia and antibodies specific for HPA-1a have lower platelet counts than affected fetuses with other antigen incompatibilities.[33]

Certain cases suggest that neonatal alloimmune thrombocytopenia is sometimes due to ABO incompatibility, but these cases have not been well documented.[32] Some people hypothesize that antibodies specific for HLA antigens cause neonatal alloimmune thrombocytopenia, but prospective studies have not shown that HLA-specific antibodies cause thrombocytopenia.[34]

Clinical Course

Neonatal alloimmune thrombocytopenia occurs in about 1 in every 2000 to 5000 pregnancies.[32] Only about 1 in 20 to 1 in 40 women with children who have incompatible platelet antigens produce platelet-specific antibodies.[35] This may in part be due to HLA Class II antigens, because almost all women who produce anti-HPA-1a express the HLA-Dw52a phenotype.[35]

Because pregnant women are not routinely screened for platelet antibodies or phenotyped for platelet-specific antigens, neonatal alloimmune thrombocytopenia is often not diagnosed until birth. Immediately after birth, affected neonates have a low platelet count, which may become even lower in the hours and days that follow. Their WBC count is usually normal, but their hemoglobin may be normal or low, because of intrauterine bleeding. Thrombocytopenia due to alloimmunization must be distinguished from other clinical conditions that can cause thrombocytopenia, including infection, disseminated intravascular coagulation, congenital leukemia, congenital immune deficiencies, and hemangiomas.

Affected neonates may be asymptomatic, but bleeding occurs in most thrombocytopenic neonates. They often have patechiae or purpura and are less likely to have gastrointestinal bleeding or hematuria. The most serious complication is intracranial bleeding, which occurs in 10% to 30% of affected children.[33] Intracranial bleeding is fatal in 7% of affected neonates. If no treatment is needed, the platelet counts usually rise to normal levels within 1 to 3 weeks.

Bleeding can occur before birth. It is estimated that one-half to one-quarter of all intracranial hemorrhages occur in utero.[33] Placental transfer of IgG can occur from week 14 of gestation, and platelet alloantigens have been shown to be expressed at 18 weeks of gestation.[36] Thrombocytopenia and intracranial hemorrhage can occur as early as week 20 of gestation.[36] Of 107 fetuses who had a sibling with neonatal alloimmune thrombocytopenia, 46% had a platelet count less than 20,000/μL before week 24 of gestation.[33]

Diagnosis

Like that of neonatal alloimmune neutropenia, the diagnosis of neonatal alloimmune thrombocytopenia is based on the detection in the mother's serum of an alloantibody that is specific to an antigen expressed on the child's and father's platelets. When an alloimmunized mother with an affected child has another child with an incompatible platelet antigen phenotype, the chance that the child will become thrombocytopenic is 80% to 100%.[32,35,36] Because of the danger of intracranial bleeding in utero and during delivery, considerable effort is put into the intrauterine diagnosis of alloimmune thrombocytopenia. Titers and subclass determinations of the platelet-specific antibodies are not predictive of fetal platelet counts, and the direct determination of fetal platelet counts is necessary for the in utero diagnosis and treatment of the thrombocytopenia.[36]

Percutaneous umbilical vein blood sampling (PUBS) is used to measure fetal platelet counts and to collect lymphocytes to determine the fetal platelet antigen genotype. While PUBS has become a critical tool for the diagnosis and treatment of neonatal alloimmune thrombocytopenia, it can cause bleeding at the cord puncture site that can lead to extensive hemorrhage and anemia. The risk of serious bleeding due to PUBS is about 1%.[32,35,36] The risk of hemorrhage may be as high as 5% in severely thrombocytopenic fetuses,[37] and some centers transfuse platelets to severely thrombocytopenic fetuses during PUBS.[35]

Treatment

If neonatal alloimmune thrombocytopenia is not diagnosed until birth, the newborn can be treated with IVIG, platelet transfusions, or both. However, because it takes several hours for IVIG to be effective, most severely thrombocytopenic newborns are given platelet transfusions. If the implicated antibody is specific for HPA-1a, many blood centers have platelets from HPA-1a-negative donors that can be transfused. If the antibody is directed toward an antigen other than HPA-1a, it is unlikely that platelets can be obtained from a blood center's pool of regular apheresis donors. However, maternal platelets can be transfused. Maternal platelets are usually collected by apheresis and must be washed to remove the alloantibody. Maternal relatives are also a potential source of compatible platelets. All platelets given to neonates must be CMV-reduced-risk, volume-reduced, and gamma-irradiated to prevent graft-vs-host disease. If a donor with compatible platelets is CMV-seropositive, their platelets can be made CMV-reduced-risk by leukocyte reduction.

Because alloimmune thrombocytopenia recurs in 80% to 90% of subsequent pregnancies and the thrombocytopenia appears to grow worse with each pregnancy, in utero treatment of thrombocytopenia is critical. Giving the mother IVIG is the most effective treatment for alloimmune thrombocytopenia.[38] Its mechanism of action is not certain, but it may block the transfer of IgG across the placenta.[32,35,36] In addition, some hypothesize that IVIG treatments may reduce the risk of intracranial hemorrhage even if the fetus remains thrombocytopenic.

Bussel and colleagues[38] found that weekly treatment of the mother with 1 mg/kg of IVIG increases the platelet counts in 62% to 85% of affected fetuses. Treating the mothers with 1.5 mg of dexamethasone in addition to weekly IVIG did not improve the response rate. But when the mothers of nonresponders were given weekly IVIG plus 60 mg of prednisone daily, the fetal platelet counts increased in 5 of 10 nonresponders.[38] Silver and colleagues[37] found that weekly maternal IVIG treatments improved platelet counts in six of eight fetuses treated. The two fetuses that did not respond to maternal IVIG treatments were treated with direct IVIG infusion into the umbilical vein, but both remained thrombocytopenic.[37] Others have found that maternal IVIG treatments are successful in only 26% of cases.[39]

A typical in utero treatment protocol involves first measuring the fetus's platelet count at 20 weeks of gestation.[35] If the fetus is thrombocytopenic, the mother is treated with IVIG at 1 mg/kg each week. A second PUBS is performed at about week 26, and, if the fetal platelet count has increased, the IVIG is continued. If the fetus remains thrombocytopenic, the mother is given 60 mg of prednisone daily in addition to the weekly IVIG treatments, and a PUBS is repeated before delivery. If the fetus remains thrombocytopenic, a platelet transfusion is given before delivery.[35]

Some sources recommend that all neonates with alloimmune thrombocytopenia be delivered by cesarean section. However, if the platelet count is greater than 50,000/μL, it appears that vaginal delivery does not place the fetus at any more risk of intracranial bleeding than does a cesarean section.[35]

Some centers recommend that weekly in utero platelet transfusions should be given along with weekly maternal IVIG treatments as long as the fetus is thrombocytopenic.[32,36] However, this requires multiple PUBS procedures, each of which places the fetus at risk of bleeding and exposes it to multiple blood transfusions.

References

1. Bux J, Jung KD, Kauth T, Mueller-Eckhardt C. Serological and clinical aspects of granulocyte antibodies leading to alloimmune neonatal neutropenia. Transfus Med 1992;2:143-9.
2. De Haas M, Muniz-Diaz E, van der Kolk K, et al. Neutrophil antigen 5b is carried by a protein, migrating from 70 to 95 kDa, and may be involved in neonatal alloimmune neutropenia. Transfusion 2000;40:222-7.
3. Bux J, Stein EL, Bierling P, et al. Characterization of a new alloantigen (SH) on the human neutrophil Fc-γ-receptor IIIb. Blood 1997;89:1027-34.
4. Huizinga TWJ, Kuijers RWAM, Kleijer M, et al. Maternal genomic neutrophil FcRIII deficiency leading to neonatal isoimmune neutropenia. Blood 1990;76:1927-32.
5. Stroncek DF, Skubitz KM, Plachta LB, et al. Alloimmune neonatal neutropenia due to an antibody to the neutrophil Fc-gamma-receptor III with maternal deficiency of CD16 antigen. Blood 1991;77:1572-80.
6. McCullough J, Clay M, Press C, Kline W. Granulocyte serology: A clinical laboratory Guide. Chicago: ASCP Press, 1988.
7. Matsuo K, Procter J, Stroncek D. Variations in genes encoding neutrophil specific antigens NA1 and NA2. Transfusion 2000;40:645-53.
8. Lernbecher T, Foster CB, Zhu S, et al. Variant genotypes of the low-affinity Fcγ receptors in two control populations and a review of low-affinity Fcγ receptor polymorphisms in control and disease populations. Blood 1999;94:4220-32.
9. Ohto H, Matsuo Y. Neutrophil-specific antigens and gene frequencies in the Japanese (letter). Transfusion 1989;29:654.
10. Trounstine ML, Peiltz GA, Yssel H, et al. Reactivity of cloned, expressed human FcRIII isoforms with monoclonal antibodies which distinguish cell type specific and allelic forms of Fc-gamma-RIII. Int Immunol 1990;2:303-10.
11. Ory PA, Clark MR, Kwoh EE, et al. Sequences of complementary DNAs that encode the NA1 and NA2 forms of Fcγ receptor III on human neutrophils. J Clin Invest 1989;84:1688-91.
12. Ravetch JV, Perussia B. Alternative membrane forms of FcγRIII (CD16) on human natural killer cells and neutrophils. Cell type-specific expression of two genes that differ in single nucleotide substitutions. J Exp Med 1989;170:481-97.
13. Stroncek DF, Shankar R, Litz C, Clement L. The expression of the NB1 antigen on myeloid precursors and neutrophils from children and umbilical cords. Transfus Med 1998;8:119-23.
14. Huizinga TW, Kleijer M, Tetteroo PA, et al. Biallelic neutrophil NA-antigen system is associated with a polymorphism on the phospho-inositol-linked Fc-γ-receptor III (CD16). Blood 1990;75:213-17.

15. Bux J, Stein EL, Santoso S, Mueller-Eckhardt C. NA gene frequencies in the German population, determinated by polymerase chain reaction with sequence-specific primers. Transfusion 1995;35:54-7.
16. Hessner MJ, Curtis BR, Endean DJ, Aster RH. Determination of neutrophil antigen gene frequencies in five ethnic groups by polymerase chain reaction with sequence-specific primers. Transfusion 1996;36:895-9.
17. De Haas M, Kleijer M, van Zwieten R, et al. Neutrophil FcγRIIIb deficiency, nature, and clinical consequences: A study of 21 individuals from 14 families. Blood 1995;86:2403-13.
18. Matsuo K, Lin A, Procter JL, et al. Variations in the expression of granulocyte antigen NB1. Transfusion 2000;40:654-62.
19. Stroncek DF, Skubitz KM, McCullough J. Biochemical nature of the neutrophil-specific antigen NB1. Blood 1990;75:744-55.
20. Goldschmeding R, van Dalen CM, Faber N, et al. Further characterization of the NB1 antigen as a variably expressed 56-62 kD GPI linked glycoprotein of plasma membranes and specific granules of neutrophils. Br J Haematol 1992;81:336-45.
21. Kissel K, Santoso S, Hofman C, et al. Molecular basis of the neutrophil glycoprotein NB1 (CD177) involved in the pathogenesis of immune neutropenias and transfusion reactions. Eur J Immunol 2001;31:1301-9.
22. Stroncek DF, Shankar RA, Plachta LB, et al. Polyclonal antibodies against NB1-bearing 58-64 kDa glycoprotein of human neutrophils do not identify an NB2-bearing molecule. Transfusion 1993;33:399-404.
23. Minchinton RM, McGrath KM. Alloimmune neonatal neutropenia—a neglected diagnosis? Med J Aust 1987;147:139-41.
24. Cartron J, Tchernia G, Celton JL, et al. Alloimmune neonatal neutropenia. Am J Pediatr Hematol Oncol 1991;13:21-5.
25. Hinkel GK, Schneider I, Gebhardt B, Leverenz S. Alloimmune neonatal neutropenia: Clinical observations and therapeutic consequences. Acta Paediatr Hung 1986;27:31-41.
26. Gilmore MM, Stroncek DF, Korones DK. Treatment of alloimmune neonatal neutropenia with granulocyte colony-stimulating factor. J Pediatr 1994;125:948-51.
27. Stroncek DF, Leonard K, Eiber G, et al. Alloimmunization following granulocyte transfusions. Transfusion 1996;36:1009-15.
28. Davis GL. Platelet specific alloantigens. Clin Lab Sci 1998;11:356-61.
29. Valentin N, Peter PJ. Human platelet alloantigens. Curr Opin Hematol 1994;1:381-7.
30. McFarland JG. Platelet and neutrophil alloantigen genotyping in clinical practice. Transfus Clin Biol 1998;5:13-21.
31. Kroll H, Kiefel V, Santoso S. Clinical aspects and typing of platelet alloantigens. Vox Sang 1998;74(Suppl 2):345-54.
32. Kaplan C, Morel-Kopp MC, Clemenceau S, et al. Fetal and neonatal alloimmune thrombocytopenia: Current trends in diagnosis and therapy. Transfus Med 1992;2:265-71.

33. Bussel JB, Zabusky MR, Berkowitz RL, McFarland JG. Fetal alloimmune thrombocytopenia. N Engl J Med 1997;337:22-6.
34. Skacel PO, Stacey TE, Tidmarsh EF, Contreras M. Maternal alloimmunization to HLA, platelet and granulocyte-specific antigens during pregnancy: Its influence on cord blood granulocyte and platelet counts. Br J Haematol 1989;71:118-23.
35. Johnson JA, Ryan G, al-Musa A, et al. Prenatal diagnosis and management of neonatal alloimmune thrombocytopenia. Semin Perinatol 1997; 1:45-52.
36. Kaplan C, Forestier F, Daffos F, et al. Management of fetal and neonatal alloimmune thrombocytopenia. Transfus Med Rev 1996;3:233-40.
37. Silver RM, Porter TF, Branch DW, et al. Neonatal alloimmune thrombocytopenia: Antenatal management. Am J Obstet Gynecol 2000;182: 1233-8.
38. Bussel JB, Berkowitz RL, Lynch L, et al. Antenatal management of alloimmune thrombocytopenia with intravenous gamma-globulin: A randomized trial of the addition of low-dose steroid to intravenous gamma-globulin. Am J Obstet Gynecol 1996;174:1414-23.
39. Kaplan C, Murphy MF, Kroll H, Waters AH. Feto-maternal alloimmune thrombocytopenia: Antenatal therapy with IVIG and steroids—more questions than answers. European Working Group on FMAIT. Br J Haematol 1998;100:62-5.

In: Herman JH, Manno CS, eds.
Pediatric Transfusion Therapy
Bethesda, MD: AABB Press, 2002

6

Additive Solutions and Product Age in Neonatal Red Blood Cell Transfusion

RONALD G. STRAUSS, MD

MANY PRETERM INFANTS, PARTICULARLY THOSE WITH a birthweight ≤1.0 kg, are given multiple red cell transfusions during the early weeks of life. Despite knowledge gained from extensive experience in prescribing red cell transfusions and from major research efforts to prevent and treat the anemia of prematurity, many controversial questions regarding the practice of neonatal red cell transfusion therapy remain unanswered—at least to the sat-

Ronald G. Strauss, MD, Professor of Pathology and Pediatrics, University of Iowa College of Medicine, and Medical Director, DeGowin Blood Center, University of Iowa Hospitals and Clinics, Iowa City, Iowa

(This work was supported by Grant P01 HL46925 from the National Institutes of Health.)

isfaction of many neonatologists. Similarly, blood banking practices pertaining to the preparation, modification, and issuance of Red Blood Cell (RBC) units for neonatal transfusion are controversial, despite a large number of published reports that offer guidance to transfusion medicine specialists. Thus, practices and policies vary widely, including the clinical and physiological indications for red cell transfusions, the choice of RBC product to be transfused, and the need for RBC product modifications such as leukocyte reduction and gamma irradiation. This chapter critically assesses information pertaining to only one of these issues—namely, the selection of RBC units stored for up to 42 days in additive solutions for transfusing neonates vs the transfusion of fresh RBCs (ie, those stored ≤7 days from the date of donation).

As is true for patients of all ages, efforts have been made to reduce the number of transfusions given to neonates and to limit donor exposures in attempts to minimize the complications of blood transfusion. A study of blood utilization for neonates at the University of Iowa illustrates changing clinical practices by comparing red cell transfusions in the years 1982, 1989, and 1993.[1] The mean number of red cell transfusions per infant (<1.5 kg birthweight) declined from 7.0 in 1982 to 5.0 in 1989 to 2.7 in 1993 ($p<0.001$). The proportion of relatively large preterm infants (birthweight 1.0 to 1.5 kg) who were managed without need for red cell transfusions increased from 17% in 1982 to 32% in 1989 and to 64% in 1993. In contrast, with rare exception, nearly 100% of extremely preterm infants (birthweight <1.0 kg) required red cell transfusions in all years.[1] The need to effectively manage the early phase of the anemia of prematurity was evident by the fact that 70% of transfusions were given during the first month of life. Unpublished data on current red cell transfusion practices at the University of Iowa document continuing similar patterns (ie, 74% and 64% of red cell transfusions given to infants with birthweight <1.5 kg and ≥1.5 kg, respectively, occurred within the first 4 weeks of life). Thus, transfusing RBCs units collected from one donor per infant and stored for up to 42 days offers a potential means to markedly reduce donor exposure, even when multiple transfusions are given.

Concerns About and Rationale for Transfusing Stored RBCs

The most frequent red cell transfusions given to preterm infants are small-volume or "booster" transfusions of 10 to 20 mL/kg of body weight of red cells suspended either in citrate-phosphate-dextrose-adenine solution (CPDA) at hematocrit of about 70% or in extended storage media [AS-1 (Adsol, Baxter Healthcare Corporation, Deerfield, IL), AS-3 (Nutricel, MedSep Corporation, Covina, CA), AS-5 (Optisol, Terumo Medical Corporation, Somerset, NJ)] at a hematocrit of 60%. Some centers prefer to centrifuge RBC aliquots before transfusion—regardless of the storage solution—to prepare a uniform RBC concentrate (hematocrit >80%) containing relatively small quantities of extracellular fluid.[2-4]

Most small-volume red cell transfusions are infused slowly over 2 to 4 hours. Because of the small quantity of extracellular fluid (storage media) infused with small-volume transfusions—particularly when the hematocrit is increased by centrifugation—plus the slow rate of transfusion, the type of anticoagulant-preservative solution in which the red cells are suspended is believed not to pose risks for the majority of premature infants.[5] Accordingly, the traditional use of relatively fresh RBCs (<7 days of storage) has been challenged by several investigators[3-10] in hopes of diminishing the donor exposure of multitransfused infants by repeated use of a dedicated unit (or part of a unit) of stored RBCs for each infant.

Neonatologists who object to transfusing stored RBCs and insist on fresh RBCs generally raise three major objections: 1) the increase in extracellular potassium (K^+); 2) the decrease in red cell 2,3-diphosphoglycerate (2,3-DPG), both of which occur in RBC units during extended storage; and 3) the safety of additives such as mannitol and relatively large amounts of glucose (dextrose) and phosphate present in extended storage preservative solutions. These concerns are quite legitimate for large-volume (≥25 mL/kg) transfusions, but likely do not apply in the small-volume setting, as discussed in the following paragraphs.

Increase in Extracellular Potassium

After 42 days of storage in extended-storage media (AS-1, AS-3, AS-5) at a hematocrit of 60%, extracellular ("plasma") K+ levels in RBC units approximate 50 mEq/L (0.05 mEq/mL), a concentration that, at first glance, seems alarmingly high. By simple calculations, however, the actual dose of bioavailable K^+ transfused (ie, ionic K^+ in the volume of extracellular fluid infused) is very small. An infant weighing 1 kg, given a 15-mL/kg transfusion of RBCs stored 42 days in extended-storage media and centrifuged to a hematocrit of 80%, will receive 3 mL of extracellular fluid containing only 0.15 mEq of K^+ that will be infused slowly. Even if the red cells are not packed by centrifugation and are infused at a hematocrit of 60% with twice as much extracellular fluid, the K^+ dose infused with red cells after 42 days storage will only be 0.3 mEq. The K^+ concentration of red cells stored in CPDA at a hematocrit of 70% will approximate 70 to 80 mEq/L after the 35 days of permitted storage, and the dose of K^+ infused with a 15-mL/kg transfusion to an infant weighing 1 kg is 0.3 to 0.4 mEq. These doses are quite small compared with the usual daily K^+ requirement of 2 to 3 mEq/kg, and they have been shown in clinical studies not to cause hyperkalemia, whether packed RBCs[3,4] or unmodified RBCs[10-12] were transfused. However, it must always be remembered that this rationale does not apply to large-volume (>25 mL/kg) transfusions in which larger doses of K^+ may be harmful, especially if infused rapidly (eg, exchange transfusions, extensive surgery, extracorporeal circuits).

Decrease in 2,3-DPG

As for the second objection, 2,3-DPG is totally depleted from the red cells by 21 days of storage, and this is reflected by a P50 value that falls from about 27 mmHg in fresh blood to 18 mmHg in stored red cells at the time of outdate. The 18 mmHg value of older transfused red cells corresponds to the physiologically low P50 value obtained from the blood of many healthy preterm infants at birth, because of the effects of high fetal hemoglobin levels in red cells of preterm infants. Thus, the low P50 of stored transfused red cells is no worse than that of red cells produced endogenously by the infant's own marrow, and both the stored red cells and those produced by the infant will have a reduced ability to offload oxygen when compared with fresh adult red cells. However, the adult red cells stored in blood bank RBC units provide an advantage over the infant's own red cells, because 2,3-DPG and the P50 of transfused adult red cells (but not endogenous infant red cells) will increase rapidly after transfusion. Although the speed of the regeneration of 2,3-DPG in red cells transfused specifically into infants has not been studied extensively, there is no reason to believe it would differ from that in adults (ie, it would increase within hours), providing that the blood of the infant being transfused contains adequate levels of glucose and phosphate to provide substrate for the metabolic pathways of the transfused red cells. In the small-volume (15 mL/kg) red cell transfusion setting, 2,3-DPG levels have been shown to be maintained in infants given stored red cells.[3] Similarly, fetuses with >80% circulating adult red cells as a consequence of intrauterine transfusions maintained normal 2,3-DPG levels when sampled by cordocentesis.[11] In the massive exchange transfusion setting, impaired oxygen offloading has been shown in infants given stored red cells by measurements of 2,3-DPG and P50. Consequently, fresh blood is used frequently in this setting.[12] However, when either stored or fresh blood was used for exchange transfusions in one comparative study, the P50 in infant blood increased from 17 mmHg 2 hours after the exchange to 23 mmHg at 24 hours after the exchange with stored blood, whereas an increase to 26 mmHg was seen at 24 hours after the exchange when fresh blood stored <24 hours was used for the exchange transfusion.[12] This difference was considered to have neither statistical nor clinical significance.

Safety of Additive Solutions

As for the third objection, the quantity of additives present in RBC units containing extended-storage media is believed not to be dangerous to neonates given small-volume (≅ 15 mL/kg) transfusions.[5] The distinction between small- and large-volume transfusions is important, because the safety of extended-storage media has not been convincingly demonstrated in large-volume settings such as exchange transfusions, cardiac bypass, or extracorporeal membrane oxygenation. A comparison of CPDA and the three types of extended-storage media (AS-1, AS-3, and AS-5) is presented in Table 6-1. Regardless of the type of suspending solution, the quantity of additives is quite small in the clinical setting in which a neonate would receive a single, small-volume red cell transfusion over 2 to 4 hours. With AS-1 and AS-3 RBCs used to illustrate (Table 6-2), the dose of extended-storage media transfused during a typical small-volume red cell transfusion is estimated to be far below levels believed to be toxic.[5] Support for this assumption was provided by prelimi-

Table 6-1. Formulation of Anticoagulant-Preservative Solutions in Blood Collection Sets[13]

Constituent	CPDA	AS-1	AS-3	AS-5
Volume (mL)	63*	100†	100†	100†
Sodium chloride (mg)	None	900	410	877
Dextrose (mg)	2000	2200	1100	900
Adenine (mg)	17.3	27	30	30
Mannitol (mg)	None	750	None	525
Trisodium citrate (mg)	1660	None	588	None
Citric acid (mg)	206	None	42	None
Sodium phosphate (monobasic) (mg)	140	None	276	None

*Approximately 450 mL of donor blood is drawn into 63 mL of CPDA. A unit of RBCs (hematocrit of about 70%) is prepared by centrifugation and removal of most plasma.

†When AS-1 or AS-5 is used, 450 mL of donor blood is first drawn into 63 mL of CPD, which is identical to CPDA, except that it contains 1610 mg of dextrose per 63 mL and has no adenine. When AS-3 is used, donor blood is drawn into CP2D, which is identical to CPD, except it contains double the amount of dextrose. After centrifugation and removal of nearly all plasma, RBCs are resuspended in 100 mL of the additive solution (AS-1, AS-3, or AS-5) at a hematocrit of 55 to 60%.

Table 6-2. Quantity (Total mg/kg) of Additives Infused During a Transfusion of 15 mL per kg of AS-1 or AS-3 RBCs at Hematocrit 60%[13]

Additive	AS-1	AS-3	Toxic Dose*
NaCl	42	7.5	137 mg/kg/day
Dextrose	129	23	240 mg/kg/hr
Adenine	0.6	0.6	15 mg/kg/dose
Citrate	9.8	12.6	180 mg/kg/hr
Phosphate	2.0	5.6	>60 mg/kg/day
Mannitol	33	0	360 mg/kg/day

*Accuracy of the toxic dose is difficult to predict for transfusions to individual infants, because infusion rates generally are slow, which permits the metabolism and distribution of additives from blood into extravascular sites. Moreover, dextrose, adenine, and phosphate enter red cells and are somewhat sequestered and not immediately "available" in the extracellular solution. Potential toxic doses taken from Luban et al.[5]

nary clinical data[14] and by a small reported study in which infants were given either AS-1 or CPDA RBCs stored <5 days under a randomized double-crossover design.[15] The quantity of additives would be even smaller when packed RBCs (hematocrit >80%) are transfused. Although multiple, rather than single, transfusions often are given to preterm infants, there is no information to document failure to metabolize or excrete additives by preterm infants (ie, no evidence of cumulative toxicity).[3-5] Thus, it is logical to assume that either single or multiple small-volume transfusions using RBC units containing extended-storage media are safe for neonatal transfusions. In fact, randomized clinical trials have established their feasibility, efficacy, and safety.

Clinical Experience Transfusing Stored RBCs

To confirm the somewhat preliminary findings and the theoretical calculations discussed in the preceding section with clinical experience, seven reports[3,4,6-10] were reviewed that have documented the successful transfusion of stored, rather than fresh, red cells for small-volume transfusion support of neonates (Table 6-3). In these reports, stored red cells were transfused safely, without increased hyperkalemia or acidosis and, in most instances, with donor exposure decreased >50% from that observed with transfusions of fresh blood. However, five of these studies[6-10] included relatively few transfusions with red cells actually stored longer than 14 days and did not address the use of extended-storage anticoagulant-preservative solutions, as are commonly used at the present time. Moreover, on the basis of in-vitro studies of AS-3, concerns have been raised again recently about levels of potassium, phosphate, glucose, and citrate in RBC units containing extended-storage media for neonatal transfusions.[16] Accordingly, data from transfusion studies of AS-1 and AS-3 RBCs stored up to 42 days and given to preterm infants at the University of Iowa Hospitals and Clinics are be summarized in detail in the following paragraphs.[2-4]

Two studies[3,4] were of a two-arm, randomized design in which nursery staff and parents were blinded to the assignment. In one study arm, infants with birthweights of 0.6 to 1.3 kg received either AS-1[3] or AS-3[4] RBCs stored up to 42 days (stored red cells); in the other study arm, infants received CPDA RBCs stored up to 7 days (fresh red cells). All transfusions were given uniformly as 15 mL/kg of centrifuged red cells (hematocrit of 85%) infused over 5 hours. To detect possible clinical transfusion reactions, nurses took seven sets of vital signs and observations during each transfusion—as it began, after 15 minutes, and hourly thereafter. To detect possible biochemical abnormalities in infant blood, pretransfusion levels of hematocrit, glucose, lactate, pH, ionized calcium, sodium, and potassium were measured when RBC units were ordered from the blood bank. Identical studies were performed on infant blood samples drawn shortly after the transfusions were completed.

Complete results, including success in reducing donor exposure, are summarized in Table 6-3 and have been reported in detail elsewhere,[3,4] and only the safety aspects of the study are reported here. None of the CPDA RBCs were stored longer than 7 days, whereas 47% of AS-1 RBCs and 50% of AS-3 RBCs were

Table 6-3. Small-Volume Transfusions of Stored RBCs Will Limit Donor Exposure Without Causing Apparent Adverse Effects

Reference	Solution	Storage	Dose	Hematocrit of Transfused RBCs	Transfusions (mean/infant)	Donors (mean/infant)
8	CPDA	≤14 days	< 60 mL/ transfusion	NR	13.4* 2.8†	4.2* 1.6†
9	CPDA	≤35 days	NR	NR	3.6	1.5
6	CPDA	≤35 days	15 mL/kg	75%	5.6	2.1
7	CPDA	≤35 days	13 mL/kg	68-75%	6.0	2.0
10	NR	≤35 days	15 mL/kg	NR	5.6	4.9
3	AS-1	≤42 days	15 mL/kg	85%	3.5	1.2
4	AS-3	≤42 days	15 mL/kg	85%	3.6	1.3

NR = Not reported.

*Infants in Cook et al[8] with birthweight <1.5 kg.

†Infants in Cook et al[8] with birthweight ≥1.5 kg.

stored 15 days or longer before transfusion. No clinical transfusion reactions were observed during 66 AS-1 RBC transfusions given to 19 infants, during 28 AS-3 RBC transfusions given to 11 infants, or during 98 CPDA RBC transfusions given to 31 infants.[3,4] No significant differences occurred in the comparative changes between pretransfusion and posttransfusion blood chemistries, whether fresh CPDA RBCs or stored AS-1 or AS-3 RBCs were transfused (Table 6-4). The hematocrit increased as expected. Changes in levels of glucose, lactate, pH, calcium, sodium, and potassium during transfusion were slight. After the randomized trials, additional safety data were generated by an open study in which 33 preterm infants (birthweight 0.6 to 1.25 kg) received all red cell transfusions as 15 mL/kg of AS-3 RBCs stored ≤42 days.[4] Of the 120 red cell transfusions given, 78 (65%) were stored 1 through 21 days and 42 (35%) were stored 22 through 42 days. When comparing pretransfusion and posttransfusion laboratory results in these two groups (ie, <22 days vs ≥22 days), no statistically significant differences were found that could be related to the length of storage (Table 6-5).

Thus, red cells from one donor stored up to 42 days in either AS-1 or AS-3 can safely provide all red cells needed by most individual preterm infants. At the University of Iowa DeGowin Blood Center, preterm infants requiring red cell transfusions are assigned to dedicated units of RBCs suspended in extended-storage (42-day) solutions. At the time the first transfusion is ordered, one-half of a freshly collected (stored ≤7 days) unit is dedicated to a preterm infant with a birthweight ≤1.0 kg. The remainder of the unit can be assigned to another infant. Thus, one complete unit can serve two very low birthweight infants simultaneously. Larger infants may be assigned to only one-third or one-fourth of a unit, depending on anticipated needs. When RBC units are ordered, aliquots are removed sterilely and issued.[2] Although units are used throughout 42 days of storage, once a unit has been stored 14 days, it has become relatively aged (ie, 14 days of its 42 days have lapsed), and no new preterm neonates are assigned to it. When infants assigned to a unit no longer require transfusions, the remainder of the unit is placed in the general

Table 6-4. Mean Changes (Delta ± SD) in Blood Chemistry Levels During RBC Transfusions[13]

	CPDA vs AS-1[8]		CPDA vs AS-3[9]	
	CPDA RBCs	AS-1 RBCs	CPDA RBCs	AS-3 RBCs
Hematocrit (%)	+ 12 ± 4	+ 12 ± 5	+ 12 ± 5	+ 11 ± 4
Glucose (mg/dL)	− 9 ± 32	− 7 ± 25	− 18 ± 40	− 17 ± 24
Lactate (mmol/L)	− 0.3 ± 0.4	− 0.1 ± 0.6	− 0.2 ± 0.3	− 0.5 ± 1.5
pH	0.00 ± 0.05	0.00 ± 0.13	− 0.01 ± 0.09	− 0.03 ± 0.06
Calcium (mg/dL)	− 0.1 ± 0.7	− 0.1 ± 0.5	− 0.1 ± 1.0	+ 0.1 ± 0.6
Sodium (mEq/L)	+ 0.5 ± 4.4	+ 0.5 ± 5.1	− 0.4 ± 5.5	+ 1.9 ± 4.7
Potassium (mEq/L)	+ 0.3 ± 0.9	− 0.2 ± 1.5	+ 0.3 ± 1.2	+ 0.4 ± 0.9

Note: For pretransfusion versus posttransfusion laboratory studies, changes (delta values) observed in infants in one study arm (fresh CPDA RBCs) were compared with those in infants in the other arm (stored AS-1 or AS-3 RBCs). Pretransfusion values were subtracted from posttransfusion results, so that a positive delta value indicated an increase of the analyte result after transfusion and a negative value indicated a decrease of the analyte result after transfusion. No statistically significant differences were found by using *t* test for values with normal distribution and Wilcoxon rank test for values with abnormal distribution.

inventory for transfusion to older patients. This plan has been shown to be cost-effective.[17,18]

Additional Potential Risks of Single-Donor Programs

As is true for all cellular blood components, RBC units should be transfused per institutional guidelines pertaining to the prevention of transfusion-associated cytomegalovirus infections and

Table 6-5. Changes in Laboratory Values (Delta ± SD) of 120 AS-3 RBC Transfusions[13]

	Days of Storage		Donor Origin of RBC Transfusions		
	1 to 21 (N = 78)	22 to 42 (N = 42)	Unrelated (N = 49)	Paternal (N = 49)	Maternal (N = 22)
Hematocrit (%)	+ 12 ± 5	+ 12 ± 4	+ 12 ± 5	+ 12 ± 5	+ 12 ± 4
Glucose (mg/dL)	– 12 ± 24	– 16 ± 28	– 12 ± 23	– 13 ± 26	– 18 ± 27
Lactate (mmol/L)	– 0.6 ± 1.1	– 0.2 ± 0.3	– 0.5 ± 1.0	– 0.4 ± 0.9	– 0.4 ± 0.6
pH	0.00 ± 0.08	0.00 ± 0.06	– 0.16 ± 0.067	+ 0.01 ± 0.08	+ 0.02 ± 0.07
Ca (mg/dL)	– 0.1 ± 0.5	0.0 ± 0.8	+ 0.1 ± 0.7	– 0.2 ± 0.5	– 0.2 ± 0.5
Na (mEq/L)	+ 0.3 ± 4.6	– 0.4 ± 4.7	+ 0.3 ± 4.7	– 0.5 ± 5.0	+ 0.8 ± 3.0
K (mEq/L)	+ 0.2 ± 0.8	+ 0.2 ± 0.6	+ 0.3 ± 0.8	+ 0.2 ± 0.7	+ 0.1 ± 0.7

Note: Changes reflect posttransfusion values minus pretransfusion values. Statistical tests used were *t* test for pH, Na, K, and glucose (normal distribution) and Wilcoxon rank sum test for hematocrit, Ca, and lactate (abnormal distribution). No statistically significant differences were found (p values all >0.05) comparing 1 to 21 days of storage and 22 to 42 days of storage. No statistically significant differences among donor groups ($p > 0.05$) except the change in calcium, which was lower ($p < 0.012$) after transfusion in paternal and maternal donors than in unrelated donors.

graft-vs-host disease. A complete discussion of these risks is presented in other chapters. However, as this is another safety issue somewhat unique to single-donor programs, it is important to discuss the type of donor selected to provide the RBC unit dedicated to serve a particular preterm infant. At the DeGowin Blood Center, volunteer group O donors who have successfully donated multiple times to the general blood bank inventory are preferred. Directed donations from family members, who often are either new or infrequent blood donors and who do not have a "pedigree" of safety established by multiple successful donations are discouraged. In addition to the infectious disease risks, believed to be greater in blood collected from new donors than from repeat donors, a potential danger of directed donations is the possibility of serologic incompatibilities between the infant recipient and the family donor.

Biological mothers, in particular, pose a potential danger, because their plasma may contain alloantibodies, stimulated by pregnancy, that are able to react with blood cell antigens inherited by the infant from the father, possibly causing hemolysis, thrombocytopenia, and leukocyte aggregation. A high frequency of alloimmunization against leukocyte antigens has been clearly established in multiparous women,[19-24] and it poses a potential risk that pulmonary infiltrates will be caused by leukocyte aggregation. Many of these antibody reports were retrospective laboratory studies of stored sera, did not contain transfusion recipient data, and did not consider the other factors that determine immunologically mediated reactions to passive antibody infusion (eg, quantity of maternal plasma transfused, titer of antibody, strength of antigen expression on neonatal blood cells, ability of the inflammatory system of preterm neonates to mediate a transfusion reaction). Thus, the genuine risks, in terms of clinically significant reactions, posed by a biological mother who wishes to donate blood components for her neonate shortly after delivery, are incompletely defined.

Accordingly, a two-arm, randomized clinical trial was conducted to systematically compare biological parents to unrelated donors in a single-donor program designed to provide AS-3 RBCs stored ≤42 days for preterm infants with a birthweight of

0.6 to 1.3 kg.[25] The feasibility of using parental donors and the clinical and laboratory assessment of immediate safety were studied by using an experimental design similar to that in the AS-1[3] and AS-3[4] reports. Briefly, all infants received AS-3 RBC transfusions as 15 mL/kg centrifuged to a hematocrit of 85% and transfused over 5 hours. To detect clinical transfusion reactions, nurses observed the infants and took seven sets of vital signs around each transfusion—immediately before it began, after 15 minutes, and hourly thereafter. At the conclusion of each transfusion, nurses placed a sticker in the medical record stating whether or not they had observed a transfusion reaction. To detect possible biochemical abnormalities, the laboratory performed pretransfusion and posttransfusion blood studies.[3,4]

Complete details have been reported elsewhere,[25] and only safety data are summarized here. Only one transfusion reaction was noted during 120 AS-3 RBC transfusions given to 40 infants, each of whom received an average of nearly four red cell transfusions more from their dedicated donor. The reaction was characterized by an increase in temperature from 36.8 to 38.3 C and by an increase in pulse rate from 146 to 180 beats per minute during the fourth transfusion of red cells (stored 28 days) obtained from the father. The infant was not distressed, the changes in vital signs were brief, the blood bank evaluation was negative (including bacterial culture of the unit), and a subsequent transfusion from the father was given without incident. Thus, the precise etiology of the episode could be neither determined nor clearly ascribed to the transfusion.

No differences of clinical importance occurred in the comparative changes of pretransfusion and posttransfusion blood chemistries, whether the red cells were from unrelated or parental donors. Because results of statistical analysis (nested analysis of variance) were similar whether parental donor data were combined or separate, paternal and maternal data are presented separately in Table 6-5. The hematocrit increased as expected in preterm infants regardless of the donor source. Changes in glucose, lactate, pH, calcium, sodium, and potassium were modest. Only calcium values were statistically significantly different, showing a slight drop after transfusion of parental red cells, compared with a slight increase after transfusion of cells from unrelated donors. This difference, although statistically different, had no apparent clinical significance.

Conclusion

All three studies[3,4,25] demonstrated that a dedicated single-donor system, in which either AS-1 or AS-3 RBCs were collected from unrelated blood donors or from biological parents and then stored up to 42 days, was capable of supplying all small-volume RBC transfusions needed by individual preterm infants, without immediate adverse effects. The results are supported by the findings of others, as cited in Table 6-3, who transfused RBCs stored up to 35 days. Only a minority of preterm infants studied at the DeGowin Blood Center[3,4] required blood components other than red cells (ie, platelet and plasma transfusions). Thus, limiting red cell donors is the key to diminishing overall blood donor exposure for many preterm infants during the neonatal period.

Although long-term risks such as transfusion-associated infections and immune modulation were not compared in studies of transfusion programs using fresh or stored RBCs,[3,4,6-10,25] the risks of infectious disease transmission and transfusion-associated immune moderation likely are reduced by limiting allogeneic donor exposure. Thus, it is logical to presume that single-donor programs should increase transfusion safety. Admittedly, safety of the blood supply has improved remarkably, and a genuine reduction in risk provided by single-donor programs beyond that of the usual blood supply cannot be proven statistically without long-term observations of very large numbers of transfused infants. These studies, however, are unlikely to be done because of their expense and the current rarity of posttransfusion infections.[26] Accepting the lack of definitive proof, it seems logical to believe that posttransfusion adverse events—however rare they might be with each donor exposure—are likely to be encountered less often when fewer risks (ie, fewer donor exposures) are taken. Thus, limiting donor exposure, when it can be done safely, is prudent for infants who are likely to receive multiple transfusions.

References

1. Widness JA, Seward VJ, Kromer IJ, et al. Changing patterns of red blood cell transfusion in very low birthweight infants. J Pediatr 1996;129: 680-7.
2. Strauss RG, Villhauer PJ, Cordle DG. A method to collect, store and issue multiple aliquots of packed red blood cells for neonatal transfusions. Vox Sang 1995;68:77-81.
3. Strauss RG, Burmeister LF, Johnson K, et al. AS-1 red blood cells for neonatal transfusions: a randomized trial assessing donor exposure and safety. Transfusion 1996;36:873-8.
4. Strauss RG, Burmeister LF, Johnson K, et al. Feasibility and safety of AS-3 red blood cells for neonatal transfusions. J Pediatr 2000;136: 215-19.
5. Luban NLC, Strauss RG, Hume HA. Commentary on the safety of red blood cells preserved in extended storage media for neonatal transfusions. Transfusion 1991;31:229-35.
6. Liu EA, Mannino FL, Lane TA. Prospective, randomized trial of the safety and efficacy of a limited donor exposure transfusion program for premature neonates. J Pediatr 1994;125:92-6.
7. Lee DA, Slagel TA, Jackson TM, Evans CS. Reducing blood donor exposures in low birth weight infants by the use of older, unwashed packed red blood cells. J Pediatr 1995;126:280-6.
8. Cook S, Gunter J, Wissel M. Effective use of a strategy using assigned red cell units to limit donor exposure for neonatal patients. Transfusion 1993;33:379-83.
9. Jain R, Jarosz CR, Myers TF. Decreasing blood donor exposure in the neonates by using dedicated donor transfusions. Transfus Sci 1997;18: 199-203.
10. Wood A, Wilson N, Skacel P, et al. Reducing donor exposure in preterm infants requiring multiple blood transfusions. Arch Dis Child 1995;72: F29-F33.
11. Soothill PW, Lestas AN, Nicolaides KH, et al. 2,3-diphosphoglycerate in normal, anaemic and transfused human fetuses. Clin Sci 1988;74: 527-30.
12. DeLivoria-Papadopoulos M, Morrow G, Oski FA, et al. Exchange transfusion in the newborn infant with fresh and "old" blood: The role of storage on a 2,3-diphosphoglycerate, hemoglobin-oxygen affinity, and oxygen release. J Pediatr 1971;79:898-903.
13. Strauss RG. Data-driven blood banking practices for neonatal RBC transfusions. Transfusion 2000;40:1528-40.

14. Gooch WM, Longhurst D, Sasich F, Laub RM. Safety of neonatal transfusions of gravity-sedimented erythrocytes following storage in CPDA-1 or Adsol (abstract). Transfusion 1986;26:562.
15. Goodstein MH, Locke RG, Wlodarczyk D, et al. Comparison of two preservation solutions for erythrocyte transfusions in newborn infants. J Pediatr 1993;123:783-8.
16. Rock G, Poon A, Haddad S, et al. Nutricel as an additive solution for neonatal transfusion. Transfus Sci 1999;20:29-36.
17. Hilsenrath P, Nemechek J, Widness JA, et al. Cost-effectiveness of a limited donor blood program for neonatal RBC transfusions. Transfusion 1999;39:938-43.
18. Wang-Rodriguez J, Mannino FL, Liu E, Lane TA. A novel strategy to limit blood donor exposure and blood waste in multiply transfused premature infants. Transfusion 1996;36:64-70.
19. Elbert C, Strauss RG, Barrett F, et al. Biological mothers may be dangerous blood donors for their neonates. Acta Haematol 1991;85:189-91.
20. Clay M, Kline W, McCullough J. The frequency of granulocyte-specific antibodies in postpartum sera and a family study of 6B antigen. Transfusion 1984;24:252-5.
21. Chardonnens X, Jeannet M. Immunobiology of pregnancy; evidence for a fetal immune response against the mother. Tissue Antigens 1980;15:401-6.
22. Neppert J, Mueller-Eckhardt G, Heine O. Reduced immune phagocytosis of monocytes from neonates whose mothers produce HLA antibodies. Vox Sang 1988;54:177-80.
23. Skacel PO, Stacey TE, Tidmarsh CE, Contreras M. Maternal alloimmunization to HLA, platelet and granulocyte-specific antigens during pregnancy: Its influence on cord blood granulocyte and platelet counts. Br J Haematol 1989;71:119-23.
24. Sharon R, Amar A. Maternal anti-HLA antibodies and neonatal thrombocytopenia (letter). Lancet 1981;1:1313.
25. Strauss RG, Burmeister LF, Johnson K, et al. Randomized trial assessing feasibility and safety of biological parents as red blood cell donors for their preterm infants. Transfusion 2000;40:450-6.
26. Finucane ML, Slovic P, Mertz CK. Public perception of the risk of blood transfusion. Transfusion 2000;40:1017-22.

In: Herman JH, Manno CS, eds.
Pediatric Transfusion Therapy
Bethesda, MD: AABB Press, 2002

7

Irradiation for Neonatal and Pediatric Transfusion

NAOMI L.C. LUBAN, MD

IN THE LAST FEW YEARS, SEVERAL ADVANCES HAVE been made in blood irradiation practice. New sources of radiation have been developed; consensus has shifted on which components should be irradiated, for which patients, and at what dose; and innovative approaches to quality assurance can confirm that the irradiation process has taken place. This chapter discusses these advances, as well as irradiated component expiration dates, and developments on the horizon.

Naomi L.C. Luban, MD, Chairman, Laboratory and Pathology, Director, Transfusion Medicine/Donor Center, Vice Chairman for Academic Affairs, Department of Pediatrics, Children's National Medical Center, and Professor, Pediatrics and Pathology, George Washington University Medical Center, Washington, District of Columbia

Overview of Transfusion-Associated Graft-vs-Host Disease

Transfusion-associated graft-vs-host disease (TA-GVHD) was first reported in the 1960s in patients with hematologic malignancies and infants with congenital immunodeficiencies.[1] Since then, the pathogenesis has been more fully described, more at-risk patient groups have been identified, and preventive strategies such as irradiation have been established. Still, many questions remain unanswered.

First, there are no risk estimates or data on disease prevalence in the United States, because no systems for collection of data are in place. Second, it is not clear why the clinical manifestations of GVHD in the setting of hematopoietic transplantation differ from those of TA-GVHD. No well-established model for TA-GVHD exists; thus investigators must extrapolate from GVHD models.

Finally, the widespread use of leukocyte-reduced (LR) blood components has diminished interest in mechanistic studies of TA-GVHD, because it is difficult to perform such studies with blood components that would simulate those being used by at-risk patients. Additional confusion is caused by some blood filter manufacturers who imply that LR components might obviate the need for attenuation of lymphocyte reactivity—a concept that remains unconfirmed by scientific studies.

Pathogenesis of GVHD and TA-GVHD

In the transplant setting, GVHD develops when the following conditions are present: 1) differences exist between donor and recipient histocompatibility, 2) immunocompetent cells are present in the graft, and 3) the recipient is unable to reject the immunocompetent donor cells. In TA-GVHD, similar situations can occur; however, if an HLA homozygous donor and an HLA heterozygous recipient share one HLA haplotype, the donor cells might not be recognized as foreign.[2,3] In both cases, the recipient's major and/or minor histocompatibility antigens stimulate

T-cell expansion and the induction of an inflammatory response with the release of cytokines. This process is responsible for development of the clinical manifestations of the disorder.

On the basis of work in a murine model, Ferrera et al[4] proposed a three-step process for the development of acute GVHD in the transplant setting.

- Radio- or chemotherapy causes tissue damage in the recipient. In turn, this causes secretion of tumor necrosis factor alpha (TNF-α) and interleukin (IL)-1, enhancing antigen recognition by donor T cells. Donor T-cell activation results in proliferation of Th1 cells and secretion of IL-2 and TNF-α, causing further T-cell activation and induction of cytotoxic T cells and natural killer (NK) cells.
- Additional donor and residual recipient phagocytes are stimulated to produce IL-1 and TNF-α. Stimulated macrophages release nitric oxide, which further damages recipient tissues, upregulates alloreactivity, and mediates the cytotoxic function of macrophages.[5]
- Lipopolysaccharides stimulate gut-associated macrophages, lymphocytes, keratocytes, and dermal fibroblasts. They also promote the inflammatory response and the end organ damage that characterize GVHD.

It is still not clear if this process is directly comparable to TA-GVHD, and more research is needed.

The pathogenesis of TA-GVHD has been studied to date by Fast et al[6] (in a murine model) and Nishimura[7] (in a patient with TA-GVHD). It is further supported by clinical correlation with human immunodeficiency virus (HIV).[8] In the mouse, CD4-cell depletion increased the number of donor cells required to induce TA-GVHD, while CD8- or NK-cell depletion had the opposite effect. In HIV/AIDS, only one case of TA-GVHD has been reported, despite profound immunosuppression in, and transfusion support of, this patient group. It is possible that early depletion of CD4+ cells may protect against development of GVHD. It is also possible that activation of CD8+ cells against HIV-infected CD4+ cells may prevent or limit the establishment of the GVHD process.

Clinical Manifestations

For the most part, GVHD and TA-GVHD exhibit the same symptoms, which include fever, anorexia, nausea, vomiting, and diarrhea. Skin manifestations may be severe, beginning as erythematous maculopapular eruptions that may proceed to bullae and frank desquamation. Gastrointestinal bleeding and hepatic dysfunction with hyperbilirubinemia are also seen. Unlike the pancytopenia of acute GVHD in allogeneic transplantation, pancytopenia in TA-GVHD is severe enough to cause death.

Diagnosis

Unfortunately, diagnosis of TA-GVHD is often made postmortem, on the basis of pathognomonic histopathogic findings of T-cell infiltration in the skin, lymph nodes, liver, and gastrointestinal track.[9] The early suspicion of TA-GVHD may prompt a skin biopsy, which may reveal vacuolization of the epidermal basal skin layer, separation of the dermal-epithelial layer, and formation of bullae. Other findings may include mononuclear cell migration into the epidermis, hyperkeratosis, and dyskeratosis.

Liver biopsy may reveal eosinophilic infiltration and degeneration of small bile ducts, peripheral inflammation, and lymphocyte infiltration. Marrow biopsies demonstrate pancytopenia, fibrosis, and lymphocytic infiltration.

Confirmation of clinical suspicion is complicated. Serologic and molecular HLA typing, karyotype analysis, restriction fragment length polymorphism analysis, and genetic fingerprinting have been used[10-14] to identify donor lymphocytes in the circulation or tissues of the recipient. Donor HLA types may need to be confirmed through use of polymerase chain reaction and sequence-specific oligonucleotide probe techniques performed on donor lymphocytes collected from the segments still attached to the donor unit.[15] Recipient HLA type can be confirmed from parental or other familial specimens.[16]

Busch and Lee[17] demonstrated a thousand-fold expansion of donor lymphocytes in the circulation of patients 3 to 5 days after they received transfusion during elective orthopedic surgery; the donor cells were cleared within 2 weeks. In another study,[18]

8 of 10 adult trauma victims who had received 4 to 18 RBC units developed microchimerism. As long as 1.5 years after transfusion, two of the eight still had microchimerism.

Wang-Rodriguez[19] observed transient microchimerism in two of six infants who received non-LR RBCs and three of eight who received LR RBCs. Vietor et al[20] discovered true microchimerism in six of seven young adults 20 years after they had received intrauterine transfusion. Reed et al[21] have identified minor chimeric populations at the 0.01% level. The establishment of microchimerism and identification of its biologic consequences are critical for pediatric patients who are expected to live to reach adulthood. The persistence of microchimerism may predispose to autoimmune disease,[22-24] chronic GVHD,[25] and recurrent abortion.[25] It may also stimulate latent virus reactivation.

At-Risk Patient Groups

In infants and children up to 1 year of age, a total of 73 cases of TA-GVHD have been well documented through 1999.[26] Because of this relative rarity of documented cases, it has been difficult to identify with certainty those patients who may be at risk for TA-GVHD. Because there is no registry of TA-GVHD, the prevalence of the disease is unknown. Cases are likely to be underreported because the clinical presentation resembles other diseases and conditions common to sick infants. Following two reports[15,27] of TA-GVHD (unrecognized at presentation) in older infants with severe combined immunodeficiency disease, the age range of susceptible patients expanded.[28,29] Even some immunocompetent patients may need irradiated components.[30] Thus, indications such as those listed in Table 7-1 use terms such as "clearly indicated" and "probably indicated."[31-33] The spectrum of patients who are at risk is likely to expand as immunosuppressive and immunomodulatory therapies are used for more than transplantation and oncology patient groups.

The Irradiation Process

Although photochemical treatment, pegylation, and ultraviolet light can prevent TA-GVHD, irradiation of whole blood and cellu-

Table 7-1. Indications for Irradiated Blood Components

	Patient Group	Indications
"Clear"	Fetus/infant	Intrauterine transfusion Premature infants Congenital immunodeficiency Exchange transfusion for erythroblastosis
	Child/adult	Congenital immunodeficiency Hematologic malignancy or solid tumor (eg, Hodgkin's disease, neuroblastoma, sarcoma) and receiving ablative chemo/radiotherapy Hematopoietic transplant Recipient of familial blood donation Recipient of HLA-matched components Conditions requiring fludaribine (eg, systemic lupus erythematosus)
"Potential"	Term infant	
	Recipient and donor pair from a genetically homogenous population	
	Patients with other hematologic malignancies or solid tumors receiving immunosuppressive agents	

lar components is the only method approved by the Food and Drug Administration (FDA).[32-37] The use of ionizing radiation inactivates T cells in the donated blood component by damaging nucleic DNA or other biologic actions. The donor T cells cannot proliferate or engraft, and TA-GVHD is prevented.[38,39] Both gamma rays and x-rays are effective in inactivating T cells.

Gamma Radiation

Gamma rays are generated during the radioactive decay process of cesium-137 (^{137}Cs) or cobalt-60 (^{60}Co). The predominant instruments for irradiation of blood components use either of these two sources. In the freestanding ^{137}Cs irradiator, a metal canister holding the blood component is placed on a rotating turntable. The gamma rays originate from one to four sources (depending on the model and manufacturer) that ensure penetration of all portions of the component. The turntable rotates continuously, at a constant speed determined by the manufacturer for each model. A lead shield encloses the irradiation chamber.

In the freestanding ^{60}Co irradiator, tubes of ^{60}Co are arranged in a circle around the entire canister, which does not rotate. All portions of the component are penetrated by the rays, which are attenuated to a lesser degree than are ^{137}Cs rays (see later discussion of attenuation).

X-Ray Radiation

Rather than being generated through a radioactive decay process, x-rays originate from the interaction of a beam of electrons and a metallic surface. Linear accelerators generate an x-ray beam over a field of a given dimension, usually projected onto a table-top structure. The blood component is "sandwiched" between two layers (each several millimeters thick) of biocompatible plastic. The top layer of plastic generates electronic equilibrium of the secondary electrons as they pass through the component container. The plastic layer under the component helps ensure that every portion is irradiated, by providing back-scattering. Typically, the component remains stationary while the total x-ray dose is delivered. In some facilities, however, the component is turned over halfway through the dose delivery, which entails turning off the instrument and starting it up again after the component has been flipped.

In 1999, the FDA licensed the first irradiator for blood components (RS3000, Rad-Source, Coral Springs, FL) that uses the principles of a standard x-ray machine. Benefits of this instrument include:

- No special floor reinforcement is needed.
- An unshielded room can be used for operation.

- There are no Nuclear Regulatory Commission licensing or reporting requirements.
- Equivalency to gamma irradiation is suggested in published abstracts.

Several reports have described the advantages and efficacy,[40-42] and the use of this type of instrument is likely to increase.

Components To Be Irradiated

For patients at risk for TA-GVHD, all components that might contain viable T cells should be irradiated. As shown in Table 7-2, these components include whole blood as well as red cells, platelets, and granulocytes (whole-blood-derived and those obtained through apheresis). It should be noted that frozen/thawed RBC units that were not irradiated before the freezing process should be irradiated after thawing, because T cells contained in those units are viable.[43-45] RBC units filtered by standard or leukocyte reduction filters should also be irradiated. Third-generation leukocyte reduction by filtration theoretically decreases the potential for TA-GVHD by decreasing the total number of white cells in the component by several logs. However, insufficient data exist on the minimum level of T cells than can cause GVHD; thus filtering is not considered an acceptable alternative to irradiation.[46]

Blood components that are homozygous for an HLA haplotype that is shared by the recipient should also be irradiated. These components typically are directed donations from first- and second-degree relatives[2,3,32,33] as well as HLA-matched platelet components from unrelated or related individuals.[47,48] As with red cells, apheresis platelets or platelets that have undergone leukocyte reduction by filtration have reduced leukocyte content. However, because the minimum number of T cells that causes TA-GVHD has not been determined, these components should be irradiated if intended for at-risk recipients.

Fresh plasma (never been frozen) should be irradiated because this component contains significant numbers of viable T cells. In contrast, Fresh Frozen Plasma does not need to be irradiated, because it is generally accepted that T cells cannot survive the

Table 7-2. Blood Components and Irradiation

All blood components (whole-blood-derived or apheresis) that might contain viable T cells should be irradiated.

- Whole blood
- Red cells (regardless of anticoagulant-preservative)
- Red cells that were frozen previously
- Platelets
- Leukocyte-reduced red cells and platelets
- Fresh plasma (non-frozen)

Components unlikely to require irradiation:

- Fresh Frozen Plasma
- Frozen Plasma
- Cryoprecipitated AHF
- Solvent/detergent-treated plasma

freezing and thawing process. However, there have been reports[49,50] suggesting that immunocompetent progenitor cells may survive the process. Therefore, some have suggested that frozen/thawed plasma may need to be irradiated.[49,50]

Dose of Radiation

Until the 1990s, no standards on the dose of radiation existed, and facilities reported using anywhere from 1500 cGy to 5000 cGy.[51] As advances in technology were made 2500 cGy was demonstrated to be the optimal dose.[52,53] The FDA has recommended that the irradiation process should deliver 2500 cGy to the internal midplane of a freestanding irradiation canister, with 1500 cGy at any other point in the canister.[37] Clonogenic T-cell inactivation can be assessed via limiting dilution analysis. With this method, there is complete inhibition of activity after a dose of 2500 cGy; with 1500 cGy, T-cell proliferation is reduced by 4 logs, but some growth is still observed.[52,53] In a study that assessed T-cell inactivation using mixed lymphocyte culture (a less sensitive assay than limiting dilution analysis) recommended a dose of 2800 to 3000 cGy.[54]

Dose Mapping

Dose mapping is the primary means of ensuring that the intended dose of radiation is being delivered to the component. It measures radiation delivery to a simulated blood component or "phantom" placed either in the canister of a freestanding irradiator or on the irradiation field of a linear accelerator. Dose mapping also measures the variation of the dose to the simulated component, thus allowing conclusions to be drawn about the minimum and maximum doses being delivered. Dose mapping should be performed with sensitive dosimetry techniques at least annually and after major repairs, especially to a turntable.

Dose Mapping with Freestanding Irradiators

For freestanding irradiators, dose mapping involves placement of dosimetry material within a canister that is filled with a simulated blood product—usually water or polystyrene.[55,56] Studies have shown that the absorbed dose at the central midplane of a canister decreased from 3100 to 2500 cGy (approximately 25%) in a ^{137}Cs irradiator (JL Shepherd and Associates, San Francisco, CA) when the canister was changed from empty (0% fill) to full (100% fill).[57] A linear relationship existed between the amount of fill and the measured dose at the central midplane; minimum and maximum levels were influenced in the same manner. Other studies have demonstrated that the variability in dose delivery is dependent on the model of a ^{137}Cs freestanding irradiator.[58,59] It has also been shown that a spacer placed in the bottom of the canister increased the minimum level of radiation in the simulated blood units.[59]

Attenuation of the radiation dose changes as the radiation passes from air to liquid. In a fully loaded canister, attenuation increases as the radiation reaches the central midplane. Thus, the edges of the canister receive a greater dose compared with the center point. In general, the attenuation with ^{60}Co is less than with ^{137}Cs.

The distributor of a freestanding irradiator provides a central dose level that has been determined in a blood-compatible environment (ie, the canister was fully loaded with a simulated blood component). However, in the 1970s and 1980s, some manufacturers provided a dose level that was determined in an unloaded canister, resulting in timer settings that did not provide an adequate dose. Therefore, on older equipment it may be necessary to adjust the irradiation times so that the attenuation effect can be taken into consideration.

Dosimetry Systems for Freestanding Irradiators

Three main types of dosimetry measurement systems are available. These routine dosimeters are calibrated against national standards, such as those provided by the National Institute of Standards and Technology (NIST). One type of routine dosimeter is a thermoluminescent dosimeter (TLD) chip, a small plastic chip with a crystal lattice that absorbs ionizing radiation. Specialized equipment is used to release the energy and measure its absorption by the TLD chip. The timer setting for the test is the same as that for routine use of the instrument.

The use of radiochromic film provides a second type of dosimetry measurement. The film darkens on exposure to radiation in linear proportion to the dose of radiation. The film is then compared with a standard film irradiated at a given dose from a calibrated source, such as NIST. In one such system (International Specialty Products, Wayne, NJ), the film is contained in a watertight casement, which is placed in a canister that is then filled completely with water. This method provides a direct readout of the delivered dose. The timer setting is the same as that used routinely for component irradiation. In a second system (Nordion International, Kanata, Ontario), a film with different radiation-sensitive characteristics is "sandwiched" between two halves of a circular polystyrene phantom component. Irradiation is then performed at several different timer settings, each of which is greater than that used routinely. The dose map produced is then normalized for a central midplane dose of 2500 cGy.

The third approach to dose mapping uses a solid-state electronic dosimeter that absorbs and stores the radiation electronically. A small number of transistors are arranged on a circuit board, which is placed between two halves of a circular polystyrene phantom that fits in the canister. The radiation causes holes in the metal-oxide layer of the circuit board, and the magnitude of the holes is evaluated by measuring voltage across the transistors. The voltages are converted to absorbed dose.

All of these dose mapping systems are associated with a degree of uncertainty or error, usually ±5% of the measured value. Thus, a measured value of 2400 cGy could be as low as 2380 cGy or as high as 2520 cGy. A measured value of 2500 cGy could be as low as 2432 cGy or as high as 2788 cGy.

Dose Mapping with Linear Accelerators

Irradiation of blood components with x-rays involves different instrument settings than those used to treat oncology patients. Because the settings are changed frequently, periodic quality control (QC) measures to assess the dose delivery to blood components are necessary. However, there are no commercially available systems for testing these instruments for use with blood components. Some facilities make their own phantom components for testing purposes.

The dose delivered to the irradiation field should be mapped with use of an ionization chamber, which is used for calibrating linear accelerators for patient use. In addition, annual dose mapping should be performed with a tissue-compatible phantom. To ensure that the instrument is being set in a consistent manner, other parameters should be evaluated on at least a quarterly basis.

- The distance between the x-ray source and the position where the blood components are to be placed. This can easily be measured with a calibrated measuring device.
- The consistency of the x-ray beam. This can be evaluated by measuring the beam current.
- The intensity of the x-ray beam. This can be evaluated by measuring the ionization current in a monitoring ionization chamber, where the number of photons delivered per square centimeter is recorded.

These parameters should be assessed routinely as part of the QC performed by radiation physicists. The Radiation Therapy Committee of the American Association of Physicists in Medicine had established guidelines for QC of linear accelerators.[60,61]

Other Quality Measures

In addition to dose mapping, other quality measures are recommended for freestanding irradiators. It is important to correct for the decay of the radiation source by periodically lengthening the time for irradiation. The half-life of ^{137}Cs is 30 years, so the timer setting should be increased annually. ^{60}Co has a half-life of 5 years, so timer settings need to be adjusted quarterly. The number of seconds of irradiation that need to be added can be determined with calculations that are available in any physics textbook. Some equipment distributors provide a chart that specifies the correct setting after passage of specific time intervals.

For irradiators with turntables, it is essential that the turntable operate at a constant speed in a circular pattern. Verification of turntable rotation should be performed daily. On some irradiator models, rotation of the turntable can be checked with the door of the compartment open. On other models, observation must be done indirectly by ensuring that an indicator light is operating properly. Proper turntable rotation on some models can also be verified by dose mapping (ie, a comparison of readings at two opposite sides of the turntable—one close to the radiation source and one on the far side).

With any source of radiation, a protective lead shield is used to prevent radioactivity from leaking. While this makes the instrument very safe to operate, periodic (at least semiannual) measurements are recommended to ensure that no leakage develops. Three methods for detecting leakage of radioactivity are in use: 1) using a Geiger counter, 2) attaching a film badge to the exterior of the irradiator, and 3) performing a wipe test (on the inside of the chamber in models that use a canister). Table 7-3 summarizes the QC intervals for irradiation equipment.

Table 7-3. Quality Control Intervals for Irradiators

Procedure	Interval
Dose mapping (freestanding irradiators)	
• ^{137}Cs	Once per year and after major repairs; using a fully filled canister with a dosimetry system to map the distribution of the absorbed dose
• ^{60}Co	Once per year and after major repairs; using a fully filled canister with a dosimetry system to map the distribution of the absorbed dose
Dose mapping (linear accelerators)	Once per year with an ionization chamber and a water phantom; more frequent evaluation of instrument conditions to ensure consistency of x-rays
Correction for radioisotopic decay	
• ^{137}Cs	Once per year
• ^{60}Co	Quarterly
Turntable rotation	Daily

Confirmation of Irradiation

It is important to have positive confirmation that the irradiation process has taken place. This evaluation will identify instrument malfunctions or operator errors that prevent irradiation. A radiation-sensitive indicator label has been developed (International Specialty Products) that is placed on the surface of the blood bag. After irradiation, the label appearance changes from clear to opaque, with obliteration of the word "NOT" in a message that reads "This unit has ___ been irradiated." The reliability of this indicator method has been documented.[62]

Two versions of this label exist, with different ranges of radiation needed to cause the film to become opaque. One version is rated for 1500 cGy, and the other is rated for 2500 cGy. Many facilities use the 1500 cGy-rated label as the most appropriate measure. On the basis of routine patterns of dose distribution in the canister of a freestanding irradiator, it can be determined that there will be spots at which the dose will be less than 2500 cGy. If the film in a 2500 cGy-rated label is located precisely at such a spot, the unit might be judged as not having been irradiated, when in fact it was. The 2500 cGy-rated label works well for linear accelerators, because the x-ray beams in these devices are more homogeneous.

Storage of Irradiated Components

Red Cells

The 24-hour recovery of irradiated red cells is reduced during storage when compared with the in-vivo viability of non-irradiated red cells.[49,50,63-65] Thus, the maximum storage time for irradiated red cells has been an issue.

Table 7-4 summarizes investigations into 24-hour recovery of red cells that have been irradiated. Most studies confirm that irradiation does reduce 24-hour recovery. The four-protocol study by Moroff et al[67] is unique because the red cells were studied after irradiation at different times during storage. In two of the protocols, the mean (±SD) 24-hour recoveries were comparable. Red cell survival in irradiated vs control red cells were comparable in all four protocols, demonstrating that despite the impact on 24-hour recovery, the long-term survival is minimally affected. While the length of storage after irradiation had a significant effect on 24-hour recovery, no effects were observed with the day of irradiation of the total storage time.

Another study[68] confirmed that adenosine triphosphate levels and the amount of hemolysis were only minimally influenced by extended storage after irradiation. There does not seem to be a correlation between irradiation and potassium leakage, as was once believed. The FDA irradiation guidelines mandate a 28-day limit for storage of red cells after irradiation. However, no re-

Table 7-4. Effect of Irradiation on 24-Hour Red Cell Recovery

Investigator	Dose (cGy)	Day of Irrad.	Length of Storage (days)	24-Hour Recovery, Mean±SD (%)	
				Irrad. RBCs	Control RBCs
Davey et al[63]	3000	0	42*	68.5±8.1	78.4±7.1
Mintz et al[64]	3000	0 or 1	35*	78.0±6.8	81.8±4.4
Friedman et al[66]	2000	1	21†	82.7	90.4
Friedman et al[66]	2000	1	28†	80.7	85.0
Moroff[67]					
Protocol 1	2500	1	1-28*	78.6±5.9	84.2±5.0
Protocol 2	2500	14	14-28*	82.3±5.6	85.2±2.3
Protocol 3	2500	14	14-42*	69.5±8.6	76.3±7.0
Protocol 4	2500	26	26-28*	81.7±6.0	82.2±4.2

*Adsol

†Nutricel

strictions are made as to when during storage the irradiation may occur. Total storage time cannot exceed that for the nonirradiated component.

Irradiation followed by storage with subsequent potassium leakage may be an issue for neonatal and pediatric practice. While the doses of potassium in small-volume (5 to 15 mL/kg) transfusion may be small, high concentrations (55 to 100 mEq/L) administered during surgery or large-volume transfusion can cause fatal cardiac arrythmias. In these settings, RBC units should be irradiated at issue or washed to ensure that hyperkalemia does not complicate the patient's clinical course, especially in those patients with complex heart disease.[69]

Platelets

In contrast to red cells, platelet properties are not changed to any extent by the irradiation process. Regardless of whether irradiation is performed before or during storage, platelet properties are retained.[68,70-75] One study has reported some differences in selected in-vitro parameters when irradiated platelets and nonirradiated controls were compared after storage.[76] On the basis of the majority of available data, however, the storage period for irradiated platelets does not need to be modified. The original expiration date (24 hours to 5 days, depending on the collection system) is retained.

New Methods to Prevent TA-GVHD

Photochemical treatment (PCT) with psoralens such as S-59 and ultraviolet A (UVA) irradiation has been used to inactivate bacteria and viruses that may contaminate platelet units. PCT is also being investigated for possible inactivation of leukocytes in platelets.

PCT inactivation of T cells has been evaluated with four different assay systems: 1) T-cell quantitation, 2) inhibition of cytokine synthesis, 3) modification of leukocyte genomic DNA by quantification of psoralen-DNA adducts, and 4) inhibition of T-cell replication using polymerase chain reaction amplification of genomic DNA sequences. Detailed studies have compared the respective abilities of PCT and 2500 cGy irradiation to inactivate T cells and prevent TA-GVHD in murine models.[32,77,78] As this line of investigation continues, PCT may one day prove to be an alternative to irradiation and provide bacterial and virus inactivation, as well as T-cell inactivation, while preserving red cell integrity and function.

References

1. von Fliedner V, Higby DJ, Kim U. Graft-versus-host reaction following blood product transfusion. Am J Med 1972;72:951-61.
2. McMilan KD, Johnson RL. HLA-homozygosity and the risk of related-donor transfusion-associated graft-versus-host disease. Transfus Med Rev 1993;7:37-41.
3. Petz LD, Calhoun L, Yam P, et al. Transfusion-associated graft-versus-host disease in immunocompetent patients. Report of a fatal case associated with transfusion of blood from a second-degree relative, and a survey of predisposing factors. Transfusion 1993;33:742-50.
4. Ferrera JM, Krenger W. Graft-versus-host disease. The influence of type 1 and type 2 T cell cytokines. Transfus Med Rev 1998;12:1-17.
5. Worrall NK, Lazenby WD, Misko TP, et al. Modulation of in vivo alloreactivity by inhibition of inducible nitric oxide synthetase. J Exp Med 1995;181:63-70.
6. Fast LD, Valeri CR, Crowley JP. Immune responses to major histocompatibility complex homozygous lymphoid cells in murine F1 hybrid recipients: Implications for transfusion-associated graft-versus-host disease. Blood 1995;86:3090-6.
7. Nishimura M, Uchida S, Mitsunaga S, et al. Characterization of T-cell clones derived from peripheral blood lymphocytes of a patient with transfusion-associated graft versus-host disease: Fas-mediated killing by CD4+ and CD8+ cytotoxic T-cell clones and tumor necrosis factor beta production by CD4+ T-cell clones. Blood 1997;89:1440-5.
8. Ammann AJ. Hypothesis: Absence of graft-versus-host disease in AIDS is a consequence of HIV-1 infection of CD4+ T cells. J Acquir Immune Defic Syndr 1993;6:122-7.
9. Brubaker DB. Immunopathogenic mechanisms of post-transfusion graft versus host disease. Proc Soc Exp Biol Med 1993;202:122-47.
10. Blundell EL, Pamphilon DH, Anderson NA, et al. Transfusion-associated graft-versus-host disease, monoclonal gammopathy and PCR. Br J Haematol 1992;82:622-3.
11. Capon SM, DePond WD, Tyan DB, et al. Transfusion associated graft-versus-host disease in an immunocompetent patient. Ann Intern Med 1991;114:1025-6.

12. Drobyski W, Thibodeau S, Truitt RL, et al. Third-party-mediated graft rejection and graft-versus-host disease after T-cell-depleted bone marrow transplantation, as demonstrated by hypervariable DNA probes and HLA-DR polymorphism. Blood 1989;74:2285-94.
13. Kunstmann E, Bocker T, Roewer L, et al. Diagnosis of transfusion-associated graft-versus-host disease by genetic fingerprinting and polymerase chain reaction. Transfusion 1992;32:766-70.
14. Depalma L, Bahrami KR, Kapur S, et al. Amplified fragment length polymorphism analysis in the evaluation of post-transfusion graft versus host disease. J Thorac Cardiovasc Surg 1994;108:182-4.
15. Wang L, Juji T, Tokunaga K, et al. Polymorphic microsatellite markers for the diagnosis of graft-versus-host disease. N Engl J Med 1994;330: 398-401.
16. Friedman DF, Kwittken P, Cizman B, et al. DNA-based HLA typing of nonhematopoietic tissue used to select the marrow transplant donor for successful treatment of transfusion-associated graft-versus-host disease. Clin Diagn Lab Immunol 1994;1:590-6.
17. Lee TH, Donegan E, Slichter S, Busch MP. Transient increase in circulating donor leukocytes after allogeneic transfusions in immunocompetent recipients compatible with donor cell proliferation. Blood 1996;85: 1207-14.
18. Lee TH, Paglieroni T, Ohto H, et al. Survival of donor leukocyte subpopulations in immunocompetent transfusion recipients: Frequent long term microchimerism in severe trauma patients. Blood 1999; 93:3127-39.
19. Wang-Rodriguez J, Fry E, Fiebig E, et al. Immune response to blood transfusion in very-low birthweight infants. Transfusion 2000;40:25-34.
20. Vietor HE, Hallensleben E, van Bree SP, et al. Survival of donor cells 25 years after intrauterine transfusion. Blood 2000;95:2709-14.
21. Reed WF, Lee TH, Trachlenberg E, et al. Detection of microchimerism by PCR as a function of amplification strategy. Transfusion 2001;41:39-44.
22. Nelson J, Furst D, Maloney S, et al. Microchimerism and HLA compatible relationships of pregnancy in scleroderma. Lancet 1998;351:559-62.
23. Arlett CM, Smith JB, Jimenez SA. Identification of fetal DNA and cells in skin lesions from women with systemic sclerosis. N Engl J Med 1998; 333:1186-91.
24. Evans PC, Lambert N, Maloney S, et al. Long-term fetal microchimerism in peripheral blood mononuclear cell subsets in healthy women and women with scleroderma. Blood 1999;93:2033-7.
25. Daya S, Gunby J, Clark DA. Intravenous immunoglobulin therapy for recurrent spontaneous abortion: A meta-analysis. Am J Reprod Immunol 1998;39:69-76.
26. Strauss RG. Data-driven blood banking practices for neonatal RBC transfusions. Transfusion 2000;40:1528-40.

27. Klein C, Fraitag S, Foulon E, et al. Moderate and transient transfusion-associated cutaneous graft-versus-host disease in a child infected by human immunodeficiency virus. Am J Med 1996;101:445-6.
28. Luban NLC, DePalma L. Transfusion-associated graft-versus host disease in the neonate—expanding the spectrum of disease (editorial). Transfusion 1996;36:101-3.
29. Ohto H, Anderson KC. Posttransfusion graft-versus-host disease in Japanese newborns. Transfusion 1996;36:117-23.
30. Ohto H, Anderson KC. Survey of transfusion-associated graft-versus-host disease in immunocompetent recipients. Transfus Med Rev 1996;10: 31-43.
31. Webb IJ, Anderson KC. Transfusion-associated graft-versus-host disease. In: Anderson KC, Ness PM, eds. Scientific basis of transfusion medicine, second ed. Philadelphia, PA: WB Saunders, 2000:420-5.
32. Williamson LM, Warwick RM. Transfusion-associated graft-versus-host disease and its prevention. Blood Rev 1995;9:251-61.
33. Kanter MH. Transfusion-associated graft-versus-host disease: Do transfusions from second-degree relatives pose a greater risk than those from first-degree relatives? Transfusion 1992;32:323-7.
34. Murad KL, Gosselin EJ, Eaton JW, et al. Stealth cells: Prevention of major histocompatibility complex class II-mediated T-cell activation by cell surface modification. Blood 1999;94:2135-41.
35. Capon SM, Sacher RA, Deeg HJ. Effective ultraviolet irradiation of platelet concentrates in Teflon bags. Transfusion 1990;30:678-81.
36. Anderson KC, Weinstein HJ. Transfusion-associated graft-versus-host disease. N Engl J Med 1990;323:315-21.
37. Food and Drug Administration. Memorandum: Recommendations regarding license amendments and procedures for gamma irradiation of blood products. (July 22, 1993) Rockville, MD: CBER Office of Communication, Training, and Manufacturers Assistance, 1993.
38. Shlomchik WD, Couzens MS, Tang CB, et al. Prevention of graft versus host disease by inactivation of host antigen-presenting cells. Science 1999;285:412-5.
39. Davey RJ. The effect of irradiation on blood components. In: Baldwin ML, Jefferies LC, eds. Irradiation of blood components. Bethesda, MD: American Association of Blood Banks, 1992:51-62.
40. Gammon RR, Prichard A, Kirk R, et al. In house x-ray irradiation of blood components, a community blood center's experience (abstract). Transfusion 2000;40(Suppl):66S.
41. Gurney NL. A simple and effective implementation of an x-ray source blood component irradiator (abstract). Transfusion 2000;40(Suppl): 154S.
42. Dinwiddie SC, Yadock W, Johnson DO, et al. X-ray radiation as an alternative to gamma radiation for irradiation of blood components (abstract). Transfusion 2000:40(Suppl):157S-158S.

43. Suda BA, Leitman SF, Davey RJ. Characteristics of red cells irradiated and subsequently frozen for long-term storage. Transfusion 1993;33:389-92.
44. Miraglia CC, Anderson G, Mintz PD. Effect of freezing on the in vivo recovery of irradiated red cells. Transfusion 1994;34:775-8.
45. Crowley JP, Skrabut EM, Valeri CR. Immunocompetent lymphocytes in previously frozen washed red cells. Vox Sang 1974;26:513-17.
46. Anderson KC. Leukodepleted cellular blood components for prevention of transfusion-associated graft-versus-host disease. Transfus Sci 1995; 16:265-8.
47. Benson K, Marks AR, Marshall MJ, et al. Fatal graft-versus-host disease associated with transfusions of HLA-matched, HLA-homozygous platelets from unrelated donors. Transfusion 1994;34:432-7.
48. Grishaber JE, Birney SM, Strauss RG. Potential for transfusion-associated graft-versus-host disease due to apheresis platelets matched for HLA class I antigens. Transfusion 1993;33:910-14.
49. Wielding JU, Vehmeyer K, Dittman J, et al. Contamination of fresh-frozen plasma with viable white cells and proliferable stem cells (letter). Transfusion 1994;34:185-6.
50. Bernvill SS, Abdulatiff M, Al-Sedairy S, et al. Fresh frozen plasma contains viable progenitor Cells—should we irradiate? (letter) Vox Sang 1994;67:405.
51. Anderson KC, Goodnough LT, Sayers M, et al. Variation in blood component irradiation practice: Implications for prevention of transfusion-associated graft-versus-host disease. Blood 1991;77:2096-102.
52. Pelszynski MM, Moroff G, Luban NLC, et al. Effect of gamma irradiation of red blood cell units on T-cell inactivation as assessed by limiting dilution analysis: Implications for preventing transfusion-associated graft-versus-host disease. Blood 1994;83:1683-9.
53. Luban NLC, Drothler D, Moroff G, et al. Irradiation of platelet components: Inhibition of lymphocyte proliferation assessed by limiting dilution analysis. Transfusion 2000;40:348-52.
54. Rosen NR, Weidner JG, Bold HD, et al. Prevention of transfusion-associated graft-versus-host disease: Selection of an adequate dose of gamma irradiation. Transfusion 1993;33:125-7.
55. Masterson ME, Febo R. Pretransfusion blood irradiation: Clinical rationale and dosimetric considerations. Med Phys 1992;19:649-57.
56. Leitman SF. Dose, dosimetry, and quality improvements of irradiated blood components (editorial). Transfusion 1993;33:447-9.
57. Perkins JT, Papoulias SA. The effect of loading conditions on dose distribution within a blood irradiator (abstract). Transfusion 1994;34(Suppl): 75S.
58. Moroff G, Luban NLC, Wolf L, et al. Dosimetry measurements after gamma irradiation with cesium-137 and linear acceleration sources (abstract). Transfusion 1993;33(Suppl):52S.

59. Luban NLC, Fearon T, Leitman SF, et al. Absorption of gamma irradiation in simulated blood components using cesium irradiators (abstract). Transfusion 1995;35(Suppl):63S.
60. Kutcher GJ, Coia L, Gillin M, et al. Comprehensive QA for radiation oncology: Report of AAPM Radiation Therapy Committee Task Group 40. Med Phys 1994;21:581-618.
61. Nath R, Biggs PJ, Bova FJ, et al. AAPM code of practice for radiotherapy accelerators: Report of AAPM Radiation Therapy Committee Task Group 45. Med Phys 1994;21:1093-121.
62. Leitman SF, Silberstein L, Fairman RM, et al. Use of a radiation-sensitive film label in the quality control of irradiated blood components (abstract). Transfusion 1992;32(Suppl):4S.
63. Davey RJ, McCoy NC, Yu M, et al. The effect of pre-storage irradiation on post-transfusion red cell survival. Transfusion 1992;32:525-8.
64. Mintz PD, Anderson G. Effect of gamma irradiation on the in vivo recovery of stored red blood cells. Ann Clin Lab Sci 1993;23:216-20.
65. Moroff G, Holme S, Heaton A, et al. Effect of gamma irradiation on viability of AS-1 red cells (abstract). Transfusion 1992;32(Suppl):70S.
66. Friedman KD, McDonough WC, Cimino DF. The effect of pre-storage gamma irradiation on post-transfusion red blood cell recovery (abstract). Transfusion 1991;31(Suppl):50S.
67. Moroff G, Holme S, AuBuchon JP, et al. Viability and in vitro properties of AS-1 red cells after gamma irradiation. Transfusion 1999;39:128-34.
68. Moroff G, George VM, Siegl AM, et al. The influence of irradiation on stored platelets. Transfusion 1986;26:453-6.
69. Brown KA, Bissonnette B, McIntyre B. Hyperkaelemia during rapid blood transfusion and hypovolaemic cardiac arrest in children. Can J Anaesth 1990;37:747-54.
70. Espersen GT, Ernst E, Christiansen OB, et al. Irradiated blood platelet concentrates stored for five days—evaluation by in vitro tests. Vox Sang 1988;55:218-21.
71. Duguid JK, Carr R, Jenkins JA, et al. Clinical evaluation of the effects of storage time and irradiation on transfused platelets. Vox Sang 1991; 60:151-4.
72. Read EJ, Kodis C, Carter CS, et al. Viability of platelets following storage in the irradiated state. A paired-controlled study. Transfusion 1988; 28:446-50.
73. Rock G, Adams GA, Labow RS. The effects of irradiation on platelet function. Transfusion 1988;28:451-5.
74. Sweeney JD, Holme S, Moroff G. Storage of apheresis platelets after gamma irradiation. Transfusion 1994;34:779-83.
75. Seghatchian MJ, Stivala JFA. Effect of 25 Gy gamma irradiation on storage stability of three types of platelet concentrates: A comparative analysis with paired controls and random preparation. Transfus Sci 1995; 16:121-9.

76. Bessos H, Atkinson A, Murphy WG, et al. A comparison of in vitro storage markers between gamma-irradiated and non-irradiated apheresis platelet concentrates. Transfus Sci 1995;16:131-4.
77. Grass JA, Hei DJ, Metchette K, et al. Inactivation of leukocytes in platelet concentrates by psoralen plus UVA. Blood 1998;91:2180-8.
78. Grass J, Delmonte J, Wages D, et al. Prevention of transfusion-associated graft vs. host disease (TA-GVHD) in immunocompromised mice by photochemical treatment (PCT) of donor T cells (abstract). Blood 1997;90 (Suppl 1):207a.

In: Herman JH, Manno CS, eds.
Pediatric Transfusion Therapy
Bethesda, MD: AABB Press, 2002

8

Cytomegalovirus Safety Issues in Neonatal Transfusion

PATRICIA T. PISCIOTTO, MD

CYTOMEGALOVIRUS (CMV) IS A UBIQUITOUS DNA-containing herpesvirus that in a normal individual is rarely associated with disease. CMV infection is identified by seroconversion or virus isolation, whereas CMV disease is identified by laboratory evidence of infection plus specific symptoms associated with the virus. In a small proportion of immunocompetent infected individuals, a mononucleosis-like syndrome consisting of fever, malaise, myalgia, liver dysfunction, and heterophile antibody-negative lymphocytosis can occur several weeks after exposure. In seronegative immunocompromised individuals CMV can cause significant morbidity and mortality.

Patricia T. Pisciotto, MD, Professor, Department of Laboratory Medicine, University of Connecticut Health Center, Farmington, Connecticut

As with other members of the herpesvirus group, CMV has the ability to cause a primary infection, remain latent in host tissue, and subsequently undergo reactivation. Primary infection occurs in seronegative individuals and is characterized by viremia, viruria, and measurable levels of antibody, IgM-specific followed by IgG-specific, to CMV. During the latency period, viruria is usually undetectable, but IgG titers persist and are readily detectable for the life of the host. If reactivation occurs there is a recurrence of virus shedding with either minimal or no increase in IgM, but an accompanied fourfold or greater increase in CMV IgG titer, representing an anamnestic response. Occasionally, virus shedding may occur without an increase in IgM or IgG. A third pattern of infection can occur in a seropositive individual, and represents a re-infection or co-infection to a strain of CMV different from the strain causing the original infection. In this setting, virus shedding as well as an IgM and IgG antibody response would be expected. The frequency of this occurrence is difficult to determine.

Transmission of CMV through blood transfusion has been recognized since the mid-1960s.[1] Direct evidence that blood transfusion transmits CMV infection occurred approximately 20 years later by demonstrating an identical restriction endonuclease pattern of DNA from CMV isolates from a blood donor and an infected neonate who received blood from the donor.[2] It is thought that latently infected mononuclear cells are the major vector of CMV transmission, although cell-free virus may also figure in transfusion-transmitted infection.[3] There are several factors that are believed to play a role in the pathogenesis of transfusion-associated CMV (TA-CMV) infection including: the volume of CMV-seropositive blood and, therefore, latently infected leukocytes; CMV reactivation from a latent state; and survival of infected donor cells for a sufficient amount of time to allow production of infectious CMV. Therefore, recipient factors as well as donor factors influence the risk of TA-CMV infection.

Congenital CMV Infection

Cytomegalovirus is one of the most common causes of congenital and perinatal infections in humans. The prevalence of congenital CMV infection ranges from 0.2% to greater than 3% among different populations.[4] It can be transmitted from mother to fetus even if the mother is not experiencing a primary infection. However, there is a greater risk of transmission (24% to 75% risk of vertical transmission) to the fetus if a pregnant woman experiences a primary infection. The infection and sequelae are more serious if the infection occurs during the first half of the pregnancy.[5] The presence of maternal antibody to CMV does not prevent transmission to the fetus, although the risk of fetal injury has been reported to be markedly reduced.[6] The majority of infected infants are asymptomatic at birth despite the occurrence of virus shedding. A follow-up study of 189 infants with congenital CMV infection showed that only infants born to mothers with primary infection were symptomatic at birth.[6] Twenty-four of 132 infants (18%) born to mothers with primary infection were symptomatic vs none of 65 infants whose mothers had recurrent infection. In long-term follow-up (approximately 4.7 years) it was found that over 25% of the children born to the mothers with primary infection showed one or more sequelae vs 8% of the children born to mothers with recurrent infection. The primary-infection group had more neurologic sequelae and no child in the recurrent-infection group had multiple sequelae. It was concluded that the presence of maternal antibody to CMV before conception provided substantial protection against damaging congenital CMV infection.

Congenital CMV disease has a broad spectrum of clinical manifestations resulting from widespread viral growth in the fetus before the immune system has had the time to develop. The more common clinical manifestations include intrauterine growth retardation, microcephaly, ventriculomegaly, intracranial calcifications, chorioretinitis, microphthalmia, hepatosplenomegaly, jaundice, petechia, purpura, and thrombocytopenia. Pneumonitis is not usually a part of the clinical presentation of congenital CMV infection but is more likely to occur in infants with perinatal CMV infection.[4] Severely affected infants have a mortality rate of approximately 30% with a high percentage of those surviving also showing severe complications.[4,5] Growing evidence has shown that a percentage of infants (5% to 15%) with subclinical or asymptomatic infection may develop long-term sequelae, the most common being sensorineural hearing deficits manifesting within the first 2 years of life as well as learning disabilities.[4,5]

Acquisition of primary CMV infection in both mother and infant has been associated with the use of blood from seropositive donors for intrauterine transfusion.[7] Few data exist, however, relating the risk of acquiring CMV infection from transfusion during pregnancy. In one prospective study of TA-CMV in 162 pregnant women who received a total of 450 cellular blood components, there was no evidence of CMV infection in the first 3 months after the transfusion. Most of the transfusions were given postpartum. It was estimated that the risk of CMV infection per unit of cellular components in a pregnant woman was less than 0.22%.[8] Because the development of a primary CMV infection during pregnancy carries such a high risk to the fetus, it has been recommended that CMV-reduced-risk blood components should be given to seronegative pregnant women requiring antenatal or intrauterine blood transfusion.[8,9] Based on epidemiologic studies in which viral DNA was analyzed by restriction enzyme techniques, endogenous CMV was more likely than reinfection to be a source of recurrent infection and intrauterine transmission in immune pregnant women.[10] Therefore, there has been no recommendation to provide CMV-reduced-risk blood to CMV-seropositive pregnant women.

Perinatal CMV Infection

Perinatal CMV infection is more prevalent than congenital infection and occurs as a result of exposure to infected maternal genital secretion at the time of vaginal delivery,[11] ingestion of infected breast milk during the postnatal period,[12-14] or receipt of blood transfusions.[15,16] The incubation period for perinatal CMV infection ranges from 4 to 12 weeks. CMV infection has been reported to occur in 40% to 65% of infants who are breast-fed by seropositive mothers and up to 40% of infants born to mothers excreting CMV in cervical secretions near delivery.[4,5,14] In the United States, on the basis of 1) the rate of seropositive mothers,

2) the prevalence of CMV excretion in the genital tract at delivery, and 3) the prevalence of breast feeding, it has been estimated that approximately 1% to 15% of infants become perinatally infected by 6 months of age.[4] The majority of full-term infants who are born to seropositive mothers and who develop perinatal CMV infection, remain asymptomatic. However, there have been reports of CMV disease being associated with protracted interstitial pneumonitis in full-term infants[17] as well as in premature infants.[18] Pneumonitis is the most common presentation for perinatally acquired CMV, which can result in rapid deterioration and death in up to 10% of the cases.[5]

Symptomatic CMV infection has been reported in premature infants who acquired CMV from a maternal source. Eighteen of 106 (17%) infants of seropositive mothers, with birthweights less than 1500 g (very low birthweight or VLBW infants) who received only RBCs from seronegative donors, acquired CMV infection. None of these infants were breast-fed; all infants received banked human milk that was either pasteurized or frozen and thawed twice. Six of the infants developed symptoms consisting of combinations of hepatosplenomegaly, thrombocytopenia, neutropenia, a relative lymphocytosis, and pulmonary morbidity.[19] The latter was associated with early excretion of CMV (less than 7 weeks of age). Five of the six symptomatic infants began excreting CMV between 4 and 6 weeks of age and one began after 6 weeks. In this prospective study there were no fatalities associated with CMV disease. The authors postulated that loss of passively acquired antibody to CMV through catabolism and iatrogenic blood loss might predispose premature infants to a higher incidence of symptomatic CMV than expected in term infants. IgG levels in infants reflect maternal transfer of antibody. The amount of measurable IgG is directly proportional to gestational age and is lower in the second and early third trimester than at term.[20] The gestational age of these VLBW infants would correlate with the period during which maternally derived IgG would be at a lower concentration. In one study[19] maternal CMV antibody levels in these premature infants fell drastically by 4 to 6 weeks after delivery and was undetectable in 32% of the premature infants studied by 7 to 9 weeks of age. Five of the six infants with symptomatic CMV had lost maternal antibody at the time of CMV shedding, supporting the belief that maternal CMV antibody may modify the course of CMV disease.

Transfusion-Associated CMV Infection in Seronegative Infants

Cytomegalovirus as a posttransfusion complication in neonates was first suggested in the late 1960s when infants of unknown serologic status who had undergone exchange transfusion for Rh incompatibility developed symptomatic CMV infection associated with fever, respiratory distress, hepatosplenomegaly, and CMV viruria within 2 months of transfusion.[21] The first study establishing the link between exchange transfusion and the acquisition of CMV was reported in 1971 by Luthardt and coworkers[22] in a prospective study to assess the incidence of CMV infection in this population of patients. Eight of 15 CMV-seronegative infants, who received blood from CMV-seropositive donors were infected vs none of 20 who received CMV-seronegative blood. Ten years later Yeager reported[23] that 10 of 74 CMV-seronegative infants (13.5%) who received blood from one or more CMV-seropositive donors acquired CMV infection; 0 of 90 infants who received blood only from CMV-seronegative donors developed CMV infection. The risk increased to 24% in infants who required 50 mL or more RBCs and were exposed to at least one CMV antibody-positive donor (10 of 41 infants). None of the 33 infants of seronegative mothers who received less than 50 mL RBCs developed CMV infection, despite being exposed to seropositive blood. Fatal or serious symptoms developed in 50% of the infected infants, all occurring in premature infants weighing less than 1200 g. Adler et al[24] described eight acquired CMV infections in 178 infants hospitalized for more than 1 month and reported similar findings. Seven of these infections occurred in newborns of seronegative mothers. All infants weighed less than 1200 g and were exposed to large numbers of donors, including multiple CMV-seropositive donors. Once again, CMV infection in these infants was associated with high morbidity and mortality.

From these early studies (prior to 1984) the risk factors identified as predisposing to the development of primary symptomatic TA-CMV infection (ie, CMV disease) were premature VLBW infants who were born to seronegative mothers and who received more than 50 mL blood, which included blood from CMV-seropositive donors. There have been case reports, however, of symptomatic TA-CMV acquired in VLBW infants after a single exposure to a relatively small amount of blood from a single seropositive donor, indicating that the infectivity of the unit is also important.[25,26] It has been demonstrated that only a subset of seropositive donors are likely to transmit CMV and has been suggested that recent or actively infected donors who are IgM positive may be responsible for TA-CMV infection.[26]

While there has been no dispute over the relationship between the exposure to CMV-seropositive blood and the development of CMV infection in seronegative VLBW infants, the reported prevalence and severity of TA-CMV infection in premature infants born to seronegative mothers has changed over time. The incidence of infection has ranged from a high of 32% in the early studies to a low of 0% in some of the more recent studies, even when seropositive blood (not processed to decrease the risk of CMV transmission) had been transfused (Table 8-1). In several of the more recent studies, the overall infection rate (rate of seroconversion and/or virus shedding) decreased, and even though morbidity continued to be high in many of these reports, the incidence of fatal infections was greatly reduced. There have been no reported long-term follow-up studies in these neonates to determine whether they suffer from late sequelae of TA-CMV.

The variability in the incidence of CMV infection and disease in these studies is not easily explained because the amount of blood transfused, donor exposure, and prevalence of CMV antibody in the donor populations were similar. Several reasons have been cited for this observed difference.[34,35] It has been postulated that the use of plasma components with the potential of passive administration of CMV antibody, which may have modified infection, could have contributed to observed differences in the rate of infection. Details regarding component use in these various studies, however, are not well documented. Differences

Table 8-1. Cytomegalovirus Infection Rates in Transfused Seronegative Low Birthweight Infants Who Received Seropositive Blood

Reference (Year Reported)	CMV Seroprevalence in Blood Donors (%)	Geographic Location	Patients Infected/ LBW Infants Studied (%)	Morbidity/ LBW Infants Infected (%)	Mortality/ LBW Infants Infected (%)	Population Birthweight (g)
Yeager[23] (1981)	45	Stanford	7/22 (31.8)	5/7 (71)	4/7 (57)	<1200
Adler[24] (1983)	34	Richmond	7/29 (24.0)	3/7 (43)	3/7 (43)	<1250
Smith[27] (1983)	68	Nashville	2/23 (8.7)	2/2 (100)	0/2 (0)	<1250
Rawls[28] (1984)	73	Ontario	1/23 (4.3)	-	0/1 (0)	<2000
Tegtemeier[29] (1985)	59	Kansas	2/29 (6.9)	2/2 (100)	0/2 (0)	<1500
Lamberson[26] (1988)	38	Syracuse	4/83 (4.8)	2/4 (50)	1/4 (25)	<1500
Preiksaitis[30] (1988)	42	Edmonton (Alberta)	1/41 (2.4)	1/1 (100)	0/1 (0)	<1250
Griffin[31] (1989)	47	Durham	0/14 (0.0)	0/0 (0)	0/0 (0)	<1250
Gilbert[25] (1989)	46	Melbourne	9/29 (31.0)	5/9 (57)	0/9 (0)	<1500
Galea[32] (1992)	-	Aberdeen (NE Scotland)	2/46 (4.4)	0/2 (0)	0/2 (0)	<1250
Syndman[33] (1995)	40	Boston	5/98 (5.1)	3/5 (60)	0/5 (0)	<1500

in indications for transfusion early in the course of care for a VLBW infant, which may have resulted in exposure to seropositive blood at a point when the immune system was most immature, may have played a factor. The methods by which blood was distributed in the nurseries, thus determining the volume of seropositive blood transfused as well as the age of the blood transfused, could also have altered the frequency of occurrence. The changes in donor deferral and testing that have taken place since 1983 may also have had an effect on the overall risk. The assays used to measure either IgG-specific or total CMV antibody in these studies varied and comparison of methods have shown difference in sensitivity and specificity.[36] This may also account for some of the differences observed. As a result of these observed differences over time and various geographic locations, the recommendations for the use of CMV-reduced-risk blood components have remained controversial.

There are other groups of term or near-term infants who receive massive transfusions, such as infants undergoing extracorporeal membrane oxygenation (ECMO) or open heart surgery in whom studies to determine the risk of serious CMV infection have not been performed. Based on the birthweight, these infants would not be considered in a high-risk category for symptomatic TA-CMV except that they sometimes have significant transfusion requirements. In the former group, a case of presumptive TA-CMV infection resulting in the death of a full-term infant has been described.[35] The child weighed 2910 g at birth and was born to a seronegative mother at 36 weeks of gestation. He received 47 RBC units, 34 platelet units, 76 plasma units, and 31 cryoprecipitate units prior to death and had evidence of disseminated CMV infection at autopsy. It has been suggested that neonates treated with ECMO may be a subgroup of patients who may benefit from the use of CMV-reduced-risk blood components.[35]

Transfusion and CMV Infection in Infants of Seropositive Mothers

The relative role of blood transfusion vs a maternal source of CMV as the etiology of symptomatic CMV infection in infants born to seropositive mothers is more difficult to discern. Similar rates of infection have been reported in infants of seropositive mothers regardless of whether they received RBC transfusions from CMV seropositive or seronegative donors. In one prospective study nine of 60 infants (15%) exposed to seropositive mothers and CMV-seropositive RBCs became infected vs 23 of 131 (17.6%) infants of seropositive mothers receiving RBCs from seronegative donors. In the latter group, 15% of infants receiving less than 50 mL of blood became infected and 20% of infants receiving more than 50 mL of blood became infected. Unlike the setting with seronegative infants, this indicated that there was no correlation with the volume of blood transfused and development of CMV infection. None of the 32 infected infants had fatal or serious disease, including the six infected infants with birthweights less than 1200 g.[23] Another prospective study that was undertaken to evaluate the role of neonatal blood transfusion and maternal exposure also showed a significant correlation between maternal antibody titers and the rate of CMV infection whether or not transfusion occurred.[28] Twenty-two of 107 infants (20.6%) born to mothers with CMV antibodies were found to be infected vs two of 65 (3.1%) infants born to mothers without CMV antibodies. An even stronger association was found between breast-feeding and CMV infection, accounting for approximately 80% of the perinatally acquired CMV infections observed. In terms of transfusion, 18.8% of the transfused infants were infected with CMV compared with 11.0% of the nontransfused infants, which was not statistically significant.

In a study[31] evaluating blood transfusion and CMV infection in 385 infants, five of 60 seropositive infants with birthweights less than 1250 g acquired CMV. Fifty of these infants, including the five infected infants, received transfusions that included blood from seropositive donors. All breast-fed infants received breast milk that was heat-treated prior to use. Four of the infants had become seronegative at the time of virus excretion; all demonstrated severe morbidity, with one fatality. The one infant who remained seropositive at the time of virus excretion had only minimal symptoms. This finding again supports the idea that passively acquired antibody may have a protective effect and that an infant may become vulnerable to CMV infection as antibody is lost. Virus excretion occurred at 4.5, 5, 6, 8, and 9 weeks of age.[37] The infant who died weighed 540 g at birth and had an initial CMV titer of 1:127. A double-volume exchange transfusion was performed with CMV-seronegative blood at 1 day of age, which would have greatly reduced the antibody titer. At 2 days of age the infant received blood from a seropositive donor and by day 4 developed persistent thrombocytopenia. The infant developed bacteremia with *Staphylococcus epidermidis* and an extensive dermatitis with *Candida*, and expired at 6.5 weeks of age, 1 week after CMV viruria was detected. Because no autopsy was performed, it was difficult to assess the role of CMV in the infant's demise. Two of the infants with symptomatic infection received only deglycerolized RBCs, known to have a decreased risk of CMV transmission. No significant difference in transfusion variables existed among the five infected infants and 39 other LBW seropositive infants who were hospitalized and followed for more than 28 days. Because viral isolates were not obtained from the infants or the mothers for comparison, it was not possible to determine the source of virus in these five infected infants. None of 147 infants of seronegative mothers [including 72 seronegative infants (38 LBW infants) who received either conventional blood (ie, not processed in any way to reduce the risk of CMV transmission) or deglycerolized blood during this same time period (July 1984–August 1985)] developed CMV infection. The overall incidence of acquired CMV infection was very low in this population, despite the use of different preparations of blood.

Another prospective study[38] evaluating acquired CMV infection in a neonatal unit followed 131 infants at 32 weeks of gestation or less for 1 month after delivery. Sixteen of 131 (12.2%) infants acquired CMV infection. Six of 65 (9.2%) seronegative infants who were transfused acquired CMV infection vs 0 of 18 seronegative infants who were not transfused. Nine of 34 (26.5%) seropositive infants who were transfused vs 1 of 14 (7.1%) seropositive infants who were not transfused developed CMV infection. These infants received up to 19 transfusions and were exposed to between zero and seven seropositive donors. All infants, however, were fed with untreated expressed maternal breast milk or breast-fed directly, which also served as a major source of CMV exposure. One infant of a seropositive mother died at 5 months of age from respiratory failure and cor pulmonale secondary to bronchopulmonary dysplasia.[39] At autopsy histologic changes characteristic of CMV infection were noted in several organs. This particular infant weighed 867 g at birth and received a total of 520 mL of blood from 19 donors, seven of whom were seropositive.

Randomized studies suggest that the use of CMV immunoglobulin (CMVIG) prophylaxis may reduce CMV disease and mortality in transplant patients.[40,41] In a multi-center study to evaluate the effect of CMV immunoglobulin on prevention of CMV disease among multitransfused premature neonates,[33] 18 of 171 (10.5%) infants followed for at least 10 days developed CMV infection, with nine symptomatic infections. CMV infection occurred in only 5.1% of seronegative infants (5/98) and 18.3% (13/71) of seropositive infants. Four of the six cases of CMV pneumonitis occurred in infants born to seropositive mothers. In the total population study the use of CMVIG did not reduce the rate of CMV infection, but in the subset of infants born to seropositive mothers only one of 31 (3.2%) infants in the CMVIG group had symptomatic disease vs five of 40 (12.5%) infants in the placebo group (not statistically significant), suggesting that passive antibody may be beneficial in these infants. A multivariate analysis for risk factors demonstrated that the total volume of CMV-seropositive RBCs transfused and birth to a CMV-seropositive mother were independently associated with development of CMV infection.

Prevention of Transfusion-Associated CMV Infections in Neonates

Various approaches have been attempted to reduce and/or eliminate TA-CMV infection in neonates (Table 8-2). The potential utility of screening blood donors for CMV antibody to prevent TA-CMV infection in all patient groups was first shown to be effective in the neonatal population.[22,23] Typically, the assays used

Table 8-2. Methods to Reduce Transfusion-Associated Cytomegalovirus in Seronegative Low Birthweight Neonates

Reference (Year Reported)	CMV Seroprevalence in Blood Donors (%)	Study Type	Methodology	Seroconversion Rate (%)	Population Birthweight (g)
Yeager[23] (1981)	45	Controlled	Unscreened IgG screen	7/22 (31.8) 0/16 (0.0)	<1200
Adler[42] (1984)	34	Historical control	Unscreened IgG screen and deglycerolized RBCs	7/25 (28.0) 0/34 (0.0)	<1250
Brady[43] (1984)	51	Uncontrolled	Deglycerolized RBCs	0/27 (0.0)	<1250
Simon[44] (1987)	58	Historical control	Unscreened Deglycerolized RBCs	2/16 (12.5) 1/26 (3.8)	<1500
Demmler[45] (1986)	51	Uncontrolled	Saline-washed RBCs	2/20 (10.0)	<1250
Luban[46] (1987)	59	Uncontrolled	Saline-washed RBCs	0/22 (0.0)	<1250
Lamberson[26] (1988)	38	Historical control	Unscreened IgM screen	7/222 (3.2) 1/141 (0.7)	Variable weight
Gilbert[25] (1989)	46	Controlled	Unfiltered Filtered	9/29 (31.0) 0/24 (0.0)	<1500

to screen for CMV status detect IgG-specific and/or total CMV antibody. In the United States the seroprevalence varies regionally with a 30% to 40% range in northern United States and a seroprevalence in excess of 65% reported in some southern regions of the United States.[47] The variability within the donor pool can make it very difficult to provide CMV-seronegative units in certain geographic areas. It has been estimated, however, that only a small percentage of these donors are truly infectious for CMV, with the probability of infectivity among blood donors ranging from 0.14% to 12%.[34] Studies have attempted to evaluate IgM CMV-positive donors as a source of truly infective units that are capable of transmitting CMV.[29,48] IgM seropositive rates in blood donors have been reported at 6%, 4%, and less than 1%, which are much less than rates for IgG seropositivity.[29,45,48] Benecke et al[48] found a significant correlation between the receipt of CMV IgM antibody-positive blood components, detected by immunofluorescence technique, and the development of CMV infection in patients undergoing open heart surgery. Lamberson et al[26] in the first of a two-phase study showed that of 222 seronegative infants seven became infected with CMV; all had received blood from at least one IgM-positive donor. The second phase of the study showed that one of 141 seronegative infants who received blood from IgM-negative donors seroconverted. Using a second assay system it was determined that the donor blood given to the infected infant was IgM-positive, again supporting the idea that actively or recently infected donors may be responsible for transmitting CMV to recipients of their blood components. Unfortunately, the positive and negative predictive values of the tests in these studies were too low to support implementation for routine testing.[40]

Breakthrough infections in seronegative patients receiving seronegative components have been reported to occur at rates ranging from 1% to 4% in the allogeneic marrow transplant setting.[40] Similar findings have not been reported in the neonatal population. This most likely represents the window period of infection prior to antibody formation or a point at which the antibody levels are too low to be detected by current serologic techniques. The length of the CMV window period remains to be determined. It has been documented, through detection of CMV DNA by polymerase chain reaction in peripheral mononuclear cells as well as in plasma, that healthy blood donors who test seronegative for CMV can still harbor the virus.[40,49] Preliminary data have shown that both seronegative and seropositive donors have detectable CMV DNA in their plasma around the time of seroconversion, which may indicate potential infectivity.[40] The latter findings may account for failure of both serologic and leukocyte reduction techniques to eliminate TA-CMV in all clinical settings.

Because CMV is highly cell-associated, the use of leukocyte-reduced components has been investigated as a means to reduce the risk of TA-CMV. Some of the first evidence that leukocyte removal would reduce the risk of TA-CMV infection appeared in a study of cardiac surgery patients in the late 1970s showing that recipients of washed red cells had a lower rate of infection compared with those receiving unwashed red cells.[50] Blood components that contain no leukocytes or very few leukocytes (fresh frozen plasma, cryoprecipitate) are not believed to carry a risk for transmission of CMV.[51] Various methods to minimize the number of leukocytes (ie, centrifugation, saline washing, freezing and deglycerolization, filtration) have been reported to reduce or eliminate TA-CMV transmission. In general, saline washing achieves leukocyte reduction of approximately 90%, freezing and deglycerolization greater than 95%, and filtration 99% to 99.9%.[52,53] The dose and subset of leukocytes necessary to transmit CMV is unknown, although components that contain $<5 \times 10^6$ leukocytes per unit are believed to be non-infectious.[52,54] In uncontrolled studies, the use of saline-washed RBCs in the neonatal setting reported a TA-CMV rate ranging from 1.3% to 16%.[45,46] The variability observed in CMV transmission may reflect the variations in protocols for washing the red cells and the efficiency for reduction of leukocytes. It is also important to realize that this process addresses CMV transmission in terms of red cells and not other cellular components such as platelets. In one of these studies, in which six of 54 infants receiving saline-washed RBCs became infected with CMV, four of six of the infants received platelets or plasma from CMV IgG-positive donors, one of whom was also CMV IgM-positive.[45] The use of frozen and deglycerolized RBCs in this setting has been more effective. In a composite evaluation of reports that included a combined 252 neonatal and adult patients only two (0.8%) seroconverted.[53] However, the preparation of these components is both time-consuming and costly and, once again, does not address other cellular components.

In 1989, a small prospective randomized controlled trial showed that RBC units that were leukocyte reduced by filtration and given to infants weighing <1500 g who were born to seronegative mothers were effective in preventing CMV transmission.[25] Nine of 42 (21%) infants receiving unfiltered blood and none of 59 infants receiving filtered blood were infected with CMV. The mean volume of RBCs transfused was greater than 50 mL with some seropositive blood transfused. No platelets were given in this study. The efficacy of leukocyte filtration was further confirmed in a study of 22 seronegative premature infants (<1200 g) who received an average of 124 mL of blood with an average of 2.9 CMV-seropositive filtered units and no evidence of seroconversion during the study period.[55] An additional 26 VLBW seronegative infants who received blood that was leukocyte reduced by a spin-cool-filter technique showed no evidence of acquired CMV. A prospective trial of more than 500 marrow transplant patients randomly selected to receive either seronegative components or components that were leukocyte-reduced by bedside filtration showed that there was a low level (<2.5%) of CMV infection and disease in seronegative recipients of leukocyte-reduced blood components.[56] This is not dissimilar to the 1%-4% CMV seroconversion rate reported with the use of CMV-seronegative components. The level of leukocyte reduction to ensure the safety of unscreened blood components in seronegative recipients has been targeted to less than 5×10^6 leukocytes per transfusion, although some experts prefer reduction to $<1 \times 10^6$ per unit.[40,52,57]

A recent randomized study of leukocyte-reduced RBCs prepared by filtration vs non-leukocyte-reduced RBCs in premature infants residing in an area where CMV was endemic (>95% of mothers seropositive) showed no difference in the acquisition of

CMV. Three of 33 infants who received leukocyte-reduced blood and one of 19 infants given non-leukocyte-reduced blood were infected with CMV as determined by IgM seroconversion and CMV DNA isolation. These infants were all born to CMV-seropositive mothers and had birthweights ranging from 736 g to 1988 g. The most immature infant (birthweight 736 g) developed symptoms of pneumonitis. There were five infants in these groups born to seronegative mothers; three received nonfiltered blood and two received filtered blood. All of these infants received some blood from CMV-seropositive donors. None of these infants became infected with CMV. The overall rate of CMV transmission was 7.7%, with the most likely source of CMV being maternal, particularly from breast milk.[58] It was concluded that provision of leukocyte-reduced components to reduce the transmission of CMV was not warranted for neonates in regions where CMV is endemic.

Another method for reducing TA-CMV infection that is undergoing investigation is pathogen inactivation by photochemical means. Photochemical treatment of blood components has been shown to inactivate viruses, bacteria, and leukocytes.[59,60] The process uses psoralen S-59 in conjunction with long-wavelength ultraviolet A light and has been shown to inactivate high levels of cell-associated human CMV in platelet concentrates.[61] This process may offer a potential alternative to the use of either CMV-seronegative units or filtered leukocyte-reduced components as a means to decrease the risk of TA-CMV infection in immunocompromised patients.

Summary

Premature infants (<1200 g) born to seronegative mothers may be at risk for TA-CMV infection and disease. However, the reported risk of TA-CMV and the associated morbidity and mortality in this group of VLBW infants have decreased over time and geographic location, making the transfusion support of these infants controversial. Once a decision has been made to provide specialized components for a patient in this group, cellular components that are transfused should either be obtained from CMV-seronegative donors or be processed to effectively remove leukocytes. In the neonatal setting it has been shown that blood that has been processed to reduce CMV transmission (CMV seronegative or leukocyte-reduced by filtration) has essentially eliminated TA-CMV in seronegative premature infants. In contrast, premature infants born to seropositive mothers have been reported to develop CMV infection as well as disease even when seronegative or leukocyte-reduced blood components have been transfused. Perinatal CMV infections from a maternal source are common, accounting for CMV infection in up to 15% of infants. Therefore, the use of CMV-reduced-risk components for neonates has varied depending on the observed risk and the availability of various blood components.

References

1. Kaarianen L, Klemola E, Paloheimo J. Risk of cytomegalovirus antibodies in an infectious-mononucleus-like syndrome after transfusion. Br Med J 1966;1:1270-2.
2. Tolpin MD, Stewart JA, Warren MS, et al. Transfusion transmission of cytomegalovirus confirmed by restriction endonuclease analysis. J Pediatr 1985;107:953-6.
3. James DJ, Sikotra S, Sivakumaran M, et al. The presence of free infectious cytomegalovirus (CMV) in plasma of donated CMV-seropositive blood and platelets. Transfus Med 1997;7:123-6.
4. Alford CA, Stagno S, Pass RF, Britt WJ. Congenital and perinatal cytomegalovirus infections. Rev Infect Dis 1990;12:745-53.
5. Brown HL, Abernathy MP. Cytomegalovirus infection. Semin Perinatol 1998;22:260-6.
6. Fowler KB, Stagno S, Pass RF, et al. The outcome of congenital cytomegalovirus infection in relation to maternal antibody status. N Engl J Med 1992;326:663-7.
7. King-Lewis PA, Gardner SD. Congenital cytomegalovirus inclusion disease following intrauterine transfusion. Br Med J 1969;2:603-5.
8. Preiksaitis JK, Brown L, McKenzie M. The risk of cytomegalovirus infection in seronegative transfusion recipients not receiving exogenous immunosuppression. J Infect Dis 1988;157:523-9.
9. Sayers MH, Anderson KC, Goodnough LT, et al. Reducing the risk of transfusion-transmitted cytomegalovirus infection. Ann Intern Med 1992;116:55-62.

10. Huang ES, Alford CA, Reynolds DW, et al. Molecular epidemiology of cytomegalovirus infections in women and their infants. N Engl J Med 1980;303:958-62.
11. Reynolds DW, Stagno S, Hosty TS, et al. Maternal cytomegalovirus excretion and perinatal infection. N Engl J Med 1973;289:1-5.
12. Stagno S, Reynolds DW, Pass RF, Alford CA. Breast milk and the risk of cytomegalovirus infection. N Engl J Med 1980;302:1073-6.
13. Dworsky M, Yow M, Stagno S, et al. Cytomegalovirus infection of breast milk and transmission with infancy. Pediatrics 1983;72:295-9.
14. Minamishima I, Ueda K, Minematsu T, et al. Role of breast milk in acquisition of cytomegalovirus infection. Microbiol Immunol 1994;38:549-52.
15. Yeager AS. Transfusion-acquired cytomegalovirus infection in newborn infants. Am J Dis Child 1974;128:478-83.
16. Ballard RA, Drew WL, Hufnagle KG, Riedel PA. Acquired cytomegalovirus infection in preterm infants. Am J Dis Child 1979;133:482-5.
17. Whitley RJ, Brasfield D, Reynolds DW, et al. Protracted pneumonitis in young infants associated with perinatally acquired cytomegalovirus infection. J Pediatr 1976;89:16-22.
18. Brasfield DM, Stagno S, Whitley RJ, et al. Infant pneumonitis associated with cytomegalovirus, chlamydia, pneumocystis, and ureaplasma: Follow-up. Pediatrics 1987;79:76-83.
19. Yeager AS, Palumbo PE, Malachowski N, et al. Sequelae of maternally derived cytomegalovirus infections in premature infants. J Pediatr 1983; 102:918-22.
20. Ballow M, Cates KL, Rowe JC, et al. Development of the immune system in very low birth weight (less than 1500 g) premature infants: Concentrations of plasma immunoglobulins and patterns of infections. Pediatr Res 1986;20:899-904.
21. McEnery G, Stern H. Cytomegalovirus infections in early infancy: Five atypical cases. Arch Dis Child 1970;45:669-73.
22. Luthardt T, Siebert H, Losel I, et al. Cytomegalievirus-Infektionen bei kindern mit Blutaustauschtransfusion in Neugeborenenalter. Klin Wochenschr 1971;49:81-6.
23. Yeager AS, Grumet FC, Hafleigh EB, et al. Prevention of transfusion-acquired cytomegalovirus infections in newborn infants. J Pediatr 1981;98:281-7.
24. Adler SP, Chandrika T, Lawrence L, Baggett J. Cytomegalovirus infections in neonates acquired by blood transfusions. Pediatr Infect Dis 1983;2: 114-18.
25. Gilbert GL, Hayes K, Hudson IL, James J. Prevention of transfusion-acquired cytomegalovirus infection in infants by blood filtration to remove leukocytes. Lancet 1989;1:1228-31.
26. Lamberson HV, McMillan JA, Weiner LB, et al. Prevention of transfusion-associated cytomegalovirus (CMV) infection in neonates by screening blood donors for IgM to CMV. J Infect Dis 1988;157:820-2.

27. Smith D, Wright P, Krueger L, et al. Posttransfusion cytomegalovirus infection in neonates weighing less than 1250 grams (abstract). Transfusion 1983;23:420.
28. Rawls WE, Wong CL, Blajchman M, et al. Neonatal cytomegalovirus infections: the relative role of neonatal blood transfusion and maternal exposure. Invest Med 1984;7:13-19.
29. Tegtemeier GE. Cytomegalovirus and blood transfusion. In: Dodd RY, Barker LF, eds. Infection, immunity and blood transfusion. New York: Alan R Liss Inc, 1985:175-99.
30. Preiksaitis JK, Brown L, McKenzie M. Transfusion-acquired cytomegalovirus infection in neonates: A prospective study. Transfusion 1988; 28:205-9.
31. Griffin MP, O'Shea M, Brazy JE, et al. Cytomegalovirus infection in a neonatal intensive care unit: Blood transfusion practices and incidence of infection. Am J Dis Child 1988;142:1188-93.
32. Galea G, Urbaniak SJ. The incidence and consequences of cytomegalovirus transmission via blood transfusion to low birth weight, premature infants in North East Scotland. Vox Sang 1992;62:200-7.
33. Snydman DR, Werner BG, Meissner HC, et al. Use of cytomegalovirus immunoglobulin in multiply transfused premature neonates. Pediatr Infect Dis 1995;14:34-40.
34. Tegtemeier GE. Posttransfusion cytomegalovirus infections. Arch Pathol Lab Med 1989;113:236-45.
35. Preiksaitis JK. Indications for the use of cytomegalovirus-seronegative blood products. Transfus Med Rev 1991;5:1-17.
36. McHugh TM, Casavant CH, Wilber JC, et al. Comparison of six methods for the detection of antibody to cytomegalovirus. J Clin Microbiol 1985;22: 1014-19.
37. Griffin MP, O'Shea M, Brazy JE, et al. Cytomegalovirus infection in a neonatal intensive care unit: Subsequent morbidity and mortality of seropositive infants. J Perinatol 1990;10:43-5.
38. de Cates CR, Gray J, Robertson NRC, Walker J. Acquisition of cytomegalovirus infection by premature neonates. J Infect 1994;28:25-30.
39. de Cates CR, Robertson NRC, Walker J. Fatal acquired cytomegalovirus infection in a neonate with maternal antibody. J Infect 1988;17:235-9.
40. Blachman MA, Goldman M, Freedman JJ, Sher GD. Proceedings of a consensus conference: Prevention of post-transfusion CMV in the era of universal leukoreduction. Transfus Med Rev 2001;15:1-20.
41. King SM. Immune globulin versus antiviral versus combination for prevention of cytomegalovirus disease in transplant recipients. Antiviral Res 1999;40:115-37.
42. Adler SP, Lawrence LT, Baggett J, et al. Prevention of transfusion-associated cytomegalovirus infection in very low-birthweight infants using frozen blood and donors seronegative for cytomegalovirus. Transfusion 1984;24:333-5.

43. Brady MT, Milam JD, Anderson DC, et al. Use of deglycerolized red blood cells to prevent posttransfusion infection with cytomegalovirus in neonates. J Infect Dis 1984;150:334-8.
44. Simon TL, Johnson JD, Koffler H, et al. Impact of previously frozen deglycerolized red blood cells on cytomegalovirus transmission to newborn infants. Plasma Ther Transfus Technol 1987;8:51-6.
45. Demmler GD, Brady MT, Bijou H, et al. Posttransfusion cytomegalovirus infection in neonates: Role of saline-washed red blood cells. J Pediatr 1986;108:762-5.
46. Luban NL, Williams AE, MacDonald MG, et al. Low incidence of acquired cytomegalovirus infection in neonates transfused with washed red cells. Am J Dis Child 1987;141:416-19.
47. Lamberson HV, Dock LD. Prevention of transfusion-transmitted cytomegalovirus infection. Transfusion 1992;32:196-8.
48. Beneke JS, Tegtemeier GE, Alter HJ, et al. Relation of titers of antibodies to CMV in donors to the transmission of cytomegalovirus infection. J Infect Dis 1984;150:883-8.
49. Larson S, Soderberg-Naucler C, Wang FZ, Moller E. Cytomegalovirus DNA can be detected in peripheral blood mononuclear cells from all seropositive and most seronegative healthy blood donors over time. Transfusion 1998;91:119-26.
50. Lang DJ, Ebert PA, Rodgers BM, et al. Reductions of postperfusion cytomegalovirus infections following the use of leukocyte-depleted blood. Transfusion 1977;17:391-5.
51. Bowden R, Sayers M. The risk of transmitting cytomegalovirus infection by fresh frozen plasma. Transfusion 1990;30:762-3.
52. Leukocyte reduction for the prevention of transfusion-transmitted cytomegalovirus (TT-CMV). Association Bulletin No. 97-2. Bethesda, MD: American Association of Blood Banks, 1997.
53. Hillyer CD, Emmens RK, Zago-Novaretti M, Berkman EM. Methods for the reduction of transfusion-transmitted cytomegalovirus infection: Filtration versus the use of seronegative donor units. Transfusion 1994;34: 929-34.
54. Strauss RG. Data-driven blood banking practices for neonatal RBC transfusions. Transfusion 2000;40:1528-37.
55. Eisenfeld L, Silver H, McLaughlin J, et al. Prevention of transfusion-associated cytomegalovirus infection in neonatal patients by the removal of white cells from blood. Transfusion 1992;32:205-9.
56. Bowden RA, Slichter SJ, Sayers M, et al. A comparison of filtered leukocyte-reduced and cytomegalovirus (CMV) seronegative blood products for the prevention of transfusion-associated CMV infection after marrow transplant. Blood 1995;86:3598-603.
57. Leukocyte reduction. Association Bulletin No. 99-7. Bethesda, MD: American Association of Blood Banks, 1999.

58. Ohto H, Ujiie N, Hirai K. Lack of difference in cytomegalovirus transmission via the transfusion of filtered-irradiated and nonfiltered-irradiated blood to newborn infants in an endemic area. Transfusion 1999;39: 201-5.
59. Lin L, Cook DN, Weisehahn GP, et al. Photochemical inactivation of viruses and bacteria in platelet concentrates using a novel psoralen and long wavelength ultraviolet light. Transfusion 1997;37:423-35.
60. Grass JA, Hei DJ, Metchette K, et al. Inactivation of leukocytes in platelet concentrates by photochemical treatment with psoralen plus UVA. Blood 1998;91:2180-8.
61. Lin L. Inactivation of cytomegalovirus in platelet concentrates using Helinx technology. Semin Hematol 2001;38(Suppl 11):27-33.

In: Herman JH, Manno CS, eds.
Pediatric Transfusion Therapy
Bethesda, MD: AABB Press, 2002

9

Donor Limitation for Neonatal and Pediatric Transfusion

ANNE F. EDER, MD, PhD

DONOR LIMITATION BROADLY encompasses strategies to minimize the exposure to allogeneic donor blood for infants and children requiring transfusion. The primary impetus for developing and implementing these approaches over the past two decades has been the risk of viral transmission with blood transfusion. The safety of the blood supply has progressively and significantly improved through the introduction of additional donor deferral criteria and improvements in infectious disease marker testing. Recent

Anne F. Eder, MD, PhD, Director, Hematology Laboratory, and Assistant Director, Blood Bank and Apheresis Service, Department of Pathology and Clinical Laboratories, The Children's Hospital of Philadelphia, Philadelphia, Pennsylvania

estimates of the residual risk of viral transmission with blood transfusion is 1 in 1,930,000 units for human immunodeficiency virus (HIV); 1 in 138,700 units for hepatitis B (HBV); and <1 in 543,000 units for hepatitis C (HCV).[1]

Any additional margin of improved safety afforded by limiting donor exposure is unknown and would be difficult to determine experimentally, given the extant probability of viral transmission. Regardless, limiting donor exposure is prudent and offers other advantages such as preventing the transmission of diseases potentially carried in blood for which screening is not performed and the psychological benefit of alleviating parental anxiety over blood transfusion. In addition, some strategies to limit donor exposure also reduce the risk of alloimmunization, optimize resource utilization, and decrease the amount of blood wasted. The latter two considerations are particularly important in light of recent blood shortages.

Different approaches to limiting donor exposure are possible depending on the age, underlying medical condition, and transfusion requirements of the child. Most efforts to minimize donor exposure focus on patients requiring red cell transfusion; however, some programs target patients requiring platelet and plasma transfusion as well. This chapter reviews clinical and blood bank practices demonstrated to be effective in minimizing exposure of infants and children to allogeneic blood, including dedicated units for multiple small-volume transfusions to newborn infants, selective use of recombinant erythropoietin in specific clinical situations, and autologous and directed blood donation prior to scheduled surgery. Intraoperative blood recovery and perioperative hemodilution provide additional opportunities to limit the use of allogeneic blood transfusion for surgical patients, and are addressed in Chapter 14.

Neonatal Transfusion

Many preterm newborn infants receive red cell transfusions, most commonly administered as multiple, small-volume (10-20 mL/kg) or "booster" transfusions, for anemia developing in the first weeks of life.[2,3] Anemia in term infants results from a physiologic decline in hemoglobin concentration that reaches a nadir of 9.0 g/L at the lower limit of the normal range by 2 months of age. In preterm infants, hemoglobin concentrations at birth are lower than those of term infants, and the decline in hemoglobin occurs earlier and is more pronounced.[4] This "anemia of prematurity" may be aggravated by disproportionately large phlebotomy losses during hospitalization. Considering that a preterm infant weighing 1 kg has a total blood volume of only about 100 mL, sampling as little as 0.5 mL/day rapidly translates into a significant loss. Not surprisingly, the probability that an infant will be transfused is inversely related to birthweight or gestational age, and directly related to the volume of phlebotomy losses. In one series, more than 95% of infants weighing 1 kg or less received red cell transfusions compared to about only 40% of infants weighing 1 to 1.5 kg.[5] In other surveys, red cells were transfused to 96% to 100% of infants born earlier than 28 weeks of gestation and 40% to 50% of infants born at 28 to 32 weeks of gestation.[4,6]

Because red cell transfusions are often given to low birthweight infants to compensate for iatrogenic phlebotomy losses in the first month of life, it is important to avoid excessive and unnecessary blood sampling. Efforts should be directed at curbing the practice of drawing more blood than required by the clinical laboratory for the requested tests and eliminating unnecessary tests. Lin et al[7] demonstrated that phlebotomy overdraw was a significant problem in the intensive care nursery, averaging approximately 20% per test and translating into 2-4 mL/kg/week. Noninvasive monitoring technology and point of care laboratory testing promise to further reduce laboratory blood requirements.[8] As an alternative to blood drawn from the infant, the blood bank can use umbilical cord red cells and maternal plasma for pretransfusion testing at birth. If no clinically significant antibodies are identified in the initial screen, AABB *Standards for Blood Banks and Transfusion Services* permits omitting crossmatch procedures for subsequent transfusions during the hospitalization, recognizing the improbability of alloimmunization in infants under 4 months of age, and the importance of minimizing phlebotomy losses in this clinical setting.[9(p48)]

Clinical Interventions

Placental blood has been identified as a source of autologous blood for infants, and placental transfusion may be accomplished by clinical maneuvers at birth or collection of placental blood for later transfusion.[6,10-15] In a randomized trial of 36 preterm infants (27 to 33 weeks of gestation), a 30-second delay in umbilical cord clamping with the infant held 20 cm below the mother's introitus resulted in a modest increase in initial hematocrit (56% vs 51%) and lower median red cell transfusion requirements (0 mL/kg vs 23 mL/kg) compared with randomly timed cord clamping within 10-20 seconds of delivery.[10] Moreover, fewer mechanically ventilated infants received multiple red cell transfusions in the regulated group (1 of 13) than in the random group (7 of 13; $p = 0.03$). The Leboyer delivery method also delays cord clamping, as the newly delivered infant is placed on the mother's abdomen and the umbilical cord is severed only after it stops pulsing, several minutes after birth. This method significantly increased mean hematocrits compared with early cord clamping (58% vs 48%; $p<0.05$), equivalent to delivering a placental transfusion of about 20 mL/kg of whole blood at birth.[11] Although excessive placental transfusion at birth increases blood viscosity and may impair blood flow and compromise oxygen supply to vital organs, moderate increments such as those accomplished with these clinical maneuvers to delay cord clamping were not associated with adverse reactions and may be beneficial to preterm infants.[6,10,11] Specific contraindications to delayed cord clamping include maternal alloimmunization to the infant's erythrocytes or platelets.

Placental blood can also be collected aseptically from the umbilical vein and used for later transfusion.[6,12-15] The volume of blood collected from placentas will vary based on gestational age at delivery and timing of cord clamping. An average of 40 to 50 mL of blood can be collected from placentas at 28 to 36 weeks' gestational age, and more than 100 mL can be collected at term. The volume of placental blood collected is predicted to be sufficient to meet the transfusion needs of most neonates of 28 weeks' gestational age or greater.[6] The overriding concern in using banked placental blood for transfusion to premature infants, however, is the potential for bacterial contamination of the collected blood and the risk of iatrogenic sepsis in infants with immature immune systems.[15] The rate of bacterial contamination is influenced by the method of collection, and unacceptably high rates of 12.5% have been reported with open collection systems.[14] Closed collection systems achieve lower rates of bacterial contamination, with reported values ranging from 0% in studies of 25 to 120 collections[12,13] to 3.3% and 8.6% in studies of 378 and 47 collections, respectively.[14,15] Other issues limiting widespread acceptance of this approach include the difficulty in predicting which infants will require transfusion in the first weeks of life, the inability to collect sufficient blood from the placentas of preterm or low- birthweight infants most likely to need transfusions, and the competing parental interest to bank placental blood for possible hematopoietic transplantation in the future.

The need for allogeneic red cell transfusion in preterm infants may be reduced by the administration of recombinant human erythropoietin (rHuEPO). Several clinical studies have demonstrated rHuEPO treatment increases reticulocyte count and hemoglobin concentration and decreases the frequency and volume of transfusion,[16] but the magnitude of the drug's effect on transfusion varies widely across studies. Possible sources of variability among the controlled studies include different patient selection criteria, dosing regimens for rHuEPO, nutritional supplementation (eg, iron, vitamin E), and transfusion criteria. Results of a meta-analysis revealed that the variation in reported findings cannot be explained by considering the effects of any single variable pertaining to the patients' clinical status or study design.[17] When the analysis was limited to a subset of four high-quality studies of infants likely to receive transfusions according to conservative transfusion practices, a significant reduction in transfusion needs was observed with rHuEPO. Treatment with rHuEPO reduced red cell transfusions by an average of 11.0 mL/kg ($p<0.001$), but exerted only a small effect on the total transfusion needs of the infants during hospitalization.

As evident in this meta-analysis and several clinical studies evaluating the efficacy of rHuEPO, conservative transfusion policies alone can decrease allogeneic blood usage and donor exposure.[16-18] In one study, the institution of strict transfusion guidelines decreased the total number and volume of transfusions by 50% in those who received a placebo compared with matched controls, without adverse consequences.[18] Conversely, less disciplined compliance with transfusion guidelines have been implicated in increased numbers of transfusions.[19] Difficulties in determining the need for red cell transfusion in preterm infants contribute to variable and sometimes liberal transfusion practices. Guidelines and audit criteria have been developed to inform transfusion decisions in neonates.[4,18,20,21] Audit criteria provide broad guidance as to when transfusions would be considered reasonable, but not mandatory, practice. The AABB has recommended red cell transfusion in patients less than 4 months of age in the following situations[20]: 1) Hemoglobin <13.0 g/dL with severe pulmonary or cyanotic heart disease or heart failure; 2) Acute loss of ≥10% of blood volume or phlebotomy for laboratory testing when cumulative amount exceeds 10% of blood volume in a 1-week period; 3) Hemoglobin <8.0 g/dL in a stable newborn infant with clinical manifestations of anemia. Transfusion guidelines such as those used in clinical trials for rHuEPO provide more specific guidance on transfusion in specific clinical instances (Table 9-1). Despite strict transfusion guidelines, careful attention to phlebotomy losses, and administration of rHuEPO, many preterm infants still require red cell transfusion, spurring development of other means to limit exposure to allogeneic blood.

Small-Volume Transfusions: Safety of Red Cells Stored in Additive Solutions

Exposure to multiple donors may result from the traditional transfusion practice of using only fresh RBC units (≤5 to 7 days

Table 9-1. Red Cell Transfusion Guidelines Used in Clinical Trials of rHuEPO in Preterm Infants[16,18]

Hemoglobin	Mechanical Ventilation or Symptoms of Anemia
≤11 g/dL	Moderate or significant mechanical ventilation requirement (MAP > 8 cm H_2O and FiO_2 > 0.4).
≤10 g/dL	Minimal mechanical ventilation requirement (any mechanical ventilation, or CPAP >6 cm H_2O and FiO_2 ≤0.4)
<8 g/dL	No mechanical ventilation requirement and one or more of the following is present: • ≥24 hours of tachycardia (HR>180) or tachypnea (RR>80) • an increased oxygen requirement from the previous 48 hours, defined as ≥ fourfold increase in nasal canula flow or an increase in nasal CPAP ≥ 20% from the previous 48 hours • an elevated lactate concentration (≥2.5 mEq/L) • weight gain < 10 g/kg/day over the previous 4 days while receiving ≥ 100 kcal/kg/day • an increase in the episodes of apnea and bradycardia (10 or more episodes in a 24-hour period, or ≥ two episodes in 24 hours requiring bag-mask ventilation) while receiving therapeutic doses of methylxanthines • undergoing surgery
<7 g/dL	No symptoms and an absolute reticulocyte count <100,000 cells/µL (RBC × % reticulocyte count)

old) for neonates, due to concerns over the biochemical changes that occur during red cell storage and the safety of extended-storage preservative solutions. The storage defects include increased extracellular potassium concentration, decreased intracellular 2,3-diphosphoglycerate (2,3-DPG), and decreased pH. The extended-storage preservative solutions (also referred to as additive solutions or AS) contain mannitol, which diminishes red cell lysis during storage, and adenine, which supports red cell metabolism.[22(p162)] Adenine, however, has been associated with renal toxicity in laboratory animals and adult humans.

Mannitol mediates osmotic diuresis that may impair cerebral blood flow, and has also been associated with renal failure in adults. Theoretical arguments based on calculation of the total amount of potassium, hydrogen and additive solutions in small-volume transfusions suggested that these constituents are present in such small quantities that they would not present substantive risk to most preterm infants.[23]

Nevertheless, a 1989 national survey of neonatal transfusion practice in 452 hospitals revealed that 73% of respondents transfused red cells stored less than 7 days to neonates, which resulted in multiple donor exposures for infants in need of prolonged transfusion support.[3] Many centers still limit the duration of storage of RBC units used for infants and question the safety of older units in extended-storage preservative solutions. However, the practice of using stored red cells for small-volume neonatal transfusions has been proven to be safe and effective in clinical trials and is more widely accepted in practice today.[24-28] Safety concerns are still valid for large-volume (>25 mL/kg) transfusions and other clinical settings. (See Chapter 6 for a more detailed discussion of additive solutions.)

Special Clinical Considerations

In contrast to small volume transfusions given slowly over 2 to 4 hours, large volumes (>25 mL/kg) of stored RBCs may not be tolerated by some infants. Rapid infusion of relatively large volumes of stored red cells has led to fatal hyperkalemia.[29] The route of administration is also an important factor influencing toxicity, and local alterations in potassium or calcium concentration may produce cardiac arrhythmia in predisposed infants if transfused through a central line directly into the atrium. Caution is also warranted if the infant has an underlying medical condition such as oliguric renal failure or tenuous cardiac function. In these cases, fresh or washed red cells may be indicated.

Another notable clinical setting is that of extracorporeal membrane oxygenation (ECMO), which is used to support neonatal patients with reversible respiratory and cardiac failure who fail to respond to maximal medical therapy. These infants require numerous transfusions of red cells, plasma, and platelets; however, donor exposures can be minimized despite these intensive blood component demands, the severity of disease and the emergent nature of the intervention. By modifying blood bank and physician practices, one ECMO program was able to substantially reduce transfusion volumes for platelet and plasma components, with corresponding reduction in donor exposures.[30] The changes in component selection and management included switching to Platelets Pheresis aliquots instead of volume-reduced Platelets and using Fresh Frozen Plasma (FFP) obtained by apheresis, divided into four aliquots at the time of component preparation ("pedi FFP"), instead of standard FFP. In contrast to these measures, extending the transfusion outdate for RBCs from 5 days to 10 days, while clinically tolerated among ECMO patients, did not result in significant changes in red cell transfusion volume or associated blood donor exposures with red cell transfusion.

Blood Bank Practices

Because most transfusions to premature infants involve RBCs and not other blood components and are given within the first 2 to 4 weeks of life, limiting donor red cell transfusions and using dedicated units to their storage expiration date are the keys to reducing donor exposures in this patient population. Donor limitation programs must first identify infants likely to require multiple transfusions during neonatal hospitalization and estimate the total volume and duration of transfusion support required. The blood bank then dedicates either a partial or an entire AS-1 or AS-3 unit to an individual infant or assigns more than one infant to a divided or full unit. For example, infants with a birthweight of less than 1 kg may be assigned to half a unit; infants with a birthweight of 1.0 to 1.3 kg to a quarter unit; and larger infants to variable fractions of units depending on their red cell requirements.[27,28] Alternatively, low birthweight infants may be assigned to a single unit but up to four larger infants may share a full or divided unit.[31] Both of these inventory management strategies have been shown to minimize waste of blood while reducing donor exposures. The donor blood on the day of dedication should be a freshly collected (≤7 days old) AS-1 or AS-3 unit that has undergone leukocyte reduction by filtration prior to storage to reduce the risk of cytomegalovirus transmission, and should lack hemoglobin S to avoid any possibility of red cell sickling in hypoxic vasculature beds. Small-volume aliquots are then prepared for transfusion to the infant from the dedicated unit until its expiration date and irradiated immediately prior to issuance.

Preparing small-volume red cell transfusions for premature or low birthweight infants presents special technical challenges,[32] with regard to minimizing both the waste of blood and donor exposures. If the hermetic seal of a unit of AS RBCs is entered or "spiked" to remove a smaller aliquot, it becomes an "open system" and the allowable storage time is drastically shortened from 42 days to 24 hours.[9(p59),22(p166)] Even if the unit is the shared source of all red cells for all infants who undergo transfusion on that day, most of the unit will be wasted. This method also virtually ensures that an infant will be exposed to a new RBC unit for every transfusion required, unless multiple small-volume transfusions are required in a 24-hour period. Pediatric quadruple ("quad-") or multipacks of red cells, composed of a primary bag of red cells with four or more integrally attached transfer bags, allow sterile removal of smaller volumes of red cells in a closed system without altering the allowable storage time. A sterile connection device can be used to attach additional transfer bags or specially designed syringes to the source unit of red cells, in a functionally closed system, without changing the storage expiration date of the component. This technique allows the preparation of multiple small-volume aliquots from a single RBC unit throughout its shelf life.

The Food and Drug Administration (FDA) does not consider pediatric aliquots of blood components prepared with the use of a sterile connection device as a new product.[33] Consequently, blood banks involved in shipping blood components across state lines do not need to obtain a biologics license application supplement for this practice, provided the following stipulations of the FDA are met: 1) the manufacturer has an approved biologics license or license supplement for the original (ie, undivided) product, 2) the labels are submitted for review and approval before distribution, and 3) the final product containers are approved for storage of the component being prepared. In contrast, pooling or mixing cellular components may represent a change in the product that requires submission and approval of a license application or application supplement to describe the manufacturing procedure and demonstrate that the new product is safe and effective for its intended use throughout the proposed dating period.

Blood components are often issued in syringes to infants, because of the widespread use and convenience of syringe infusion pumps. At the Children's Hospital of Philadelphia, the use of a syringe to prepare small-volume aliquots of blood components streamlined preparation, and reduced both red cell waste and donor exposures in multitransfused infants. (See Chapter 10 for a more detailed discussion of syringes.)

Efforts to limit donor exposures for individual infants may fail for technical or clinical reasons, including inaccurate estimation of transfusion needs, unexpected medical complications, or problems encountered in preparing small-volume aliquots. Because the average hematocrit of CPDA RBC units is higher than AS RBC units (70% vs 57%), centrifugation prior to aliquotting may be performed to provide red cells with a uniformly high hematocrit (about 85%) and to minimize the supernatant volume. This practice is not universal, however, and introduces the potential for units to break during centrifugation. Loss of dedicated units during centrifugation resulted in additional donor exposures for several infants in one clinical study.[27] This problem was eliminated by reducing the speed and duration of centrifugation, and may also be avoided by using gravity sedimentation for concentration of red cells prior to transfusion.[34] Several other infants were exposed to more than one donor because clinical circumstances prevented timely collection of a second RBC unit from the directed donor.[27,28] On six occasions, the infants' transfusion needs extended beyond the expiration date of the dedicated unit, but the dedicated donors (volunteer unrelated donors) returned to donate second units, necessitating collection more frequently than the 56-day interval allowed by AABB standards.[9(p64)] The institution's investigational review board approved the protocol for research purposes, provided that the donor hematocrit was greater than or equal to 33% and consent had been obtained.

Parents may inquire about being a directed donor for their infant or about designating a relative or friend as a directed donor because of their perception that they or someone they know would be the safest source of blood for their infant. However, there is no evidence that directed donors are safer than volunteer community donors.[35,36] On the contrary, concerns have been raised regarding the possibility that directed donors may feel pressured to give blood under these circumstances and may not be truthful about their risk factors. Infectious disease risk is not eliminated with directed donation; HIV has been transmitted via directed donation, and HBV and HCV serologic markers were more prevalent in directed donations than volunteer allogeneic donations in one study, although this difference did not reach statistical significance.[35,36]

Moreover, blood from biologic relatives may not be appropriate for transfusion to the infant because of serologic incompatibility. Plasma from biologic mothers may contain alloantibodies stimulated by pregnancy, capable of reacting with blood cell antigens inherited from the father and causing hemolysis, thrombocytopenia, or leukocyte aggregation in the infant. A clinical study compared biologic parents to unrelated donors as the source for small-volume red cell transfusions for preterm infants.[37] As described in Table 6-5, a total of 40 preterm infants received 120 AS-3 RBC transfusions from either maternal, paternal, or unrelated donors, and none experienced clinical transfusion reactions or significant laboratory disturbances, regardless of the relationship of the donor to the patient. Biologic parents, especially mothers, experienced several donor eligibility problems, but once enrolled as donors were able to supply all the red cells needed by their infants. Because the red cell aliquots were prepared from centrifuged units in this study, they were relatively devoid of plasma. Consequently, the authors could not exclude the possibility that transfusions may not be tolerated if there are clinically significant serologic incompatibilities and cautioned against transfusing plasma-rich blood components from maternal donors to their infants.

Pediatric Transfusion

Beyond the neonatal period, options for reducing a child's exposure to allogeneic blood also include use of rHuEPO, autologous blood transfusion, and directed donor programs for chronically transfused patients. Clinical trials involving small numbers of pediatric patients with solid tumors have demonstrated that rHuEPO is effective at increasing the hemoglobin concentration and reducing transfusion requirements of anemic cancer patients receiving concomitant chemotherapy.[38-43] Erythropoietin has also been evaluated as a means to reduce transfusion requirements in the postoperative period for children undergoing orthopedic, cardiac, or craniofacial surgery.[44,45] Clinical challenges using erythropoietin most effectively include predicting which patients will benefit from adjunctive erythropoietin therapy, and determining the optimal dose of erythropoietin in various clinical settings, as well as appropriate iron supplementation during erythropoietin treatment. As with premature infants, erythropoietin reduces but does not eliminate the need for allogeneic red cell transfusion in most clinical settings.

Preoperative Donation of Autologous Blood

Autologous blood transfusion may decrease or eliminate the need for allogeneic blood transfusion, and reduce the risk of infectious disease transmission, alloimmunization, and immune suppression.[46] Autologous blood transfusion involves any one or a combination of strategies, including preoperative donation of blood, the exclusive focus of this section, or perioperative blood recovery and hemodilution, topics addressed separately in Chapter 14. Although most clinical experience with autologous donation is with adults, there is no minimum age requirement for autologous donation mandated by regulatory agencies in the United States. Children can donate autologous blood prior to elective surgery provided the following AABB requirements are met: 1) the patient's physician and medical director of the blood bank establish alternative requirements for donor selection and collection; 2) the hemoglobin concentration of the donor's blood should be no less than 11 g/dL (33% hematocrit); 3) the phlebotomy does not occur within 72 hours of the time of anticipated surgery unless approved by the medical director; 4) collection does not occur if the donor has bacteremia or a significant bacterial infection that could be associated with bacteremia, and 5) the unit must be reserved for autologous use.[9(p19-20)]

In several clinical case series of preoperative donation, autologous blood has been collected safely from children within the current AABB guidelines and with low rates of adverse reactions and collection failures (Table 9-2).[47-58] Candidates for preoperative autologous donation in most studies were children greater than 6 years old, weighing more than 25 kg, although smaller children and even infants have also been case subjects. Adverse reactions are usually transient and minor, with the most common being nausea, lightheadedness, and vasovagal symptoms. The most common reasons for failure to collect autologous units are patient or parental anxiety, inadequate venous access, or low hemoglobin. When used for surgical procedures expected to result in significant acute blood loss and transfusion in 60% to 80% of patients, preoperative autologous donation reduced the allogeneic transfusion rate to 10% to 30%.[53-55]

Unique practical considerations and technical challenges in collecting blood from young children include predicting the number of units that will be required in the postoperative period, securing adequate venous access, dealing with restlessness of the pediatric donor and the anxiety and apprehension of both the donor and parents, and processing volumes of whole blood smaller than a standard blood donation. The 16-gauge needle in a standard whole blood collection set may be too large for phlebotomy of a young child. Because sets with smaller needles are not commercially available, a sterile connection device can be used to attach a 20-gauge needle to the set. This caliber needle facilitates phlebotomy in small children; smaller needles may

Table 9-2. Preoperative Autologous Blood Donation in Pediatric Patients

Ref	Patients (n)	Age Range	Weight Range (kg)	Surgery Type	Allogeneic Transfusions (% patients)*	Adverse Reactions [% patients or procedures (P)][†]	Collection Failures [% patients or procedures (P)][‡]
47	147	7-20 years	25-76	Orthopedic	34% (50/147)	12% (43/352 P)	5% (8/147)
48	180	8-18 years	NR [26 pts <45 kg]	Orthopedic; plastic	12% (21/180)	2% (4/180)	<1% (2/415 P)
49	118	6-20 years	30-45.4	Orthopedic	37% (20/118)	3% (9/306 P)	1% (3/309 P)
50	29	8-25 years	NR [Avg 46 kg]	Orthopedic	11% (3/27)	0 (0)	30% (8/27)
51[§]	175	10-21 years	NR [44 pts <45.5 kg]	Orthopedic	27% (48/175)	8% (14/175)	11% (19/175)
52[§]	13	9 months-10 years	7.3-33.6	Gastro-intestinal; tumors	15% (2/13)	0 (0)	0 (0)
53	59	3-15 years	13-70	Cardiac; orthopedic	6% (3/53)	2% (1/59)	3% (2/59)
54[§]	80	3-15 years	12.3-69	Cardiac	6% (5/80)	2% (2/80)	9% (7/80)

(continued)

Table 9-2. Preoperative Autologous Blood Donation in Pediatric Patients (continued)

Ref	Patients (n)	Age Range	Weight Range (kg)	Surgery Type	Allogeneic Transfusions (% patients)*	Adverse Reactions [% patients or procedures (P)][†]	Collection Failures [% patients or procedures (P)][‡]
55	116	10-18 years	20-95	Orthopedic	11% (13/116)	22% (26/116)	4% (6/147)
56[§]	24	1-13 years	8-25	Urological; orthopedic	12% (3/24)	0 (0)	13% (6/46 P)
57	163	NR 12.6±2.3 years	NR [51.6±16.5 kg]	Orthopedic	9% (15/163)	— NR	3% (5/163)
58	173	8-18 years	23.2-120	Orthopedic	27% (46/173)	‖	‖

Abbreviations: NR = not reported; P = phlebotomy attempts.

*The allogeneic transfusion rate is the percentage of patients who received allogeneic blood in addition to autologous blood.

[†]Reported adverse reactions included nausea, vomiting, and vasovagal symptoms. The adverse reaction rate was extracted from the published data as the percentage of patients who experienced adverse reactions, unless otherwise noted at the percentage of phlebotomy procedures (P) during which patients experienced adverse reactions.

[‡]Collection failures resulted from low predonation hemoglobin, inadequate venous access, or an uncooperative or anxious patient that prevented phlebotomy. The collection failure rate was extracted from the published data as the percentage of patients who had at least one failed attempt, unless otherwise noted at the percentage of all phlebotomy procedures (P) that failed.

[§]All patients donated autologous blood prior to surgery, but intraoperative blood recovery and/or hemodilution was also performed for some patients.

[‖]The authors reported a 19.6% rate of "noncompliance" defined as the inability to collect the total number of units requested by the surgeon, due to either collection failure or adverse events.

not permit sufficient flow rates during the collection, and may result in clotting and waste. Because the units collected from small children are only a fraction of the 500 mL or more collected from adults, the anticoagulant/whole blood ratio must be adjusted prior to collection.[46] Children can donate on a weekly schedule, permitting collection of 2 to 4 units of autologous blood in the month prior to the scheduled surgery; alternatively, units may be collected further in advance of the surgery and cryopreserved,[54] although this processing adds to the expense and decreases the yield of red cells for transfusion.

The success of preoperative autologous donation programs is often measured in terms of the allogeneic transfusion rate and the autologous utilization rate, because the failure to collect sufficient autologous blood results in allogeneic blood exposure and overcollection is costly and wasteful. Accurate prediction of the number of autologous units required by individual patients to avoid allogeneic transfusion is crucial, yet often not achieved. In one study, surgeons accurately predicted the blood requirements of only about half of the patients; for the remainder, transfusion needs were more commonly overestimated than underestimated.[58]

Furthermore, few studies of preoperative donation explicitly audit the appropriateness of transfusion of either autologous or allogeneic blood or define transfusion criteria for when transfusions should be given. When transfusion criteria are given, autologous blood is transfused more liberally than allogeneic blood,[50] or with an acknowledgment that transfusion may not have been given at all had autologous blood not been available.[48] Simpson et al[51] reported that 55 (40%) autologous and allogeneic transfusions were administered to children in clinical circumstances that failed to meet generally accepted criteria for transfusion. Transfusion of all donated autologous units to two patients in another study resulted in "polycythemia."[54] Although autologous transfusion is generally safe, it is not without risk. Autologous blood transfusion does not prevent clerical, laboratory, or administration errors, septicemia from bacterially contaminated units, volume overload, or nonhemolytic transfusion reactions caused by accumulation of cytokines during storage. For these reasons, transfusing autologous units simply because they are available is not appropriate.

Finally, a rational approach to pediatric autologous blood donation is advocated. Subjecting an infant or young child to the risks and discomfort of phlebotomy must be carefully considered. The clinical studies that enrolled children under 5 years old, or weighing less than 25 kg, resorted to measures of restraining a crying child,[56] using local anesthesia and collecting blood through an external jugular vein[56] or an arterial or central venous line,[52] or collecting blood during another invasive procedure (eg, cardiac catheterization).[54] In some cases where the reported surgical blood loss was less than 15 mL/kg or 10% to 15% of the total blood volume, it is possible that red cell transfusions need not have been given at all or the use of hemodilution or intraoperative blood recovery may have been sufficient to meet the child's transfusion requirements.[51,52,56] Consequently, preoperative autologous donation should be reserved for children with adequate peripheral venous access who are old enough to understand the procedure and cooperate fully. Furthermore, it should be offered as an option only if the surgical procedure has been documented to result in an acute loss of more than 20% of the total blood volume in a majority of patients.

Single or Committed Directed Donor Programs

If allogeneic red cell transfusion is highly probable and autologous donation is not possible for children undergoing elective surgery, some practitioners have advocated limiting exposure to as few donors as possible by using single or committed dedicated donors. In 1990, Brecher et al[59] reported parental committed donors provided 48%, 64%, and 14% of red cells, platelets, and FFP, respectively, that were needed by 50 pediatric patients undergoing cardiac surgery. In 1992, Strauss et al[60] reported one dedicated donor could provide all the red cell transfusions required by a patient in 83% of the cases. The collection schedule was more frequent than AABB standards allow for volunteer donation, occurring once a week with at least 3 days between collections, but the minimum predonation hematocrit value was ≥33%, which is consistent with current regulations. Committed donor programs may offer advantages other than infectious disease considerations, such as decreasing the risk of alloimmunization. Pediatric cancer patients often require platelet support following marrow transplantation and may be less likely to become refractory to platelet transfusion if one or a small number of matched donors provide apheresis platelets during the hospitalization. Patients requiring chronic red cell transfusion also are at decreased risk of red cell alloimmunization if a relatively small pool of racially or phenotypically similar donors supply the units they need over time. Directed donation programs may also increase the volunteer blood donor base. Although most hospitals and blood centers offer directed donation programs, dedicated allogeneic units generally account for a minority of total red cell and platelet transfusions. At the Children's Hospital of Philadelphia, less than 10% of the total inventory of red cells and platelets represents directed donations.

Conclusion

The blood supply is safer today than it has ever been, but allogeneic transfusion still carries finite risk of transmitting known viruses and potential risk of transmitting other infectious agents for which screening is not performed. Limiting allogeneic blood donor exposures is prudent and may offer other advantages in certain clinical settings, such as decreasing the risk of alloimmunization, reducing blood wastage, and optimizing resource utilization. Strategies to limit donor exposure depend on the age, underlying medical condition, and transfusion requirements of the infant or child and may involve one or a combination of strategies such as dedicated units and donors, recombinant erythropoietin, and autologous blood transfusion.

References

1. Dodd RY. Germs, gels, and genomes: A personal recollection of 30 years in blood safety testing. In: Stramer SL, ed. Blood safety in the new millen-

nium. Bethesda, MD: American Association of Blood Banks, 2001: 92-122.
2. Strauss RG. Transfusion therapy in neonates. Am J Dis Child 1991; 145:904-11.
3. Levy GJ, Strauss RG, Hume H, et al. National survey of neonatal transfusion practices: I. Red blood cell therapy. Pediatrics 1993;91:523-9.
4. Hume H, Bard H. Small volume red blood cell transfusions for neonatal patients. Transfus Med Rev 1995;9:187-99.
5. Widness JA, Seward VJ, Kromer IJ, et al. Changing patterns of red blood cell transfusion in very low birth weight infants. J Pediatr 1996; 129:680-7.
6. Bifano EM, Curran TR. Minimizing donor blood exposure in the neonatal intensive care unit. Current trends and future prospects. Clin Perinatol 1995;22:657-69.
7. Lin JC, Strauss RG, Kulhavy JC, et al. Phlebotomy overdraw in the neonatal intensive care nursery. Pediatrics 2000;106:E19.
8. Widness JA, Kulhavy JC, Johnson KJ, et al. Clinical performance of an in-line point-of-care monitor in neonates. Pediatrics 2000;106:497-504.
9. Gorlin JB, ed. Standards for blood banks and transfusion services, 21st ed. Bethesda, MD: American Association of Blood Banks, 2002.
10. Kinmond S, Aitchison TC, Holland BM, et al. Umbilical cord clamping and preterm infants: A randomized trial. Br Med J 1993;306:172-5.
11. Nelle M, Zilow EP, Kraus M, et al. The effect of Leboyer delivery on blood viscosity and other hemorheologic parameters in term neonates. Am J Obstet Gynecol 1993;169:189-93.
12. Ballin A, Arbel E, Kenet G, et al. Autologous umbilical cord blood transfusion. Arch Dis Child 1995;73:F181-3.
13. Bifano EM, Dracker RA, Lorah K, Palit A. Collection and 28-day storage of human placental blood. Pediatr Res 1994;36:90-4.
14. Bertolini F, Lazzari L, Lauri E, et al. Comparative study of different procedures for the collection and banking of umbilical cord blood. J Hematother 1995;4:29-36.
15. Eichler H, Schaible T, Richter E, et al. Cord blood as a source of autologous RBCs for transfusion to preterm infants. Transfusion 2000; 40:1111-17.
16. Ohls RK. The use of erythropoietin in neonates. Clin Perinatol 2000; 27:681-96.
17. Vamvakas EC, Strauss RG. Meta-analysis of controlled clinical trials studying the efficacy of rHuEPO in reducing blood transfusions in the anemia of prematurity. Transfusion 2001;41:406-15.
18. Ohls RK, Osborne KA, Christensen RD. Efficacy and cost analysis of treating very low birth weight infants with erythropoietin during their first two weeks of life: A randomized, placebo controlled trial. J Pediatr 1995;126:421-6.

19. Hilsenrath P, Nemechek J, Widness JA, et al. Cost-effectiveness of a limited-donor blood program for neonatal red cell transfusions. Transfusion 1999;39:938-43.
20. AuBuchon JP, ed. Guidelines for blood utilization review. Bethesda, MD: American Association of Blood Banks, 2001.
21. Calhoun DA, Christensen RD, Edstrom CS, et al. Consistent approaches to procedures and practices in neonatal hematology. Clin Perinatol 2000; 27:733-53.
22. Brecher ME, ed. Technical manual, 14th ed. Bethesda, MD: American Association of Blood Banks, 2002.
23. Luban, NLC, Strauss RG, Hume HA. Commentary on the safety of red cells preserved in extended-storage media for neonatal transfusions. Transfusion 1991;31:229-35.
24. Liu EA, Mannino FL, Lane AT. Prospective, randomized trial of the safety and efficacy of a limited donor exposure transfusion program for premature neonates. J Pediatr 1994;125:92-6.
25. Lee DA, Slagle TA, Jackson TM, Evans CS. Reducing blood donor exposures in low birth weight infants by the use of older, unwashed packed red blood cells. J Pediatr 1995;126:280-6.
26. Wood A, Wilson N, Skacel P, et al. Reducing donor exposure in preterm infants requiring multiple blood transfusions. Arch Dis Child 1995;72: F29-33.
27. Strauss RG, Burmeister LF, Johnson K, et al. AS-1 red cells for neonatal transfusions: A randomized trial assessing donor exposure and safety. Transfusion 1996;36:873-8.
28. Strauss RG, Burmeister LF, Johnson K, et al. Feasibility and safety of AS-3 red blood cells for neonatal transfusions. J Pediatr 2000;136: 215-19.
29. Hall TL, Barnes A, Miller JR, et al. Neonatal mortality following transfusion of red cells with high plasma potassium levels. Transfusion 1993; 33:606-9.
30. Rosenberg EM, Chambers LA, Gunter JM, Good JA. A program to limit donor exposures to neonates undergoing extracorporeal membrane oxygenation. Pediatrics 1994;94:341-6.
31. Wang-Rodriguez J, Mannino FL, Liu E, Lane TA. A novel strategy to limit blood donor exposure and blood waste in multiply transfused premature infants. Transfusion 1996;36:64-70.
32. Butch SH. Preparation of components for pediatric patients: "Boutique" blood components. In: Chambers LA, Issitt LA, eds. Supporting the pediatric transfusion recipient. Bethesda, MD: American Association of Blood Banks, 1994:15-64.
33. Food and Drug Administration. Guidance for industry: Use of sterile connecting devices in blood bank practices. (November 2000) Rockville, MD: CBER Office of Communication, Training, and Manufacturers Assistance, 2000.

34. Sherwood WC, Donato T, Clapper C, Wilson S. The concentration of AS-1 RBCs after inverted gravity sedimentation for neonatal transfusions. Transfusion 2000;40:618-19.
35. Pink J, Thomson A, Wylie B. Infectious disease markers in autologous and directed donations. Transfus Med 1995;4:135-8.
36. Yomtovian R. Is directed blood transfusion a good idea? Med Lab Observer 1992;24:31-4.
37. Strauss RG, Burmeister LF, Johnson K, et al. Randomized trial assessing the feasibility and safety of biologic parents as RBC donors for their preterm infants. Transfusion 2000;40:450-6.
38. Porter J, Leahey A, Polise K, et al. Recombinant human erythropoietin reduces the need for erythrocyte and platelet transfusions in pediatric patients with sarcoma: A randomized double-blind placebo-controlled trial. J Pediatr 1996;129:656-60.
39. Leon P, Jimenez M, Barona P, Sierrasesumaga L. Recombinant human erythropoietin for the treatment of anemia in children with solid malignant tumors. Med Pediatr Oncol 1998;30:110-16.
40. Bolonaki I, Stiakaki E, Lydaki E, et al. Treatment with recombinant human erythropoietin in children with malignancies. Pediatr Hematol Oncol 1996;13:111-21.
41. Varan A, Buyukpamukcu M, Kutluk T, Akyuz C. Recombinant human erythropoietin treatment for chemotherapy-related anemia in children. Pediatrics 1999;103(2):E16.
42. Vitale MG, Stazzone EJ, Gelijns AC, et al. The effectiveness of preoperative erythropoietin in averting allogeneic blood transfusion among children undergoing scoliosis surgery. J Pediatr Orthop B 1998;7:203-9.
43. Csaki C, Ferencz T, Schuler D, Borsi JD. Recombinant human erythropoietin in the prevention of chemotherapy-induced anemia in children with malignant solid tumours. Eur J Cancer 1998;34:364-7.
44. Helfaer MA, Carson BS, James CS, et al. Increased hematocrit and decreased transfusion requirements in children given erythropoietin before undergoing craniofacial surgery. J Neurosurg 1998;88:704-8.
45. Shimpo H, Mizumoto T, Onoda K, et al. Erythropoietin in pediatric cardiac surgery: Clinical efficacy and effective dose. Chest 1997;111:1565-70.
46. Thompson HW, Luban NL. Autologous blood transfusion in the pediatric patient. J Pediatr Surg 1995;30:1406-11.
47. Cowell HR, Swickard JW. Autotransfusion in children's orthopedics. J Bone Joint Surg [Am] 1974;56:908-12.
48. Silvergleid AJ. Safety and effectiveness of predeposit autologous transfusions in preteen and adolescent children. JAMA 1987;257:3403-4.
49. MacEwen GD, Bennett E, Guille JT. Autologous blood transfusions in children and young adults with low body weight undergoing spinal surgery. J Pediatr Orthop 1990;10:750-3.
50. Flynn JM, Cintron K, Canals RM. The use of autologous blood transfusions in pediatric orthopaedic surgery. Bol Asoc Med P R 1991;83:192-5.

51. Simpson MB, Georgopoulos G, Orsini E, Eilert RE. Autologous transfusions for orthopaedic procedures at a children's hospital. J Bone Joint Surg [Am] 1992;74:652-8.
52. Kemmotsu H, Joe K, Nakamura H, Yamashita M. Predeposited autologous blood transfusion for surgery in infants and children. J Pediatr Surg 1995;30:659-61.
53. Tasaki T, Ohto H, Noguchi M. Autologous blood donation in elective surgery in children. Vox Sang 1994;6:188-93.
54. Masuda M, Kawachi Y, Inaba S, et al. Preoperative autologous blood donations in pediatric cardiac surgery. Ann Thorac Surg 1995;60:1694-7.
55. Moran MM, Kroon D, Tredwell SJ, Wadsworth LD. The role of autologous blood transfusion in adolescents undergoing spinal surgery. Spine 1995;20:532-6.
56. Mayer MN, de Montalembert M, Audat F, et al. Autologous blood donation for elective surgery in children weighing 8-25 kg. Vox Sang 1996; 70:224-8.
57. Murray DJ, Forbes RB, Titone MB, Weinstein SL. Transfusion management in pediatric and adolescent scoliosis surgery. Efficacy of autologous blood. Spine 1997;22:2735-40.
58. Letts M, Perng R, Luke B, et al. An analysis of a preoperative pediatric autologous blood donation program. Can J Surg 2000;43:125-9.
59. Brecher ME, Taswell HF, Clare DE, et al. Minimal-exposure transfusion and the committed donor. Transfusion 1990;30:599-604.
60. Strauss RG, Wieland MR, Randels MJ, Koerner TAW. Feasibility and success of a single-donor red cell program for pediatric elective surgery patients. Transfusion 1992;32:747-9.

In: Herman JH, Manno CS, eds.
Pediatric Transfusion Therapy
Bethesda, MD: AABB Press, 2002

10

Pediatric Blood Collection and Transfusion Technology

SUSAN D. ROSEFF, MD

Mr. McGuire: "Ben – I just want to say one word to you – just one word."
Ben: "Yes, sir."
Mr. McGuire: "Are you listening?"
Ben: "Yes I am."
Mr. McGuire: "Plastics."
Ben: "Exactly how do you mean?"
Mr. McGuire: "There is a great future in plastics. Think about it. Will you think about it?"
—The Graduate" (1967)[1]

IMPROVEMENTS IN MEETING THE transfusion needs of neonates have come about through a variety of avenues, but mostly through innovations in how blood and blood components can be collected, stored, and delivered. Critically ill neonates are among the most heavily transfused hospitalized patients and, with improvements in survival, are among those with the greatest overall lon-

Susan D. Roseff, MD, Assistant Professor of Pathology, Virginia Commonwealth University School of Medicine, and Medical Director, Transfusion Medicine, Virginia Commonwealth University Health Systems, Richmond, Virginia

gevity. Therefore, improving the safety of the blood delivered to these infants will have a substantial impact.

Overall transfusion safety has been the focus of the blood industry since blood was first banked, and this pursuit has increased in intensity since the first case of transfusion-transmitted AIDS was identified. Pediatric transfusion medicine specialists have long recognized the unique and different needs of transfused infants. By decreasing exposure to multiple allogeneic donors through the use of new delivery systems, employing anticoagulant-preservative solutions with longer shelf lives, and applying autologous blood-collection principles used in adult patients, great strides have been made in improving transfusion safety in neonates. This chapter outlines the changes that have been made and looks at the pros and cons of available strategies.

It is important to note that there is a dearth of published, randomized, controlled trials evaluating the safety and efficacy of each technology, as well as all the permutations in use. Therefore, a plethora of practices exists, each with its own historical beginnings at different institutions and each with its own advantages and disadvantages.

Sterile Connection Devices

The ability to weld plastic tubing together, while maintaining its sterility, has increased the number of available options for delivering small-volume transfusions. Sterile connection devices were being used, in the early 1980s, by Baxter Healthcare (Deerfield, IL) to transfer sterile solutions, and by the DuPont Corporation (Wilmington, DE) for performing intraperitoneal dialysis. The devices were difficult to use and required great care, which limited their potential value and acceptability in other settings. Further refinements in the technology used by the DuPont model led the way for the current generation of sterile connection devices.[2]

Sterile connection devices have added a great deal of flexibility to blood manufacturing and transfusion. They can be used for a variety of processes, to both join and remove blood and blood components. With this technique, the primary component as well as its "satellites" can retain the original outdate and maintain sterility. Some of these applications include:

- Addition of leukocyte-reduction (LR) filters to accomplish prestorage leukocyte reduction, after the component is collected in its primary bag.
- Addition of a smaller needle to a collection set, before initiation of the procedure.
- Addition of more bags to collection sets.
- Removal of samples from the primary bag for culture, quality control (QC), or pretransfusion testing, as long as the variables listed on the bag, such as volume or cell count, are not altered. If an alteration occurs, the label should change to reflect the new values.[3]
- Removal of aliquots from the primary bag for small-volume transfusion, without wasting the remaining components.
- Pooling of individual platelet units, possibly decreasing the risk that bacterial contaminants may enter through spikes or ports during routine pooling.[3]

For two pieces of tubing to be joined, they are placed next to each other in parallel grooves on the sterile connection device. Each of the pieces is then cut with a piece of metal, called a wafer, that has been heated to 260 F. After the cut has been made, one piece of tubing is slid over so it meets the other piece of tubing. The wafer retracts and the two pieces are heat-sealed together.[2] This is illustrated in Fig 10-1.

A recently published paper describes a new sterile connection device (Fresenius NPBI Transfusion Technology, Hamburg, Germany) that does not use the welding wafer to make cuts. Instead, the ends of the tubing that will be joined are placed in blocks and are sealed by using a high-frequency electric field. These pieces of tubing are moved into an area where a heating element is present. The seals are heated, which causes them to melt and open. The heating element is then retracted and the two ends are pushed toward each other, causing them to weld to each other.[4]

Sterile connection devices in use are able to weld both dry tubing and tubing that contains fluid. For adequate weld

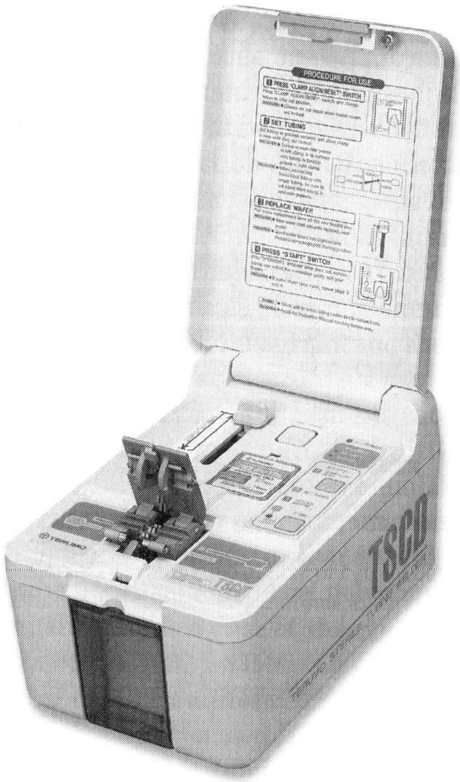

Figure 10-1. Terumo TSCD® sterile tubing welder. Reproduced with permission from Terumo Medical Corp., Somerset, NJ.

strength to be achieved, the average of three welds must maintain 70% of the tensile strength of the tubing being welded, with no weld being less than 50%. Weld strength is dependent upon weld inclusions and misalignments that may occur.[2] After a weld is made, the lumen of the tubing is opened by rolling the weld site gently between the thumb and index finger. At this point, the operator should inspect the site for any openings or misalignments. If the integrity at the welding site is not maintained, such a fault can be a source of contamination of the system.[3,5]

A variety of studies have evaluated the sterility of sterile connection device components. By directly applying bacteria to the tubing of components to be welded together and by aerosolizing bacteria, van der Meer et al[4] showed that sterility could be maintained. AuBuchon et al[5] did similar studies and found a few positive cultures for bacteria. It is unclear whether bacteria isolated in platelet pools that were prepared using a sterile connection device are from the welding site or, more likely, from bacteria that were introduced into the component during donor phlebotomy.[2,5,6] Sterility testing is not recommended as a part of routine QC, because it is known that a certain number of components collected will contain bacteria introduced during collection.[2]

The Food and Drug Administration (FDA) has provided written guidance regarding the use of FDA-approved sterile connection devices. The use of sterile connection devices must be incorporated into standard operating procedures (SOPs) and include record keeping, component tracking, tube weld QC, and maintenance of the lot numbers of disposables. QC procedures should include a test for the integrity of each weld, as discussed above, and procedures should outline the steps taken if the component has air bubbles or leakage. In addition, there should be written procedures for labeling aliquots that allow for tracking the final disposition of the component, especially in the event of a component recall or withdrawal. The appropriate blood unit number and ABO/Rh type must be present on the transfer pack, and all records should allow transfer packs to be traced back to the primary bag.[3] If it is possible, it is best to automate this process through the transfusion service's computer system, but if the computer cannot support this function, it must be done manually.

When a pooled platelet component is made by using a sterile connection device, the outdate period is 4 hours. To prepare a pool with a longer outdate period, a license application must be submitted to the FDA and approved. Despite the fact that the sterile connection device does not change the outdate period for other components, it is believed that pooling may increase the risk of bacterial contamination of platelets, by increasing the volume of the inoculum if bacteria are present in one unit. Increasing the inoculum might in turn allow increased replication of the bacteria.[3]

The FDA does not require additional licensure of components altered by use of a sterile connection device, if its use is consistent with authorized labeling. If, however, a new component is created or a component is changed, so that there are no supporting safety and efficacy data, FDA licensure may be required. Failure to obtain approval may result in the creation of a misbranded component.[3]

Providing Aliquots

RBCs

Traditionally, an aliquot of RBCs was removed by spiking a port on the primary bag and using a transfer bag that would be sent to the floor for transfusion. The remainder of the bag was assigned a 24-hour expiration. When the infant needed another transfusion, frequently >24 hours later, the aliquot would have to come from a different unit. Because the primary bag's volume was reduced after the aliquot was withdrawn, it was unlikely that the primary bag could be used for another patient in that 24-hour period. In this manner, neonates were usually exposed to multiple donors in a short time, and there was considerable waste of the remaining unit.[7] In multiple studies, the use of aliquots prepared from a single unit has been shown to decrease donor exposure.[8-13] (See Chapters 6 and 9 for related discussions on additive solutions and donor exposures.)

Advantages and Disadvantages

In the late 1980s and early 1990s, the concept of decreasing donor exposure for infants, through the provision of aliquots, was becoming popular. With the availability of the sterile connection device, in combination with the data showing that AS-1 was a safe RBC preservative for small-volume transfusion, providing multiple transfusions from a single unit over the entire 42-day storage period became feasible. There was also increasing evidence that, for most indications, the advantages of decreasing donor exposure outweighed the benefits of fresher blood. Another advantage of using a sterile connection device was that the component left in the satellite bag could be used for other infants, which minimized waste. Most transfusion services will assign multiple infants to a single bag of RBCs; usually, a smaller number of sicker infants will be assigned to a unit, with the expectation that they will require more transfusions. Conversely, with larger, less ill infants, more patients can be assigned to an individual unit.[14]

Despite all the advantages cited, concerns over the increase in expense with this method, specifically the costs for specialized bags, welders and wafers, and technologist time, have been raised. Because of the decrease in waste and the proven benefit to patients, this has not been an impediment to implementation. In fact, there is some evidence that these programs can be cost-effective.[15] Another theoretical disadvantage of the use of multiple transfusions from one donor has been possible disease transmission. There has been speculation that an undetected infectious agent in the donor could be transmitted to multiple patients, as one unit of blood is usually assigned to two to four infants.[16(p524)] Additional theoretical concerns about increases in bacterial contamination due to frequent manipulation of these units have not been borne out.[17]

Methods and Options

A variety of systems have been designed specifically for the purpose of providing aliquots for infant transfusion. Some systems are best suited for use in the manufacturing facility, while others can be used in the transfusion service. Whichever method is used, all aliquots must be labeled with their contents and ABO/Rh type and in such a manner that they can be traced back to the original unit. It is important to remember that syringes and transfer bags are meant only as temporary containers for RBCs and should not be used for long-term storage.

The first generation of aliquots was actually produced during manufacturing from blood collected in quadruple-bag collection sets. Using such sets, whole blood is collected into the primary bag with three integrally attached satellite bags. At the time of component production, the plasma is separated and diverted into one bag, leaving three bags for RBC storage. In this manner, the original expiration date is maintained. The transfusion service can then divide the aliquots as needed, using either a heat sealer or metal clips (grommets). For a hospital without a sterile connection device, this will allow the provision of three transfusions as aliquots from a single donor. The disadvantages are the expense of the bags and the fact that the three satellite bags are of larger volume than may be required for a single small-volume transfusion. There might, therefore, still be significant waste.

Another option for hospitals without access to a sterile connection device but that still hope to use small aliquots is the use of "pedipacks," which are six small bags that can be attached in the blood center to a unit of RBCs by use of a sterile connection device. As described in the previous paragraph, the transfusion service can then separate the aliquots, as needed, using metal clips or a heat sealer. This approach maintains the original dating of the unit and gives a larger number of small aliquots for transfusion, in contrast to quadruple-bag sets.

The hospital transfusion service has additional options. There are now a variety of systems available in which primary RBC units can be connected either to transfer packs, small-volume bags, or tubing with integrally attached syringes. There is a system (PEDI-PAK, National Hospital Specialties, Hackensack, NJ) with four 75-mL bags that can be attached to a primary bag. The set can be purchased with or without a 195-micron filter in the tubing, placed between the primary bag and the aliquots. As aliquots are drawn off the main bag, blood passes through the filter. The aliquot is then removed using the sterile connection device. The main bag remains attached to the filter along with the unused bags. Each aliquot is removed in a similar fashion, as needed. If more than four aliquots are needed, a new quadruple-bag PEDI-PAK can be connected using a sterile connection device. Individual labels are affixed to each satellite bag by the manufacturer. This is illustrated in Fig 10-2.

The inability to measure exact volumes is a disadvantage of this system. Volumes are usually measured using weight (1 g = 1

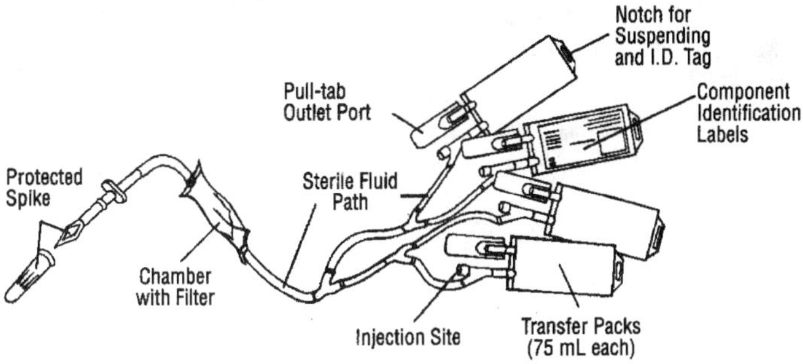

Figure 10-2. Diagram of PEDI-PAK® (reproduced with permission of National Hospital Specialties, Hackensack, NJ).

mL), and they cannot be tailored for individual transfusions, as each aliquot is roughly the same size. Moreover, many nurseries like to use syringe pumps for delivery of the component, which requires nursing staff to transfer the blood from the bag into a syringe before transfusion.[18]

Charter Medical, Ltd. (Winston-Salem, NC) has a variety of bags, syringes, and transfer packs, specifically designed for neonatal transfusion. A plastic syringe [30- or 60-mL (Becton Dickinson, Franklin Lakes, NJ); 35- or 60-mL (Kendall Healthcare, Mansfield, MA)] with integral tubing and a 150-micron in-line filter can be connected to the primary unit using a sterile connection device. The desired amount is drawn out of the primary bag, passing through the filter, by using the syringe. In this manner, the syringe is filled with the required volume and then disconnected by use of the sterile connection device. For subsequent transfusions, additional syringe sets can be added. This is shown in Fig 10-3.

Syringe sets offer a variety of advantages over the use of transfer bags, primarily their flexibility, by allowing the desired volume to be measured precisely each time. Once prepared by the transfusion service, they can be transported to the nursing unit and placed directly into infusion pump devices. This eliminates the intermediate steps of transferring the blood from the bag into a syringe for transfusion. With this step performed in the transfusion service, the extra processing done by busy clinical

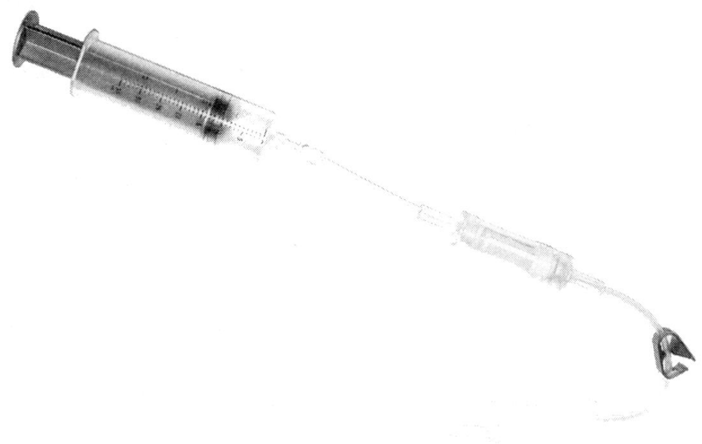

Figure 10-3. Syringe with filter (reproduced with permission from Charter Medical, Ltd, Winston-Salem, NC).

nurses is avoided, as well as the possibility of spilling or losing blood, mislabeling at the bedside, or introducing contaminants. It is important to realize that different infusion systems may need to be adjusted, depending on the brand of syringe used.

A disadvantage of using these products is that they usually cost more when compared to other systems. Another potential problem may be encountered if blood is distributed by a tube-transport system. In some institutions, the transfusion service and many clinical services are spread out over a considerable distance. Most of the blood dispensing at these institutions is done through a tube system. There has been concern that syringes might discharge their contents while traveling through the tubes. Charter Medical reports that it has customers who use the company's products in conjunction with tube-transport systems. If this were a concern, it would probably be prudent to test the integrity of the syringe using other colored solutions.

Each institution should have SOPs that outline how infants are assigned to individual units and what mechanism is used to keep track of the process, to ensure that infants repeatedly receive transfusions from the same bag. As mentioned earlier, it would be ideal to use the computer system, but, if this is not possible, manual tracking is necessary.

Additive Solutions

A discussion of the safety of different anticoagulant-preservative solutions can be found in Chapter 6. Some technical matters should be considered when using blood collected in additive solutions.

Because of the addition of an AS, the hematocrit of an AS unit is lower than that of a unit collected in CPDA-1, 55 to 60% versus 70 to 75%. Therefore, to obtain an equivalent rise in hematocrit with AS, the volume of the transfusion might have to be adjusted.[19] Some blood banks concentrate RBCs given to neonates to achieve a consistent hematocrit of ≥80%.[20] This can be accomplished by storing the unit in an inverted position, with the tubing and ports down, which allows the red cells to concentrate at the bottom of the bag for dispensing. Another possibility is to centrifuge the unit at 1000 × *g* for 4 minutes before preparing the aliquot, to concentrate the red cells.[8,20,21] This is especially helpful if there are volume constraints requiring a smaller volume for each transfusion. It is important to realize that, once a volume-reduced aliquot is prepared, it should be transfused as quickly as possible, as it now lacks the nutrients from the anticoagulant-preservative solution present in the primary bag.[17,22]

Evaluating the effects of centrifugation upon RBC units stored in AS-3, Strauss et al[17] showed that repeated centrifugation itself was not deleterious. There was, though, a greater efflux of potassium into the extracellular fluid of units that had been centrifuged at 5000 × *g* for 5 minutes, with a hematocrit of 90%, and stored in inverted position. By remixing the RBCs after centrifugation, extracellular potassium, hemoglobin, and lactate dehydrogenase were not higher than in units prepared without concentration. The authors concluded that nutrients contained in the storage media are necessary for long-term storage.[17] Transfusion of RBCs that are stored in AS-1 or CPDA-1 and have undergone gravity sedimentation does not appear to cause biochemical or physiologic changes in neonates.[23]

Because of concerns about high levels of supernatant potassium, it is best to irradiate RBCs as close as possible to the time of issue. There are no studies of the safety of transfusing RBCs to infants when they have been irradiated early in their shelf life and are used up by their 28-day outdate. On the basis of calculations of the amount of potassium that is present on various days of storage, in combination with the amount in a simple transfusion, it is probably safe to use irradiated Red Blood Cells up to 28 days, although this has not been demonstrated in clinical trials (R. Strauss, personal communication). Even with the conservative approach of using a 14-day outdate, there is still a demonstrated reduction in donor exposure.[19]

Although studies have shown the safety and efficacy of AS for small-volume transfusion to neonates, there are no data on safety and efficacy in the setting of massive transfusion. A letter from the University of Zurich to the editor of *Pediatrics* in 1990 described an exchange transfusion using AS-1.[24] The authors concluded that exchange using AS-1 resulted in depletion of plasma coagulation protein, as there is very little plasma left in the unit, but there is no mention of any other adverse effects.[24] Likewise, some large transfusion services use AS for large-volume transfusions, without reports of adverse effects.[23] Most transfusions in this setting are still accomplished by using a unit of RBCs stored in CPDA-1, although it is comforting to know that some anecdotal data exist to support the use of additives if there are no alternatives available.

A cautionary note: any time there is acute decompensation after transfusion, there should still be a high degree of suspicion for hyperkalemia. A case report from 1998 describes an infant with complex congenital anomalies who experienced a hyperkalemic arrest after a 10 mL/kg transfusion of RBCs.[26] The implicated unit of blood was at Day 19, or 14 days after leukocyte reduction and irradiation were performed. This blood was transfused through an arterial line, which raises the possibility that transfusion through a central line might increase the risk of severe hyperkalemia.[26] The dynamics of a transfusion through a central line may differ from those of transfusion through a peripheral intravenous line.

As new technologies are introduced, the likelihood increases of more components being collected in new anticoagulant-preservative solutions. As an example, RBCs collected by apheresis using one of the current technologies are preserved in AS-3. Many collection facilities that are incorporating red cell apheresis into their manufacturing processes will target O– and O+ donors for double RBC components. Because many neonates use type O blood, their transfusion needs may be met with RBCs collected by apheresis. This approach may also allow the use in larger children of two different components from the same donor. As new methods of prestorage leukocyte reduction or other changes in manufacturing are introduced, the use of different anticoagulant-preservative solutions will become more common, and it is important to ensure that each can be used safely in sick premature infants.[27,28] Because most blood collection facilities collect the majority of their RBC units in extended storage media, CPDA-1 units are not as readily available, and they might require a special request, which could affect the turnaround time of orders.

Platelets and Fresh Frozen Plasma

Platelets and Platelets Pheresis

After the RBCs are separated from whole blood, Platelets can be prepared from the remaining platelet-rich plasma by using a light spin. The platelets are then resuspended in approximately 50 to 70 mL of plasma. Platelets prepared in this manner are referred to as random-donor platelets (RDPs) or whole-blood-derived platelets. This terminology differentiates them from Platelets Pheresis, which are prepared by apheresis technology and from single-donor platelets (SDPs). Because of their smaller volume, Platelets are more suitable than Platelets Pheresis for use in neonates. Platelets are given in doses of 5 to 10 mL/kg.

Because of the 5-day outdate of platelets and the small volume of a Platelet unit, it is usually not necessary to make sterile aliquots. Moreover, donor exposure is not as much of a concern as it is in red cell transfusion, because most infants do not receive as many platelet transfusions as red cell transfusions. For ease of transfusion, some hospitals will draw the required amount in a labeled syringe and send it to the floor. In other institutions, the unit is sent to the nursing unit and drawn into the syringe before transfusion. The same concerns regarding component manipulation on the nursing unit that are discussed in the section on red cell transfusion apply here.

To deliver a higher dose of platelets per volume transfused, some practitioners choose to volume-reduce platelets. This is accomplished by centrifugation to concentrate the platelets and then by expression of the supernatant plasma. Different facilities have different speeds and times of centrifugation, but, as a general rule, the higher the speed, the less time is required. After centrifugation and plasma removal, the platelets are allowed to rest before being gently resuspended. The harder the spin, the longer the platelets should rest before resuspension. Volume reduction is most important for patients with volume constraints, and it can be especially useful for intrauterine transfusions. Platelets must be washed and volume-reduced when maternal platelets are used to treat neonatal alloimmune thrombocytopenia, to remove the immunizing antibody.[16(p512)] Apheresis technology also has the capability of producing a more concentrated platelet component.[29]

For routine transfusions, it is not necessary to remove excess plasma. With a dose of 10 mL/kg, a standard transfusion has the potential to raise the platelet count of a 1-kg infant by 100,000/μL.[30] It has been commonly believed that manipulation of platelets might cause activation, possibly leading to a suboptimal clinical response.[31] In-vitro studies have shown that degranulation and p-selectin expression, which are markers of activation, increase with manipulation.[32] On the other hand, there is also evidence that volume reduction can be done without harm to the function or later efficacy of the platelets.[33,34] Because there are no studies of posttransfusion survival of washed platelets in neonates, it is best to limit these types of manipulations to clinical situations in which the plasma can be harmful. Of greater concern is the risk of entering the unit and introducing bacteria, which would increase the risk of a septic transfusion reaction. In addition, the outdate of the product is reduced to 4 hours, which is a further complication, especially if the process occurs at a blood center at a distance from the transfusion facility. Any manipulations done at the blood center or in the transfusion service can cause delays in transfusion.

Some blood establishments are collecting an increasing percentage of platelets by apheresis. As a consequence, many hospitals have begun to use these large-volume components (about 300 mL) for neonates by splitting them into aliquots. With rare-blood donors, such as those supplying blood to a thrombocytopenic infant with antibody-negative platelets, having a high-volume component that can be used daily for its entire shelf life is desirable to reduce donor exposure.

When a transfusion service uses a component collected by apheresis for small-volume transfusion, a sterile connection device can be used to weld a transfer pack onto the primary platelet bag, as is done for red cell transfusions. Because no small-volume bags are currently licensed for platelet storage, RBC transfer bags are commonly used. As a consequence, these transfer packs are used only to aliquot, dispense, and transfuse platelets. Platelets should not be stored in these bags for any length of time, as the plastics used for RBC storage will not allow the proper diffusion of gases necessary for optimal platelet survival for the full shelf life. Though in-vitro studies show that platelets remain viable for 4 to 6 hours in syringes, they should be transfused as soon as possible once they are aliquoted.[35,36] The lack of a licensed bag is also a disadvantage for transfusion services without a sterile connection device and whose blood supplier collects most platelets by apheresis. Because of regulatory requirements, blood manufacturers may not be able to attach bags to Platelets Pheresis as the small-volume bags are not approved for platelets.

At the time this chapter is being written, sales representatives from both Baxter and Charter Medical say their companies are working on small-volume platelet bags. Baxter has a working prototype that is being prepared for FDA approval.

Fresh Frozen Plasma

Fresh frozen plasma (FFP) is prepared from plasma that has been separated from whole blood and frozen within 8 hours. It is stored in a frozen state and then thawed for transfusion. For neonates, it is given at a dose of 10 mL/kg. The usual volume of a unit of FFP, which depends on the donor's plasmacrit, is about 200 mL. Plasma that has been thawed can be used for up to 24 hours if refrigerated.

Pediatric FFP is produced so the plasma from one donor is divided into two to three bags of 75 mL each, depending on the volume available. The set of aliquots is connected by using a sterile connection device at the blood manufacturing site. The individual aliquots are usually divided and sent as a group, with the same whole-blood number. Plasma that is collected but not frozen within 8 hours to be labeled as FFP can also be divided into aliquots.

Intrauterine Transfusion

Blood prepared for intrauterine transfusion can be divided into aliquots as described above. It may be difficult to limit donor exposure unless a designated donor is used, as fetal transfusions are usually spread out over time. Volume constraints may be more of a limitation and a challenge in this setting, which makes it important to concentrate components that will be used for transfusion. Knowing that both intrauterine monitoring and transfusion have inherent risk, it is important to transfuse the maximum amount of component while access is available. Moreover, if the patient's mother is used as a source of antigen-negative platelets or red cells, her component must be washed to remove harmful antibody directed against antigens on the infant's cells.

All blood used for intrauterine transfusion should be irradiated, and after delivery the infant should continue receiving irradiated blood components.[16] Because of the special requirements for blood components used for fetal transfusion, it is important to discuss any needs with the transfusion service well in advance of the need. This will facilitate the process if special arrangements have to be made with the local blood center to provide the appropriate components, such as recruiting a particular donor. This can ensure that the component is available at the time of the procedure.

Irradiation and Filtration

As discussed earlier, it is best to irradiate components immediately before transfusion, because irradiation accelerates the RBC storage lesion. If the transfusion service irradiates its own blood, this can be accomplished easily. Syringes, though, present a challenge in that they are hard to fit into some irradiator canisters when the plunger is maximally withdrawn. Charter Medical, LTD, has a product, illustrated in Fig 10-4, that can help solve this problem—a syringe with a 150-mL transfer pack attached. Blood can be drawn into the syringe and then dispensed into the transfer pack for irradiation. This allows the plunger of the syringe to be fully depressed, so the set can fit into the irradiator. Once the irradiation is complete, the blood can be transferred back into the syringe and dispensed to the patient. Of course, transfusion services without their own irradiator will receive a unit of RBCs that has been irradiated before storage, which limits its outdate to 28 days. It is interesting to note that there is currently no dose mapping available for irradiation performed in syringes, although this is a common practice.

Filtration of units dispensed as aliquots has been a controversial topic. In accordance with the standards of the American Association of Blood Banks, blood and components shall be transfused through a sterile, pyrogen-free transfusion set that has a filter designed to retain particles potentially harmful to the recipient (5.18.8).[37] Because of the logistics of small-volume transfusion and the system used in the particular institution, bedside filtration is not always possible for small-volume transfusions. Many transfusion services chose to consider the filtra-

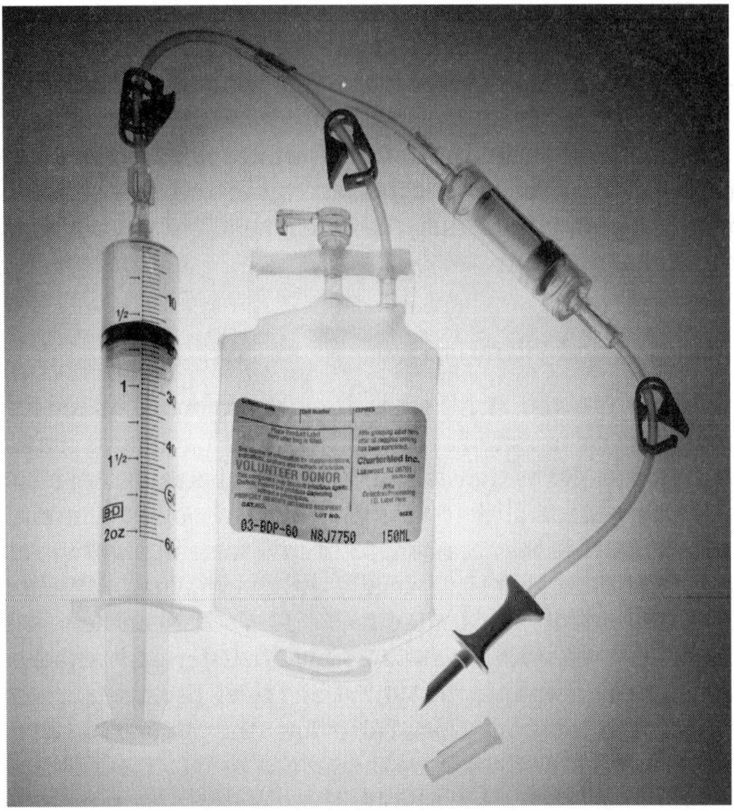

Figure 10-4. Syringe with filter and attached transfer bag (reproduced with permission from Charter Medical, Ltd., Winston-Salem, NC).

tion performed in the blood bank at the time of dispensing as the final filtration step. Concern about whether this practice was in violation of the standards led to extensive discussion, with later clarification in the final edition of the *Accreditation Requirements Manual*[38] of the AABB. This publication states that only one filtration step is necessary for infant transfusion, and it can occur either between the syringe and the infant or between the blood container and the syringe.[38] This is quite simple when the syringe and bag sets described previously are used. There is no conclusive evidence that microaggregates are detrimental to neonatal recipients, although some theorize this could become a problem when RBCs are used up to their outdate.[22]

Leukocyte reduction has not been proven to be necessary for blood transfused to neonates.[39,40] Some hospitals that exclusively use leukocyte-reduced components also use them in neonates. This makes inventory management simpler and may be necessary because of the component mix provided by their blood supplier. In addition, leukocyte reduction has been accepted as a means of decreasing the risk of cytomegalovirus (CMV) transmission and is used by some in lieu of CMV-seronegative blood.[16(p522),41] Although not all of the benefits of universal leukocyte reduction are universally accepted, some neonatologists feel the removal of leukocytes makes empirical sense, and they use leukocyte-reduced blood in neonates for that reason.

Current Good Manufacturing Practice

It is important to remember that manufacturers of blood and blood components are required to follow current good manufacturing practice (cGMP), in accordance with FDA rules and regulations. Whereas, in the past, many product manipulations could be performed by blood centers to meet highly specialized needs, this is no longer possible. The manufacturer must have a written SOP, with documented, up-to-date staff training and proficiency, for each product and variation in production.

Autologous Blood Collection

Autologous donation evolved as an early strategy designed to decrease the risks of transfusion transmission of disease. As testing for infectious diseases improves and knowledge about blood safety grows, leading to better donor screening, the necessity for autologous donation and transfusion is questioned. It is also increasingly recognized that there are complications that can result from autologous transfusion; neither the donation process nor subsequent transfusion is risk-free. Because of the perception that autologous donation and collection are unequivocally safe, autologous blood is commonly over-collected. The autologous donor, however, should be thought of as a patient, who is more likely to have undergone an invasive procedure in preparation for surgery and who may be at higher risk of donating a unit of blood that contains occult bacteria. There have been numerous reports of asymptomatic autologous donors whose death was the direct result of receiving their own blood that was later found to contain bacterial contaminants.[42]

Autologous donation itself has also been found to render the patient anemic at the time of surgery, possibly increasing the risk of ischemia and in turn creating the need for transfusion.[43] To justify some of the risks associated with collection, it is important that autologous blood be collected only if there is a great likelihood that it will be used.[44,45] Medical contraindications to autologous donation include any underlying condition that could be worsened by hypovolemia (eg, heart disease), bacterial infection, and an uncontrolled seizure disorder, as donation can trigger seizure activity[16(p107)] (see Table 10-1).

Table 10-1. Autologous Transfusion in Children

Advantages	Disadvantages
Decreased risk of viral infection	Risk of donation, depending on underlying illness
Decreased risk of alloimmunization	Risks of occult bacteremia
Decreased risk of graft-vs-host disease	Risks of hypovolemia in young children and infants
Decreased risk of transfusion-related acute lung injury	Risk of anemia with lower iron stores
Supply own antigen-negative blood	Problems with venous access
	Lack of cooperation

On the other hand, because of long potential life spans and the unlikelihood of a zero-risk blood supply, a child who can reap the benefits of getting back his or her own blood may be even better served by autologous transfusion than an adult. Studies of the quality-adjusted life year or the economic cost-effectiveness of medical treatment would probably be more favorable if calculations were done for children who donate and receive their own blood rather than for adults.[46] In addition, a healthy child undergoing an elective procedure is far more likely to make a complete recovery than an older adult with underlying medical disease. For children who are severely alloimmunized, there might be situations in which autologous blood is the only means of providing compatible blood. This may be especially important in children with hemoglobinopathies.[47]

Many studies document the safety of autologous donation, as well as its ability to markedly decrease the use of allogeneic blood, in infants and children. Studies have evaluated donations during infancy, from as early as 3 months of age, and have also evaluated safety during intraoperative recovery and acute normovolemic hemodilution. Several references cite some of these studies.[48-57]

Infants and small children represent a different group of autologous donor-patients than their adult counterparts. The major differences are in the decreased ability in young children and infants to compensate for volume changes, to cooperate, and to understand the procedure; problems with venous access; and their smaller blood volume.

In small children and infants, the lack of cooperation may make obtaining autologous blood difficult. An interesting study by Masuda et al[48] outlined the process of collecting autologous blood during cardiac catheterization before surgery. Because the children (including an infant 6 months of age) were sedated for catheterization, cooperation was not a problem. In addition, vascular access used for the catheterization was used for the first collection. Blood (10 mL/kg) was collected from the arterial access while lactated Ringer's solution was infused through the venous access.[48] In this study, as well as others, the use of sedatives and topical anesthetics was found to be helpful.[49]

An abstract presented at the Annual Meeting of the AABB in 1997 reported on an evaluation of the safety of autologous donation in the pediatric population.[50] In this study, autologous blood was collected from 106 children, ranging in age from 3 months to 10 years. Donation and subsequent transfusion appeared to be well tolerated, with the exception of the practical logistics of obtaining the blood. According to discussions during the presentation at the meeting, some infants required sedation. Despite the fact that allogeneic transfusion was avoided in 95.2% of surgical procedures performed, the risks and benefits must be carefully weighed in very small children.

It is also important to remember that donors below legal age of majority cannot give their own informed consent. The parents or legal guardians must also understand the risks and benefits of autologous donation and transfusion and must be available to give consent.

Though no consensus appears on the use of volume replacement, smaller children and infants are sometimes given crystalloid solutions during or after autologous donation, to decrease the risks of hypovolemia. This is more common when the child is under the age of 4 years, because of concerns that there might be a decreased ability for the cardiovascular system of persons in this age range to compensate for volume loss. It appears that the rate of vasovagal reaction reported in autologous donation in these settings is lower than the rates reported in adult populations.[49] Programs that collect blood from small children may benefit from additional skilled medical personnel, with the ability to set up an intravenous line and infuse fluids. This is a population who may do better when distraction techniques are used and extra attention is given by the phlebotomy staff.[49,56] Many programs also advocate the use of iron supplementation, as children have lower stores of iron.[49]

Another consideration is the size of the needle used. Standard adult blood bags are equipped with a 16-gauge needle, which might be too large for a child's veins. A smaller needle, between 17- and 20-gauge, can be attached using a sterile connection device, before the collection process. It is important to realize that, the smaller the needle, the greater the concern for hemolysis occurring during the collection process. Therefore, it is best to use needles with the largest gauge lumen that can be tolerated.[51]

Obviously, the greatest risks of autologous donation in small children include volume depletion during the collection, with concerns of increased autonomic lability. A recent study of healthy volunteer whole-blood donors might have some applicability for teenagers who donate autologous blood.[49] Using logistic regression analysis, the authors found that younger age, lower weight, and first-time donor status were associated with higher rates of vasovagal reaction during blood donation.[58]

Any donor weighing less than 110 lb (50 kg) is considered a small-volume donor. When a unit of RBCs is collected from a small-volume donor, the volume collected must not exceed 10.5 mL/kg of the donor's weight.[16(p93)] Moreover, the volume of anticoagulant must be adjusted in proportion to the decreased collection volume. This will prevent the side effects of excess citrate that can occur on reinfusion. Anticoagulant can be removed while sterility is maintained by the use of a sterile connection device. A standard adult collection set can be used for volumes as low as 300 mL without having to change the amount of anticoagulant.

For collections less than 300 mL, the anticoagulant can be reduced by expressing the desired amount into a satellite bag and then sealing the tubing using a sterile connection device. These calculations are shown in Table 10-2.[16(p94)] The Terumo Medical Corporation (Somerset, NJ) makes a bag that is used for collection of a maximum volume of 250 mL. It is composed of AS-5 (42-day outdate) with a 17-gauge needle attached. For donors with smaller blood volume, this decreases the need to remove excess anticoagulant. Baxter also makes a small-volume bag for 250-mL collections. The bag has a 16-gauge needle and uses CPD as the anticoagulant-preservative (21-day outdate period). There is no sampling pouch, which makes removal of samples for testing difficult. Baxter also has a CPDA-1 (35-day outdate) quadruple-bag unit with a primary bag of 250 mL and three empty 150-mL transfer packs, a 17-gauge needle, and a sampling site.

Table 10-2. Calculations for Drawing Blood from Low-Volume Pediatric Blood Donors (<110 lb or 50 kg)

A = Volume to Draw =	(Donor's weight in kg ÷ 50) × 450 mL*
B = Amount of Anticoagulant* Needed =	(A ÷ 100) × 14
C = Amount of Anticoagulant to Remove =	63 mL – B

*1 mL = 1 g.
†CPD or CPDA-1. Optimal anticoagulant:blood ratio is 1.4:10
Adapted with permission from Brecher.[16(p96)]

Directed Donors

The use of directed donors, or patient-selected donors, became popular in the late 1980s, because of heightened concern about transfusion transmission of disease. When a patient was medically unable to donate blood for himself or herself, or when there wasn't enough time before surgery to collect autologous units, the patient might ask friends or relatives to provide blood. It has never been proven that blood from directed donors is safer than blood from volunteer donors. There are, in fact, concerns that blood from directed donors might be less safe than blood from the general population, theoretically because of the risk that they feel coerced to provide blood when asked and thus may not be totally honest about their risk behavior.[59] With regard to the pediatric population, however, parents are usually very motivated to try to help support their infants, so they may represent a different population from other directed donors and might be an appropriate choice for transfusion support.[60]

With regard to the neonatal population, there are additional immunologic factors that must be considered. If a mother has been immunized by an antigen inherited by the infant from its father, maternal plasma products containing the antibody are not an appropriate choice for the infant's transfusion. Furthermore, the father and his relatives would not be a good choice for cellular transfusion needs in this circumstance, as passively acquired maternal antibodies may still be present in the infant's circulation after birth. Both these scenarios could increase the risk of destruction of neonatal blood components. When taking these concerns into account, relying on parents as the sole source of blood for their infants may not be practical.[61]

Umbilical Cord Blood

Another approach that has been explored to meet transfusion needs of infants is the use of umbilical cord blood (UCB). Because placental vessels contain anywhere from 75 to 125 mL of blood, it has been postulated that this otherwise wasted resource could serve for autologous transfusion.[62] A variety of methods for collection employ withdrawal of blood from the umbilical vein.[62,63] The umbilical vein is usually "sterilized" with betadine and/or alcohol swabs and then entered with a sterile needle. Usually, this is done after delivery and cord clamping. Collection can also be done after the infant is delivered but before cord clamping, using the placental contractions to aid in the process. Special collection sets are now available that have CPD in the primary bag and integrally connected satellite bags. There are also sets that are configured for freezing progenitor cells, available from Pall Corporation (East Hills, NJ).

Studies of in-vitro characteristics of UCB as well as in-vivo transfusion experience have yielded variable results. In a study by Ballin et al[62] a 1250-g triplet was successfully transfused with two 10-mL aliquots of UCB with good clinical response and without any adverse consequences reported. After collection of 120 UCB samples, with a mean volume of 44 mL from premature infants and a mean volume of 86 mL from full-term infants, all samples were sterile.[62] This is contrast to other studies that report significant rates of bacterial contamination of 9.7%[64] and 8.6%.[65] The most common organisms cultured reflect vaginal flora. The bacterial contamination rate will most likely be higher when chorioamniotitis or neonatal sepsis is present.[66] As a result, it is recommended that UCB should be quarantined for 3 to 5 days, pending results of bacterial culture.[64-66]

Despite the fact that UCB transfusion is feasible and has not resulted in complications, various questions still exist. Because the amount of blood collected is not large, an infant may receive only one to three transfusions, at most, of UCB. Whether this results in a true benefit and greatly reduces overall donor exposure has not been proven. In addition, concerns about bacterial contamination rates, the viability and quality of red cells in comparison with those from adult banked blood, and the true efficacy of such transfusions remain unresolved.[67,68] With the improving safety of blood, more conservative transfusion practices, and the decrease in donor exposure obtained by assigning units of blood stored until their outdate, the overall yield in safety of using UCB may not justify its use.[67,69] As pointed out by Eichler et al,[65] the smallest infants and most heavily transfused infants, those weighing <1000 g, are the most difficult from whom to collect UCB for transfusion. On the other hand, infants weighing over 1400 g at birth are unlikely to receive any transfusions.[65]

Some of the unique benefits of cord blood transfusion must also be weighed. With a source of UCB, it is true that the infant has a ready source of dedicated blood with decreased risk of allogeneic pathogen and immunologic exposures. In addition, reinfusing the progenitor cells contained in UCB may result in an increase in marrow erythropoiesis and an enhancement of host defenses to combat infection.[62]

An ethical concern about the timing of clamping the umbilical cord has been underscored. In an attempt to collect UCB, the cord may be clamped early, at a time that is not ideal for the infant. By delaying the clamping of the cord, a generous fetal-placental transfusion can take place, increasing the infant's postdelivery red cell mass. This transfer of blood to the infant at the time of the delivery is usually well tolerated. The disadvantages are the increased volume and viscosity, as well as risks that arise if the mother is immunized and transfers additional antibody to the infant.[22,69,70] In any event, this method of transfusion may have a place in meeting the needs of select infants requiring transfusion support.

Conclusion

Recognizing the unique needs of neonates and older children has led to the development of novel approaches to meeting their transfusion requirements. By the use of sterile connection devices to maintain the integrity of the primary bag of a blood component, donor exposure has been significantly reduced in the neonatal population. Autologous transfusion has also reduced children's exposure to allogeneic blood. In smaller patients, however, the logistics required to collect these units may not outweigh the risks they incur. Finally, thanks to creative and innovative thinking, new approaches to meeting these needs continue to unfold. Just as Dustin Hoffman's character was told in "The Graduate"—plastics, they're the future.

Acknowledgments

The author thanks the following persons who provided technical assistance during the preparation of this chapter: Valli R. Criss, MT(ASCP)SBB, Children's National Medical Center; Amy Graham, NHS; Maria Milani, Charter Medical Limited; Cheryl Jones, MT(ASCP), American Red Cross Biomedical Services, Tennessee Valley Region; Gene Propst, Baxter Healthcare; Patricia Reilly, MT(ASCP)SBB, Terumo Medical Corporation; Ann Marie Southers, MT(ASCP)SBB, Virginia Commonwealth University Health Systems; Katherine H. Tinsley, MT(ASCP)SBB, American Red Cross Biomedical Service, Appalachian Region; and Judith S. Wolfe, MS, MT(ASCP)SBB, American Red Cross Biomedical Services, National Testing and Reference Laboratory.

References

1. Webb CI, Willingham C, Henry B, writers; Levine JE, executive producer. "The Graduate." Hollywood, CA: Embassy Pictures Corporation, 1967.
2. Kothe FC, Platenkamp GJ. The use of the sterile connecting device in transfusion medicine. Transfus Med Rev 1994;8:117-22.
3. Food and Drug Administration. Guidance for industry: Use of sterile connecting devices in blood bank practices. (November 22, 2000) Rockville, MD: CBER Office of Communication, Training, and Manufacturers Assistance, 2000.

4. Van der Meer PF, Biekart FT, Pietersz RNI, et al. Compodock, a new device for sterile docking. Transfusion 2000;40:682-6.
5. AuBuchon JP, Pickard C, Herschel L. Sterility of plastic tubing welds in components stored at room temperature. Transfusion 1995;35:303-7.
6. Mertens G, Muylle L, Goossens H. Possible implication of sterile connecting device in contamination of pooled platelet concentrates. Transfus Sci 1997;18:387-92.
7. Strauss RG, Sacher RA, Blazina JF, et al. Commentary on small-volume red cell transfusions for neonatal patients. Transfusion 1990;30:565-70.
8. Strauss RG, Burmeister LF, Johnson K, et al. AS-1 red cells for neonatal transfusions: A randomized trial assessing donor exposure and safety. Transfusion 1996;36:873-8.
9. Cook S, Gunter J, Wissel M. Effective use of a strategy using assigned red cell units to limit donor exposure for neonatal patients. Transfusion 1993;33:379-83.
10. Wang-Rodriguez J, Mannino FL, Liu E, et al. A novel strategy to limit blood donor exposure and blood waste in multiply transfused premature infants. Transfusion 1996;36:64-70.
11. Liu EA, Mannino FL, Lane TA. Prospective randomized trial of the safety and efficacy of a limited donor exposure transfusion program for premature neonates. J Pediatr 1994;125:92-6.
12. Bednarek FJ, Weisberger S, Richardson DK, et al. Variations in blood transfusions among newborn intensive care units. J Pediatr 1998; 133:601-7.
13. Maier RF, Sonntag J, Walka MW, et al. Changing practices of red blood cell transfusions in infants with birth weights less than 1000 g. J Pediatr 2000;136:220-4.
14. Strauss RG. Practical issues in neonatal transfusion practice. Am J Clin Pathol 1997;107(S1):S57-S63.
15. Hilsenrath P, Nemechek J, Widness JA, et al. Cost-effectiveness of a limited-donor blood program for neonatal red cell transfusions. Transfusion 1999;39:938-43.
16. Brecher ME, ed. Technical manual. 14th ed. Bethesda, MD: American Association of Blood Banks, 2002.
17. Strauss RG, Villhauer PJ, Cordle DG. A method to collect, store and issue multiple aliquots of packed red blood cells for neonatal transfusions. Vox Sang 1995;68:77-81.
18. Chambers LA. Evaluation of a filter-syringe set for preparation of packed cell aliquots for neonatal transfusion. Am J Clin Pathol 1995;104:253-7.
19. Strauss RG. Routinely washing irradiated red cells before transfusion seems unwarranted (editorial). Transfusion 1990;30:675-7.
20. Strauss RG. Blood banking issues pertaining to neonatal red blood cell transfusions. Transfus Sci 1999;21:7-19.

21. Sherwood WC, Conato T, Clapper C, et al. The concentration of AS-1 RBCs after inverted gravity sedimentation for neonatal transfusions (letter). Transfusion 2000;40:618-19.
22. Hume H, Bard H. Small volume red blood cell transfusions for neonatal patients. Transfus Med Rev 1995;9:187-99.
23. Gooch WM III, Longhurst D, Sasich R, et al. Safety of neonatal transfusion of gravity-sedimented RBC's following storage in CPDA-1 or Adsol (abstract). Transfusion 1986;26(Suppl):562.
24. Tuchschmid P, Mieth D, Burger R, et al. Potential hazard of hypoalbuminemia in newborn babies after exchange transfusions with Adsol red blood cell concentrates (letter). Pediatrics 1990;85:234-5.
25. Brecher ME, ed. Collected questions and answers. 6th ed. Bethesda, MD: American Association of Blood Banks, 2000:73-5.
26. Harris V, Lumadue J, Luban NLC, et al. Transfusion-related hyperkalemic arrest from irradiated packed red blood cells (abstract). Transfusion 1998;38(Suppl):69S.
27. Elfath MD, Whitley P, Jacobson MS, et al. Evaluation of an automated system for the collection of packed RBCs, platelets, and plasma. Transfusion 2000;40:1214-22.
28. Högman CF, Knutson F. Standardized units of RBCs: Is it time for implementation? Transfusion 2000;40:330-4.
29. Dumont LJ, Krailadsiri P, Seghatchian J, et al. Preparation and storage characteristics of white cell-reduced high-concentration platelet concentrates collected by an apheresis system for transfusions in utero. Transfusion 2000;40:91-100.
30. Strauss RG. Transfusion therapy in neonates. Am J Dis Child 1991;1145:904-11.
31. Pineda AA, Zylstra VW, Clare DE, et al. Viability and functional integrity of washed platelets. Transfusion 1989;29:524-7.
32. Holme S, Sweeney JD, Sawyer S, et al. The expression of p-selectin during collection, processing, and storage of platelet concentrates: Relationship to loss of in vivo viability. Transfusion 1997;37:12-17.
33. Moroff G, Friedman A, Robkin-Kline F, et al. Reduction of the volume of stored platelet concentrates for use in neonatal patients. Transfusion 1984;24:144-6.
34. Simon TL, Sierra ER. Concentration of platelet units into small volumes. Transfusion 1984;24:173-5.
35. Pisciotto PT, Snyder EL, Napychank PA, et al. In vitro characteristics of volume-reduced platelet concentrate stored in syringes. Transfusion 1991;31:404-8.
36. Werch J, Banez EI, Crump L, et al. CD61 and CD 62 studies for in vitro evaluation of viability of syringe aliquots of platelet concentrates (abstract). Transfusion 1997;37(Suppl):67S.
37. Gorlin JB, ed. Standards for blood banks and transfusion services. 21st ed. Bethesda, MD: American Association of Blood Banks, 2002:53-4.

38. Sazama K, ed. Accreditation requirements manual. 6th ed. Bethesda, MD: American Association of Blood Banks, 1995:126.
39. Strauss RG. Selection of white cell-reduced blood components for transfusion during early infancy. Transfusion 1993;33:352-7.
40. Strauss RG, Johnson K, Cress G, et al. Alloimmunization in preterm infants after repeated transfusions of WBC-reduced RBCs from the same donor. Transfusion 2000:40:1463-8.
41. Gilbert GL, Hayes K, Hudson H, et al. Prevention of transfusion-associated cytomegalovirus infection in infants by blood filtration to remove leukocytes. Lancet 1989;1:1228-31.
42. Haditsch M, Binder L, Gabriel C, et al. *Yersinia enterocolitica septicemia* in autologous blood transfusion. Transfusion 1994;40:907-9.
43. Cohen J, Brecher ME. Preoperative autologous blood donation: Benefit or detriment? A mathematical analysis. Transfusion 1995;35:640-4.
44. Kanter MH, van Maanen D, Anders KH, et al. A study of an educational intervention to decrease inappropriate preoperative autologous blood donation: Its effectiveness and the effect of subsequent transfusion rates in elective hysterectomy. Transfusion 1999;39:801-7.
45. Linden JV, Kruskall M. Autologous blood: Always safer? (editorial). Transfusion 1997;37:455-6.
46. Etchason J, Petz L, Keeler E, et al. The cost effectiveness of preoperative autologous blood donations. N Engl J Med 1995;332:719-24.
47. Chaplin H, Mischeaux JR, Inkster MD, et al. Frozen storage of 11 units of sickle cell red cells for autologous transfusion of a single patient. Transfusion 1986;26:341-5.
48. Masuda M, Kawachi Y, Inaba S, et al. Preoperative autologous blood donations in pediatric cardiac surgery. Ann Thorac Surg 1995;60:1694-7.
49. Murto KTT, Splinter WM. Perioperative autologous blood donation in children. Transfus Sci 1999;21:41-62.
50. Hoshi Y, Maki N, Asai O. Predeposit autologous blood transfusion in infants and children (abstract). Transfusion 1997;37(Suppl):66S.
51. Thompson HW, Luban NLC. Autologous blood transfusion in the pediatric patient. J Pediatr Surg 1995;30:1406-11.
52. Novak RW. Autologous blood transfusion in a pediatric population. Safety and efficacy. Clin Pediatr 1988;27:184-7.
53. Spain DA, Miller FB, Bergamini TM, et al. Quality assessment of intraoperative blood salvage and autotransfusion. Am Surg 1997;63:1059-63.
54. Hishon ML, Ryan A, Lithgow P, et al. An evaluation of changes in composition and contamination of salvaged blood from the cardiopulmonary bypass circuit of pediatric patients. Heart Lung 1995;42:307-11.
55. Velardi F, DiChirico A, DiRocco C, et al. "No allogeneic blood transfusion" protocol for the surgical correction of craniosyntoses, II. Clinical application. Childs Nerv Syst 1998;14:732-9.
56. Silvergleid AJ. Safety and effectiveness of predeposit autologous transfusions in preteen and adolescent children. JAMA 1987;257:3403-4.

57. Tasaki T, Ohto H, Abe R, et al. New "leap-frog" technique for autologous blood donation. Transfus Sci 1991;12:307-10.
58. Trouern-Trend JJ, Cable RG, Badon SJ, et al. A case-controlled multicenter study of vasovagal reactions in blood donors: Influence of sex, age, donation status, weight, blood pressure, and pulse. Transfusion 1999;39:316-20.
59. Starkey JM, MacPherson JL, Bolgiano DC, et al. Markers for transfusion-transmitted disease in different groups of blood donors. JAMA 1989;262:3452-4.
60. Luban NLC, Criss VR, Coles-Bell S. Use of parental directed donations for pediatric transfusion (abstract). Transfusion 1987;27:574.
61. Elbert C, Strauss RG, Barrett F, et al. Biological mothers may be dangerous blood donors for their neonates. Acta Haematol 1991;85:189-91.
62. Ballin A, Arbel E, Kenet G, et al. Autologous umbilical cord blood transfusion. Arch Dis Child 1995;73:F181-3.
63. Armitage S. Collection and processing of cord blood units. In: Cohen SBA, Gluckman E, Rubinstein P, Madrigal JA, eds. Cord blood characteristics: Role in stem cell transplantation. Malden, MA: Blackwell Science, 2000:129-48.
64. Golden SM, O'Brien WF, Lissner C, et al. Hematologic and bacteriologic assessment of autologous blood for neonatal transfusions. J Pediatr 1980;97:810-12.
65. Eichler H, Schaible T, Richter E, et al. Cord blood as a source of autologous RBCs for transfusion to preterm infants. Transfusion 2000; 40:1111-7.
66. Surbek DV, Glanzmann R, Senn HP, et al. Can cord blood be used for autologous transfusion in preterm neonates? Eur J Pediatr 2000;159: 790-1.
67. Strauss RG. Autologous transfusions for neonates using placental blood, a cautionary note (editorial). Am J Dis Child 1992;146:21-2.
68. Horn S, Mazor D, Zmora E, et al. Storage-induced changes in human newborn red cells. Transfusion 1987;27:411-14.
69. Beattie R, Stark JM, Wardrop CAJ, et al. Autologous umbilical cord blood transfusion (letter). Arch Dis Child 1996;74:F221.
70. Kinmond S, Aitchison TC, Holland BM, et al. Umbilical cord clamping and preterm infants: A randomized trial. Br Med J 1993;306:172-5.

Appendix 10-1. Suggested Internet Resources

www.baxter.com
www.chatermed.com
www.nhsusa.com
www.pall.com
www.terumo.com

In: Herman JH, Manno CS, eds.
Pediatric Transfusion Therapy
Bethesda, MD: AABB Press, 2002

11

Alloimmunization in Patients with Sickle Cell Disease

KIM SMITH-WHITLEY, MD

RED CELL TRANSFUSIONS ARE COMMON in the management of sickle cell disease (SCD) because they reduce disease-related morbidity and mortality. However, the benefits of transfusion therapy must be weighed against the frequent development of transfusion-related complications such as iron overload and red cell alloimmunization. Red cell alloimmunization in patients with SCD is primarily due to disparities between red cell antigens in the blood donor population, predominantly those of European ancestry, and in the patient population, predominantly those of African ancestry. The complications of red cell alloimmunization

Kim Smith-Whitley, MD, Assistant Professor, Department of Pediatrics, University of Pennsylvania School of Medicine, Division of Hematology, The Children's Hospital of Philadelphia, Philadelphia, Pennsylvania

can lead to obstacles that limit safe, lifesaving red cell transfusion therapy in alloimmunized patients with SCD. Subsequently, transfusion practices that reduce the development of red cell alloantibodies could have a major impact on the medical management of patients with SCD.

This chapter provides an update on alloimmunization and its complications in patients with SCD. An overview of transfusion therapy is followed by a discussion of the epidemiology, complications, and management of red cell alloimmunization and immune-mediated hemolysis in patients with SCD. Then, transfusion programs to increase Red Blood Cell (RBC) unit availability and to decrease alloimmunization are analyzed. Controversies regarding appropriate RBC unit selection to prevent alloimmunization are discussed. The chapter concludes with a section on future directions in transfusion therapy for patients with SCD.

Red Cell Transfusion Therapy in Patients with SCD

SCD, a hemoglobinopathy in which sickle hemoglobin (Hb S) predominates, is characterized by chronic hemolytic anemia and complications caused by vaso-occlusion. Red cell transfusions benefit patients with SCD by increasing oxygen-carrying capacity, suppressing sickle erythropoiesis, and reducing the percentage of red cells containing primarily Hb S by increasing the concentration of those containing primarily Hb A. Acute or episodic transfusions are administered to prevent the occurrence of acute complications or to reduce the morbidity of acute complications once they develop. Long-term transfusion (chronic transfusion therapy) are administered to prevent the development or recurrence of acute complications or to reduce the morbidity of chronic complications. The following sections address transfusion methods and specific clinical indications for transfusion in patients with SCD.

Methods of Red Cell Administration

Two methods of red cell administration—simple and exchange transfusion—are used routinely in patients with SCD. In the short term, simple transfusions increase the hemoglobin level and provide a mild or moderate decrease in the relative proportion of Hb-S-containing red cells, depending on the volume of red cells administered. Frequently repeated, simple transfusions can maintain a low Hb S percentage. If these transfusions are administered over the long term, as in chronic transfusion therapy, iron overload is inevitable. In comparison, acute exchange transfusions rapidly and significantly decrease the relative proportion of Hb-S-containing red cells with or without an increase in the hemoglobin level. Chronic exchange transfusions can reduce iron overload while maintaining a low Hb S percentage. Compared with simple transfusions, exchange transfusions require larger volumes of red cells, thereby increasing donor exposure.

Indications for Red Cell Transfusion Therapy

The following provides a brief overview of the clinical indications for transfusion therapy in patients with SCD. For detailed discussions on these indications, the reader is referred to recent reviews.[1-4]

Acute red cell transfusions reduce the morbidity and mortality associated with acute chest syndrome[5-7] and severe exacerbation of anemia due to transient red cell aplasia[8] or acute splenic sequestration episodes.[9] Transfusions for acute stroke may reduce extension of cerebral infarction but whether they improve long-term neurologic outcome is unproven.[10] Complications related to general anesthesia[11,12] and hyperionic radiographic contrast media can be prevented by transfusions in this patient population. In these situations, many clinicians agree that transfusion therapy is the standard of care for patients with SCD. However, reports vary on the benefits of episodic transfusions for other clinical complications such as transient ischemic attacks or priapism. Here, the indication for transfusion therapy is controversial.

Chronic transfusion therapy lowers stroke risk in children with abnormal transcranial Doppler (TCD) ultrasound results,[13] a risk factor for primary stroke in patients with SCD, and reduces stroke recurrence in those with a history of infarctive stroke.[14-17] Other complications such as painful episodes, acute chest syndrome, and priapism are reduced as well.[18,19] The use of chronic transfusion therapy to manage pregnant patients with SCD[20,21] or those with neurologic complications other than overt stroke is controversial.[3] Table 11-1 summarizes the standard and controversial indications for transfusion therapy in patients with SCD.

Frequency of Red Cell Transfusions

Because red cell transfusions have benefited patients with SCD, the majority of patients have received not only one, but multiple, red cell transfusions in their lifetimes. In the Cooperative Study of Sickle Cell Disease (CSSCD), which enrolled over 3000 patients with SCD, 50% of adults had received red cell transfusions at the time of study entry and 5.2% were receiving chronic transfusion therapy.[23] Nearly 60% received blood transfusions by 20 years of age and over 80% received transfusions in their lifetimes. Smaller studies reported a range of 13 to 23 transfusions in the first four decades of life.[24]

Since 1988, the end of study enrollment for adults in the CSSCD, the indications for transfusion therapy have broadened and the life expectancy of patients with SCD has improved. Subsequently, the number of RBC units administered to patients with SCD has improved over the last two decades. As the use of red cell transfusions increases in this patient population, so will transfusion-related complications such as alloimmunization.

Epidemiology of Alloimmunization in Patients with SCD

Red cell transfusion therapy is complicated by alloimmunization in 18% to 47% of patients with SCD[21,23-37] compared with 2.6% in the general population.[38] Although these data primarily represent prevalence estimates, similar discrepancies between the population of patients with SCD and the general population are reported on the incidence of alloimmunization. The CSSCD is the only report to measure the incidence of alloimmunization in a large population of patients with SCD transfused primarily with non-antigen-matched RBC units.[23] During the course of the study, 908 patients who were not previously alloimmunized re-

Table 11-1. Indications for Red Cell Transfusion Therapy in Patients with Sickle Cell Disease[1-3,22]

	Consensus Group	Other Investigators

Episodic or acute	Standard
	• Acute exacerbation of anemia
	  • Acute splenic or hepatic sequestration
	  • Transient red cell aplasia (aplastic crisis)
	  • Symptomatic anemia of unknown etiology
	• Acute chest syndrome
	• Stroke
	• Pre-general anesthesia
	• Pre-administration of hyperionic radiographic contrasts
	Controversial
	• Priapism
	• Transient ischemic attacks
		Controversial
		• Priapism
		• Acute painful episodes
		• Preadministration of radiographic contrasts (gadolinium)

Chronic	Standard
	• Stroke
	  • Primary prevention(repeatedly abnormal transcranial Doppler ultrasound results)
	  • Secondary prevention
	• Acute chest syndrome
	• Pain
	• Acute splenic sequestration in young children
	• Priapism
	Controversial
	• Pregnancy
	• Transient ischemic attacks
		Controversial
		• Priapism
		• Silent cerebral infarcts
		• Neurocognitive defects
		• Leg ulcers
		• Growth and developmental delays
		• Early renal disease
		• Early retinopathy

ceived red cell transfusions. New alloantibodies formed in 15.5% of patients who had a history of transfusion and in 18.2% of patients who had no history of transfusion. In comparison, the incidence of new red cell antibody formation in transfused patients in the general population ranges from 0.2% to 2.8%.[39-42]

Although alloimmunization rates in patients with SCD are higher than in the general population, reported rates may be underestimates for two major reasons. Alloantibody formation is often transient in patients with SCD (see Table 11-2). In the CSSCD, 37% of alloantibodies were not detected at subsequent testing.[23] This value does not reflect the true prevalence of transient alloantibodies, as follow-up testing was not obtained shortly after transfusion. In fact, many study protocols did not include screening for antibodies until months after transfusion; therefore, alloimmunization may have been missed. Second, methods for improved alloantibody detection were not used universally in these studies. Recently, polyethylene glycol (PEG) direct antiglobulin tests (DATs) have demonstrated improved detection of Duffy group alloantibodies, common in patients with SCD.[43] These tests used alone or in combination with standard DATs may be superior to the use of a standard DAT alone.

Multiple alloantibodies are common once alloimmunization is detected in patients with SCD.[23,27,37] Forty-five percent of alloimmunized patients develop new alloantibodies.[23] Data from the general population suggest that once one alloantibody forms, the risk of further antibody development increases.[39] This observation implies that methods to reduce alloimmunization in patients with SCD should be started prior to alloantibody formation or after one alloantibody has formed. This may prevent multiple alloantibody development and decrease the risk for hemolytic transfusion reactions.

Pathogenesis of Alloimmunization in Patients with SCD

Alloimmunization rates are high in patients with SCD due to heavy utilization of red cells and possibly due to HLA antigen inheritance and altered immunologic responses in patients with

Table 11-2. Racial Red Cell Antigen Characteristics and the Frequency of Alloantibodies in Patients with Sickle Cell Disease

Blood Group	Phenotype	Antigen Frequency: European-Americans	Antigen Frequency: African-Americans	Alloantibody Frequency in Patients with SCD[22]	Transient[22]
Rh	D	85	92	13.0	26.3
	E	30	19	42.3	32.0
	C	70	30	30.2	40.7
Kell	K	9	2	28.1	30.6
	Kp^a	2	< 0.1	2.1	
Duffy	Fy^a	66	10	18.3	47.1
	Fy^b	83	23	4.7	
	Fy(a–b–)	< 0.01	68		
Kidd	Jk^a	77	92	1.8	42.9
	Jk^b	74	49	10.7	
MNSs	M	78	70	7.7	37.5
	N	72	74	1.5	40.0
	S	55	31	9.2	
	s	89	97	1.5	
	U	>99.9	99	0.6	
Lewis	Le^a			24.6	53.9
	Le^b			12.4	40.0

SCD. However, the primary cause of alloimmunization in patients with SCD is disparate red cell antigens between the blood donor and patient populations. Many of the red cell antigens found frequently in people of primarily European heritage are absent in people of primarily African heritage. Because most of the blood donors in the United States are European-American and the majority of patients with SCD are African-American, patients with

SCD are exposed to transfused red cells expressing antigens that are unlike their own.

Several blood group systems demonstrate this disparate red cell antigen frequency between racial and ethnic groups. Table 11-2 lists common red cell alloantibodies in patients with SCD and the different frequencies of responsible red cell antigens between European- and African-Americans. As this table illustrates, the majority of red cell alloantibodies in patients with SCD are to antigens in the Rh blood group system, primarily C and E. In the Rh blood group system, the presence of D antigen in European-Americans is associated with the presence of either the C or E antigen. However, the presence of the D antigen in African-Americans is rarely associated with the presence of the C or E antigen. Because more African-Americans are D-positive than European-Americans, the fact that many patients with SCD develop anti-C and anti-E is not unanticipated. Another common alloantibody in patients with SCD is anti-K. Again, the frequency of the Kell antigen in European-Americans is 9% compared with 2% in African-Americans. Although the difference in prevalence appears small for Kell and other red cell antigens, these antigens tend to be more immunogenic.

Although alloantibodies in the Rh and Kell blood groups account for almost two-thirds of the clinically significant alloantibodies found in transfused patients with SCD, other alloantibodies in the Duffy, MNSs, and Kidd systems are frequent as well and include anti-Fy^a, -Jk^b, and -S.[23] The frequencies of these offending antigens are lower in African-Americans than in European-Americans, emphasizing again the major role these disparities play in the development of alloantibodies in patients with SCD.

The Rh and Duffy blood group systems deserve further discussion, as clinicians are capitalizing on variances in antigen frequencies between people of European and African ethnicity to select blood for transfusion in patients with SCD. As many as 68% of African-Americans lack the Duffy antigen, Fy(a–b–). However, this phenotype is rare in European-Americans. Rather than using this blood solely for Fy(a–b–) patients with SCD, this pool of Fy(a–b–) blood could be used primarily as a source of blood from African-Americans. Blood suppliers would be more likely to find C-, E-, and K-negative RBC units within this group. These C-, E-, and K-matched units could be used for transfusions in patients with SCD, thereby decreasing exposure to potentially immunogenic red cell antigens.

Using racial antigenic differences in the Rh blood group system to select RBC units for patients with SCD may be more problematic. Some clinicians advocate the use of D-negative blood for transfusions in patients with SCD.[28] This practice is supported by the philosophy that D-negative blood is more likely to be C- and E-negative as well. This transfusion practice could prevent exposure to Rh blood group antigens that account for the majority of alloantibodies in patients with SCD. Although the Rh blood group system encodes the C, c, D, E, and e antigens, other antigen variants occur due to genetic changes in the *RH* locus. For example, variants of the e antigen are more frequently seen in African-Americans than in European-Americans. Therefore using D-negative units for patients with SCD requiring transfusion would expose these patients to an e antigen from European-Americans that differs from their own, because most D-negative blood donors in the United States are of European ancestry.

Other possible factors causing alloimmunization in patients with SCD are immunologic and genetic. Two observations support the theory that mechanisms other than disparate red cell antigens between the donor and recipient may be responsible for alloimmunization in this patient population. Certain patients develop alloantibodies after receiving a small number of transfusions, while others do not, despite a larger donor exposure. Patients who develop alloantibodies often develop multiple antibodies and they may be at greater risk for developing autoantibodies. This subgroup of patients (responders) seems to be at higher risk for alloantibody development than others (nonresponders). Responders may be genetically predisposed to alloantibody formation. Another explanation could be that certain patients with SCD have an altered immune response to red cell antigens, while others do not. However, data supporting these theories are minimal.

One study has reported the possible association of HLA phenotypes and the tendency to form red cell alloantibodies.[44]

HLA-B35 frequency was higher in the group of patients who formed red cell alloantibodies than in those who had not formed alloantibodies. However, the study size was relatively small. Further studies are required to investigate this association further.

Patients with SCD have altered immune responses including those related to splenic dysfunction and the alternative complement activation pathway. The role of these altered immune responses in alloantibody formation has not been investigated. However, once alloimmunization occurs, defects in complement-mediated hemolysis previously reported in patients with SCD may be important.[45]

Factors Affecting Alloimmunization in Patients with SCD

The wide range of alloimmunization rates in patients with SCD is due in large part to the composition of patients being studied. Transfusion burden, age, and gender are patient characteristics that affect alloimmunization. Race and ethnicity of the blood donor population and the degree of minor blood group antigen-matching are important factors as well. In addition, screening for alloantibodies shortly after transfusion and using sensitive screening tests may increase alloantibody detection. These factors are discussed in detail in the following section.

Alloimmunization rates in patients with SCD depend significantly on the number of units transfused per patient.[23,27,46] Rates increase directly with the number of RBC unit received. This rate does not appear to plateau even after a large number of RBC unit exposures. Although alloimmunization rates are greatest with the first transfusions received, these rates continue to increase even after transfusion of 100 or more RBC units.[23,46]

Adults with SCD generally have received more RBC units than children have received. Therefore, studies including a large number of children report lower rates than those with large adult populations.[23,32] Although the number of units transfused seems to be the primary determinant of alloimmunization in patients with SCD, age seems to be an independent factor. Red cell transfusion early in life leads to lower alloimmunization rates. Children under 10 years of age have a lower alloimmunization rate per number of units exposed than children over 10 years of age.[23] This observation is supported by alloimmunization data from young children with thalassemia.[47] These observations imply that exposure to allogeneic RBC units early in life may induce immune tolerance, resulting in lower alloimmunization.

Adult females with SCD have higher alloimmunization rates than adult males.[26] Originally this was thought to be due to alloantibodies acquired during pregnancy. However, it has been observed that women were transfused more frequently than men. Historically, many females with SCD received blood transfusions for treatment or prevention of disease-related complications during pregnancy. When the number of RBC units received was taken into account, this gender difference no longer remained statistically significant.[23]

Because the major cause of alloimmunization in patients with SCD is due to disparities in red cell phenotypes between patients and blood donors, the proportion of the blood donor population that is racially or ethnically similar to those with SCD will affect the overall alloimmunization rate. When patients with SCD receive RBC units from racially similar donors, the rate of alloimmunization is lower than the rate in studies where the donor population is racially dissimilar. Transfused children with SCD in Jamaica develop alloantibodies at a 2.6% rate compared with a 76% rate in affected children residing in the United Kingdom.[33] Alloimmunization rates in Brazilian patients with SCD are 1.15% per unit of blood transfused.[35] Investigators have examined red cell antigen disparities in other racial or ethnic groups that support the observations in African-Americans with SCD. First-generation African children residing in the United States have more dissimilar red cell antigen frequencies to European-Americans than to African-Americans.[34] Seventy-five percent of Asian-Americans with thalassemia develop alloantibodies, again due to disparate red cell antigen frequencies between the donor and patient populations.[48]

The greatest difficulty in assessing the frequency of alloimmunization in patients with SCD is the lack of persistent red cell antibody detection in this patient population mentioned previously. Studies using protocols to screen patients several days to a week after RBC unit exposure may report higher alloimmunization rates than those using protocols that screen patients weeks after exposure.

Complications of Alloimmunization in Patients with SCD

The complications of red cell alloimmunization in patients with SCD fall within four major categories: 1) decreased availability of compatible RBC units, 2) delayed hemolytic transfusion reactions (DHTRs), 3) acute hemolytic transfusion reactions (AHTRs), and 4) autoantibody formation.

Decreased Availability of Compatible RBC Units

The presence of alloantibodies in patient sera necessitates the exclusion of RBC units specific for the offending red cell antigen or antigens. The difficulty in finding a compatible unit depends also on the specificity and number of alloantibodies involved. RBC unit availability in a particular donor group depends on the frequency of the antigen in that population. Because blood donors in the United States are more likely to be of European as opposed to African ancestry, this limits the availability of compatible RBC units for alloimmunized patients with SCD. As the number of alloantibodies increase, the ability to find specific antigen-negative units will decrease.

If labeling blood with the racial identification of the donor were possible, the probability of finding a compatible unit would increase and associated costs would decrease. However, this is not presently practiced in the United States for political, societal, and cultural reasons. As discussed in the previous section, various red cell antigens with lower frequencies in African-Americans than in European-Americans can be used to select RBC units for patients with SCD. For example, monoclonal antibodies to Fy3 have been used to identify Fy(a–b–) blood donors, more likely African-American, in the general blood donor pool.[49] This Fy(a–b–) pool of blood can be used to find compatible RBC units for alloimmunized patients with SCD or to support transfusion programs designed to supply partially or extended antigen-matched blood. Unfortunately, this practice has not received much attention.

Presently, because of the continued under-representation of African-Americans in the general blood donor pool, patients with SCD remain the most frequent patient population using blood obtained through the American Rare Donor Program.[50] This source is available if compatible units cannot be obtained locally or regionally. Blood banks servicing highly alloimmunized patients with SCD, patients with rare red cell phenotypes, or patients requiring extended antigen-matched blood for other reasons, often request frozen compatible units for storage. In this manner, compatible units will be available locally when needed.

Delayed Hemolytic Transfusion Reactions

Delayed hemolytic transfusion reactions are more common in patients with SCD than in the general population. This increased frequency may be due to a number of reasons. First, patients with SCD are transfused episodically. Therefore, years may pass between transfusions. Because red cell alloantibodies are transient in this patient population,[23] they may not be detected by screening tests prior to the next red cell transfusion. Second, patients with SCD are transfused frequently; therefore, exposure to potentially immunogenic red cell antigens is common. Finally, red cell antigen disparities between the donor and recipient populations increase the likelihood of alloimmunization and hemolytic transfusion reactions.

Hemolytic transfusion reactions may be immediate, but are more likely to be delayed reactions in patients with SCD. After the first exposure to a red cell antigen, alloantibodies may not be detected for many weeks. A second exposure to the same foreign antigen usually leads to a rapid increase in alloantibodies that peaks in 7 to 10 days. These alloantibodies cause donor red cell sensitization and may lead to their destruction through IgG-mediated mechanisms. This resulting extravascular hemolysis, a DHTR, clinically manifests as fever, hyperbilirubinemia, and anemia 5 to 14 days following transfusion. However, if complement-mediated hemolysis occurs, hemoglobinuria and hemoglobinemia may develop due to intravascular hemolysis. Direct and indirect antiglobulin tests often provide serologic evidence of immune-mediated hemolysis.

The incidence of DHTRs is 1% to 6%, with a higher incidence in patients receiving a larger number of RBC units.[11] Prevalence rates of DHTRs in patients with SCD range from 4% to 22%.[21,24,27,32,51] However, obtaining epidemiologic data on DHTRs in patients with SCD is difficult. Most information is provided by case reports and case series.[27,51-65] Few authors provide required information in order to determine frequency rates.

A greater concern with the epidemiologic data on DHTRs is that published data may represent underestimates. Clinicians may not suspect DHTRs in patients with SCD, as DHTR-related symptoms may mimic a painful episode. In addition, many of the laboratory tests useful in documenting DHTRs are abnormal in patients with SCD because of chronic hemolysis. Increased hemolysis in these situations may not be ascribed to a DHTR, but classified as a hyperhemolytic episode of unknown etiology. The observation that the Hb A level is lower than expected in a recently transfused patient or the detection of a red cell alloantibody will guide the clinician in the correct diagnosis. However, red cell alloantibodies may be difficult to detect in patients with SCD. Therefore, the diagnosis of DHTRs in patients with SCD is based highly on clinical suspicion.

The clinical course of DHTRs in patients with SCD differs from other patient populations:

- Pain appears to be a significant component of DHTRs; therefore, affected patients may be misdiagnosed as having an SCD-related painful episode.[51]
- Frequently, posttransfusion hemoglobin levels will drop below pretransfusion values, indicating bystander hemolysis or suppressed erythropoiesis.[58,66]
- An absolute reticulocytopenia develops frequently during the course of the DHTR.
- New alloantibodies are difficult to detect; either they appear late in the course of a DHTR or they are never detected.
- The DAT is negative frequently.

These and other atypical features have led some clinicians to adopt the term "sickle cell hemolytic transfusion reaction syndrome" to describe DHTRs in patients with SCD.[66] If widely adopted, this description may lead to earlier or more accurate diagnosis of immune-mediated hemolysis in patients with SCD.

Several of the above features merit further discussion. DHTRs may mimic painful episodes in patients with SCD.[51] In fact, pain has been reported in 87% of DHTRs in patients with SCD.[45] This association may be due to cytokines released during immune-mediated red cell destruction. Close observation and laboratory studies to evaluate a DHTR should be performed on any patient with SCD and pain who has received a recent red cell transfusion.

DHTRs are generally mild in other patient populations but severe, life-threatening anemia is common in patients with SCD. Posttransfusion hemoglobin levels drop below pretransfusion levels in 83% of DHTRs reported in this patient population.[45] The term "hyperhemolysis" is frequently used to describe this clinical feature. Although the most likely etiology of this exaggerated decrease in hemoglobin levels after transfusion in patients with SCD is multifactorial, there are two leading controversial theories to explain this phenomenon.

The first theory is that of "bystander hemolysis."[58] In this situation, immune-mediated hemolysis of cells negative for the offending antigen occurs. This theory is further supported by the observation that sickle cells are susceptible to complement-mediated lysis initiated by mechanisms not including the autologous sickle cells. Garratty[45] has suggested that complement activation occurs by the reaction of red cell alloantibodies with transfused cells.

The second theory is that of "suppressed erythropoiesis" due to acute illness or recent red cell transfusion. Petz et al[66] presented five cases of DHTR in patients with SCD. They demonstrated through scientific calculations of red cell production and senescent destruction that "suppressed erythropoiesis" accounts for the decrease in hemoglobin below pretransfusion levels in most cases. Most likely, bystander hemolysis, suppressed erythropoiesis, and autoantibody formation (discussed below) contribute in various extents to the severe, often life-threatening anemia observed in patients with SCD and DHTRs.

Although serologic investigations in some DHTRs in patients with SCD never identify the offending alloantibody, many are successful in alloantibody identification. The majority of red cell alloantibodies identified in patients with SCD and DHTRs are similar to those causing red cell alloimmunization. Therefore, most alloantibodies are anti-C, -E, -Jk^a, -Jk^b, -Fy^a, -Fy^b, -S, -s, and -K, although anti-C, -E, and -Jk^b predominate.[27,52,55,56,58,60,61,63,66-68] However, rare alloantibodies including anti-Fy5, anti-Rh46, anti-W^r, anti-Do^a, and anti-Go^a have been reported.[55,59,65]

The clinical outcome of patients with SCD and DHTRs is a concern. While many DHTRs are clinically manageable without transfusion, sometimes the severe anemia associated with DHTRs leads to additional transfusion. Often these repeat transfusions are unsuccessful or worsen the hemolysis. Subsequently, fatalities are not infrequently reported in the literature. Renal failure, disseminated intravascular coagulation, and stroke have occurred as well.[60]

Acute Hemolytic Transfusion Reactions

Isolated acute hemolytic transfusion reactions (AHTRs), as previously mentioned, are rare in patients with SCD. However, cases of AHTRs in patients with SCD involving anti-Do^a, anti-Do^b, and anti-IH have been reported.[65,69,70] Acute hemolysis following a transfusion during a DHTR without alloantibody identification has been discussed in the previous section.

Autoantibody Development

Posttransfusion autoantibody development occurs in patients with SCD at a rate of 3% to 8%.[24,32] The clinical spectrum varies widely from absent to severe exacerbation of anemia. A large pediatric study reported a 7.6% red cell autoantibody prevalence in 184 previously transfused children with SCD.[71] Although the majority of patients with autoantibodies did not have clinical evidence of hemolysis, one of four developed fatal hemolysis. Case reports of red cell autoantibodies in patients with SCD support this observation that autoantibody formation in patients with SCD can lead to severe hemolysis.[65,72-75]

Although red cell autoantibodies are detected in some patients without alloimmunization, most occur in patients with alloantibodies.[24,29,32,71] The pathophysiology of red cell autoantibody formation in patients with SCD may be directly linked to alloimmunization. If red cell alloantibodies cause conformational changes in red cell antigens by binding to the cell surface, then autoantibody development may be stimulated.[22] However, other possible mechanisms of autoimmunization include a genetic predisposition to autoantibody formation.

Management of Alloimmunization and Immune-Mediated Hemolysis in Patients with SCD

Tailored Transfusion Therapy

The management of DHTRs and autoimmune hemolysis in patients with SCD depends on the degree of cardiovascular compromise caused by a rapid decrease in hemoglobin. If the patient requires a blood transfusion to avoid cardiovascular collapse or to manage a life-threatening complication of SCD, the least incompatible RBC unit should be selected. However, if red cell transfusion is not urgent clinically, the clinical course of DHTR may be better if red cell transfusion can be avoided acutely. In these situations, pharmacologic therapy should be instituted and extended antigen-matched blood should be given if the patient deteriorates clinically.

Pharmacologic Therapy

Many case reports of DHTRs and autoimmune hemolysis in patients with SCD describe patients who improve after receiving steroids during the clinical course.[27,51,57,60,63,76-78] However, the length of steroid therapy, ranging from one dose to multiple doses over 5 days, was often not reported. A conservative approach would include the intravenous administration of high-dose methylprednisolone for 5 days followed by a slow taper over 1 to 2 weeks. Intravenous gammaglobulin (1 g/kg) in single and repeated doses has been used in an attempt to prevent further antibody-mediated destruction of red cells.[76,78] Erythropoietin therapy may also be beneficial in DHTRs in patients with SCD.[78,79] This is supported by the observation that erythroid progenitor cells are quite responsive to erythropoietin in vitro. Combined pharmacologic therapy may be required for severe DHTRs.

Discontinuation of Chronic Transfusion Protocols

Given the severe nature of hemolytic transfusion reactions in patients with SCD, the decision to discontinue chronic transfusion therapy and to limit episodic transfusions whenever possible seems rational for heavily alloimmunized patients. However, whenever chronic transfusion therapy is discontinued, the patient assumes the risk that SCD complications may recur. Other therapies that reduce SCD-related complications may be used to decrease complication recurrence after transfusion therapy is discontinued. Hydroxyurea therapy has demonstrated success at decreasing SCD complications such as pain, acute chest syndrome, and the need for transfusion therapy.[80] Recently, Ware et al[81] reported a low stroke recurrence rate in a small group of patients receiving hydroxyurea after discontinuation of transfusion therapy because of red cell alloantibodies or autoantibody development. Phlebotomy decreased iron accumulation in these patients. The authors recommended continuing transfusion therapy until a response to hydroxyurea is noted to further decrease stroke recurrence in this group of patients.

Prevention of Alloimmunization in Patients with SCD

Red Cell Antigen Phenotyping in Patients with SCD

Extended red cell antigen phenotyping of patients with SCD is necessary to prepare for primary or secondary alloantibody development. The extended phenotype determination should include, at the minimum, analysis of the red cell antigens commonly causing alloimmunization in patients with SCD. This includes antigens in the following blood group systems: ABO, Rh, MNSs, Kell, Kidd, Duffy, Lewis, and P_1. Phenotyping other blood group systems such as Lutheran, Colton, and Dombrock may be useful if they can be performed. However, these phenotypes are often difficult to obtain.

Because extended red cell antigen-matched blood may be recommended or indicated throughout the lifetime of the patient with SCD, the red cell phenotype analysis performed before the institution of transfusion therapy is preferred. However, if antigen phenotyping is required in a patient with SCD who has been transfused recently, methods are available for accurate typing.[82,83] One method exploits the fact that red cells containing Hb S are resistant to lysis with hypotonic solutions, while those containing Hb A are not. Once the patient's cells are washed in 0.3% saline, the remaining cells are typed using routine procedures.[82] Extended red cell typing is also available by molecular DNA technology. These technologies are based on variations of techniques for polymerase chain reaction amplification of targeted gene sequences.[84] Peripheral white cells are used as a DNA source. This technique has been successful in typing blood groups in multitransfused patients with SCD[83] and in populations of highly diverse ancestry.[85]

Transfusion of Partially or Extended Red Cell Antigen-Matched Red Cells

Studies have demonstrated reduced alloimmunization in patients with SCD who receive RBC units matched for specific antigens.[1,28,29,74,86] Red cell antigen matching in these studies has been as limited as three antigens—primarily E, C, and Kell—and as extensive as 17 antigens.

The benefits of red cell antigen matching are clear when comparing alloimmunization rates to historical controls where patients did not receive partial or extended antigen-matched RBC units. However, it is difficult to determine what extent of red cell antigen matching is best for patients with SCD. This limitation is due to the lack of randomized controlled trials designed to compare the rate of red cell antibody formation in previously untransfused patients with SCD who receive red cell transfusions matched for specific antigens. Until these studies are performed, clinicians must rely on comparing data from published reports. However, these comparisons are troublesome, because factors that influence the development or detection of red cell antibodies vary between studies. Critical variables include subject age and gender, the number of RBC units received at study entry, the methods of antibody detection, the timing of antibody testing after exposure to the RBC unit, and the number of subjects previously alloimmunized. In addition, newer transfusion practices such as leukocyte reduction, could potentially affect the development of red cell as well as platelet alloimmunization, although no published data exist to support this theory.

The first report of a transfusion program for patients with SCD using extended antigen-matched blood was by Ambruso et al[29] in 1987. All patients had received transfusions in the past and 66% were alloimmunized at a rate of 3.5/100 units transfused. Twelve patients received antigen-matched blood from 1200 donors, the majority of whom were African-American. RBC units were matched for A, B, and D as well as C, E, Le^a, Le^b, Fy^a, Fy^b, Jk^a, Jk^b, M, N, S, and P_1. Four new alloantibodies developed in three patients at a rate of 0.3/100 units transfused. Two patients developed anti-Kp^a and anti-C, while the third patient developed anti-C and anti-Kell. This latter patient was exposed to these antigens due to technical error. The cost of maintaining this program was $50,000 per year.

Wayne[1] reported a reduction in alloimmunization in 117 children with SCD using extended antigen-matched red cell transfusions. The alloimmunization rate was 6.4% compared with 17% when non-antigen-matched units were transfused. The alloantibodies produced in previously unexposed patients were anti-C (accidental exposure) , -Jk^b, -S, -Fy^a, -Kp^a, -V, and -Bg. The cost of an antigen-matched RBC unit at this center was 60% higher than standard RBC units.

Tahhan et al[86] were successful in reducing alloimmunization rates in 40 patients with SCD by transfusing leukocyte-reduced RBC units matched for C, E, K, S, and Fy^a or Fy^b antigens. Patients who received red cell antigen-matched transfusions did not develop alloantibodies, while 34.8% of 46 patients who received both antigen-matched and non-antigen-matched transfusions developed clinically significant antibodies. However, the cost of providing antigen-matched transfusions was 1.5 to 1.8 times that of a standard transfusion protocol, relatively lower than in other published reports.

A recent report by Vichinsky et al[74] described the use of partial red cell antigen-matched blood in chronic transfusion programs for children at increased risk for stroke. Eighty percent of those randomly assigned to receive transfusion therapy had received transfusions in the past and 6% were alloimmunized. Sixty-one children with repeatedly abnormal transcranial Doppler ultrasound studies received RBC units matched for C, E, and Kell. All patients were screened for antibody development prior to routine monthly transfusion using enzymatic and direct antiglobulin techniques. Five (8%) subjects developed clinically significant alloantibodies: anti-E (2), anti-Kell (2), and multiple alloantibodies including anti-Fy^a, -Le^a, -Le^b, and -S (1). Three patients developed warm autoantibodies: anti-e (2) and a panagglutinin (1). The immunization rate in this study was 0.5% when including clinically significant and clinically insignificant alloantibodies and autoantibodies. Two (3.3%) patients developed hemolytic transfusion reactions at a rate of 0.11% per unit transfused.

Controversies Surrounding Appropriate RBC Unit Selection for Patients with SCD

Although many clinicians agree that red cell antigen phenotyping is beneficial to patients with SCD,[32,87,88] few agree as to the best blood for patients with SCD.[23,28,30,32,34,37,68,87,89-92] Most of the controversy is related to the following: 1) disagreement on the clinical significance of alloimmunization in patients with SCD; 2) cost of minor red cell group antigen matching; 3) availability of blood from African-Americans in the general blood donor pool; and 4) the possibility of developing rare red cell alloantibodies when racially matched blood is used for patients with SCD. Many express the concern that the majority of transfused patients with SCD will never become alloimmunized. However, failure to adopt programs to prevent alloimmunization in this group of patients comes at the expense of those patients who develop multiple alloantibodies once the first alloantibody has been formed or those who develop severe hemolytic transfusion reactions after minimal blood donor exposure.

Because of lack of agreement on blood selection for patients with SCD, many different recommendations have been published.[4,23,24,26,28,32,34,37,87,89,91] These specific recommendations can be grouped into three general categories for discussion:

- Red cell antigen matching, partial or extended, on all patients with SCD prior to alloantibody development.
- No red cell antigen matching until a patient with SCD forms an alloantibody or develops a HTR.
- Both scenarios above using blood from people of African ethnicity.

Many believe that red cell antigen-matched blood should be provided for patients with SCD before alloimmunization develops. The philosophy behind this approach is that alloimmunization will be prevented, thereby decreasing hemolytic transfusion reactions and difficulties in finding compatible blood. These benefits may balance the increased costs associated with providing partial or extended red cell antigen-matched blood. However, a major drawback to this approach, if widely adopted, would be the utilization of rare antigen-negative blood for patients who have not developed alloimmunization. This approach would be more acceptable if those of African ethnicity represented a larger portion of the general blood donor pool.

Others advocate reserving red cell antigen-matched blood only for those patients who are at great risk of developing alloantibodies or hemolytic transfusion reactions. Specifically, patients with one or more alloantibody, those with autoantibodies, pregnant females, or those that have experienced hemolytic transfusion reactions would be transfused with partial or extended antigen-matched RBC units. The limitations of this approach have been discussed previously.

Many are beginning to recognize the benefits of obtaining blood for patients with SCD from similar racial or ethnic groups. Because the majority of patients with SCD in the United States are of African ancestry, African-Americans should be recruited actively as members of the general blood donor pool or as members of a designated donor pool to provide blood preferentially to patients with SCD. If included in the general blood donor pool, antibody screening should be performed to detect a phenotype common in African-Americans and uncommon in European-Americans, such as Fy(a–b–). Then these units can be directed toward patients with SCD or to the American Rare Donor Program. Involuntary labeling of blood from African-Americans is distasteful and politically unwise. However, voluntary labeling may be very practical, inexpensive, and culturally acceptable.

Recently, a group of hematology physicians, nurses, and psychologists gathered to discuss the controversies surrounding blood transfusion in patients with SCD. The result was a consensus document published in 2001.[88] Their recommendations regarding RBC unit selection for this patient population are summarized in Table 11-3. Generally, many researchers and clinicians do agree that at a minimum, partial antigen matching should be strongly considered when selecting RBC units for patients with SCD and that partial antigen matching should include C, E, and K.[37,74,86] Partial matching for these antigens that most frequently cause alloimmunization and hemolytic transfusion reactions seems practical and feasible, particularly if combined with increased African-American donor recruitment. Because extended antigen matching is very expensive, reserving the use of extended antigen-matched blood for patients with multiple alloantibodies or those with hemolytic transfusion reactions may be more appropriate.[28,29,32]

Programs Designed to Increase Availability of Blood for Patients with SCD

Providing RBC units from African-Americans to patients with SCD seems to be a rational approach to lowering alloimmunization, autoimmunization, and hemolytic transfusion reaction rates in this patient population. Many advocate increasing African-American blood donor recruitment to achieve this outcome.

Table 11-3. Consensus Group Recommendations for Blood Component Use in Patients with SCD[88]

- All patients with SCD should have extended red cell antigen phenotyping (ABO, Rh, Kell, Kidd, Duffy, Lewis, and MNSs systems) prior to the initiation of transfusion therapy.
- Patients should receive RBC units that are phenotypically matched for ABO, C, c, D, E, e, and K, k.
- Patients with red cell alloantibodies should receive more extensively matched units:
  - Fy^a- and Fy^b-negative at a minimum.
  - Negative for the antigen(s) to which the patient has developed alloantibodies in the past.
- Programs to increase African-American donor recruitment are needed.
- Transfusion of blood components from related donors should be avoided in potential marrow transplant recipients unless family members are needed to obtain compatible units.
- Blood from individuals with sickle cell trait is safe for patients with SCD but should be avoided when monitoring posttransfusion hemoglobin S levels.

Several centers that provide medical care to a large number of patients with SCD have developed innovative programs to support the transfusion needs of this patient population.

Special transfusion programs to provide RBC units from African-American donors to patients with SCD can be divided into three donation groups: 1) direct, 2) designated, 3) general donor pool. Table 11-4 outlines the positive and negative characteristics of these programs. A designated donation program is described below.

A program to direct blood from African-American donors to children with SCD, beginning in 1997, has been developed at the author's affiliated institution, The Children's Hospital of Philadelphia (CHOP), in a cooperative effort with the Penn-Jersey Region American Red Cross and the Philadelphia-Delaware Valley Chapter of the Sickle Cell Disease Association of America.[93] African-American donors are recruited during program blood drives

Table 11-4. Comparison of Directed, Designated, and Traditional Blood Donation Programs Designed To Meet Transfusion Needs of Patients with Sickle Cell Disease

Variables for Program Comparison	"Directed" Donation Program	"Designated" Donation Program*	Traditional Donation Program (Using General Donor Pool)
Program blood unit supply meets "unscheduled" (acute/episodic) and "scheduled" (elective/chronic) transfusion needs	"Scheduled" transfusion needs only	"Scheduled" and "unscheduled" transfusion needs	"Scheduled" and "unscheduled" transfusion needs
Level of program administrative effort	High level of administrative effort to arrange donations based on the scheduled transfusion needs of patients	Minimal to moderate administrative effort, depending on the size of the designated donor pool	Minimal administrative effort
Costs beyond traditional program	High	Moderate to low	NA
Contributions to general donor pool	None to minimal	Can vary from low to high depending on the needs of patients with SCD and the size of the designated donor pool	NA
Degree of difficulty in identifying partial or extended antigen-matched blood for patients with SCD	Low, depending on the structure of the direct donation program	Low	Moderate to high, depending on the racial composition of the general donor pool

*Designated donation program refers to the preferential use of selected donated units for patients with sickle cell disease, but not a specific patient.

as well as during routine blood collection in the region. Information on the program and special blood tie tags are available at all collection sites. Program participants voluntarily agree to have their blood sent to CHOP for a child with SCD. If screened program units are not used within 3 weeks, they are released to the general blood donor pool.

Since November 2000, this program has averaged 800 RBC units per month. After routine screening, the "program" units are sent to CHOP. Units that are leukocyte reduced and lacking Hb S are used for patients with SCD after matching for C, E, and K antigens. This program supplies over 85% of RBC units needed to transfuse patients with SCD at CHOP, both episodically and chronically. Fewer units of "program" blood than units from the local general donor pool are screened to identify C-, E-, and K-matched units. The development of new alloantibodies is infrequent in the CHOP patient population, but present alloimmunization rates have not been estimated. This program demonstrates that providing units of blood from a racially similar blood donor pool is feasible, practical, and economically sound in a large urban area servicing a large population of patients with SCD.

Platelet Alloimmunization in Transfused Patients with SCD

Friedman et al[36] reported increased platelet alloimmunization in patients with SCD who had received red cell transfusions. Eighty-five percent of the patients who had received 50 or greater red cell transfusions and 48% of patients who had received less developed platelet alloimmunization. No platelet alloantibodies were found in untransfused patients with SCD. Because marrow transplant is a potential cure for patients with SCD, if transplanted, platelet-alloimmunized patients may be at greater risk for platelet refractoriness during marrow transplantation. The authors recommend leukocyte-reduced blood components for patients with SCD who are potential marrow transplant recipients.

Future Directions

Alloimmunization is a frequent complication of red cell transfusion therapy in patients with SCD. Although adverse consequences of alloimmunization may be infrequent, when they do occur, they are often life-threatening. Unless efforts are made to reduce alloimmunization, the number of alloimmunized patients with SCD will increase as indications for transfusion therapy in this patient population broaden. As programs to recruit blood donors of African ethnicity for patients with SCD in the United States expand, other options for safe transfusion therapy should be explored.

Two optional blood products presently under investigation may be beneficial to patients with SCD. Blood substitutes are in the advanced stages of clinical trials in the United States. Unfortunately, these substitutes are cleared from the circulation rapidly by the kidneys and remain intravascularly for only 6 to 12 hours.[94] However, these products may provide short-term benefit to severely alloimmunized patients with SCD in life-threatening clinical situations until compatible blood can be obtained. A modification of red cells that masks surface antigens using PEG has been shown to have good in-vivo survival and function.[95,96] However, there are no published reports at this time on safety and efficacy in humans. If PEG-coated red cells are safe in early human trials, then patients with SCD should be considered for later studies.

Clinical studies are needed to identify patients at high risk for RBC alloimmunization and clarify appropriate blood selection for patients with SCD in general. Immunologic and genetic factors that predispose patients with SCD to allo- and autoantibody formation should be investigated. If these high-risk patients could be identified, then extended antigen-matched RBC units could be reserved primarily for this patient population. Randomized, controlled trials should be performed to address the clinical question of what extent of antigen matching is most effective at reducing alloimmunization and transfusion-related hemolysis in patients with SCD. Previously untransfused patients would be the best subjects for these studies, given the high rate of transient alloantibodies in this patient population. The impact on red cell alloimmunization of transfusing leukocyte-reduced RBC units should be explored simultaneously. Economic, societal, and clinical aspects of transfusion programs for patients with SCD should be considered as well.

National registries providing red cell antigen profiles as well as transfusion and alloimmunization histories of patients with SCD to treating physicians are required. The transient nature of red cell alloantibodies and the frequency with which these patients require transfusions outside of their primary hospitals are justifications for this approach. The Internet can be used to extend the availability of this information, although methods to ensure patient confidentiality will be necessary. This approach must be combined with efforts to educate patients with SCD and their families about the risk of alloimmunization and DHTRs. Updated alloantibody information should be provided to patients and their families on a regular basis. This should improve communication between primary and treating physicians particularly in emergent situations.

Innovative approaches to recruit African-American blood donors should be expanded. Programs allowing for voluntary "labeling" of RBC units donated from a person of African ethnicity may overcome the past and present societal, cultural, and political barriers to blood donation classically attributed to African-Americans. These programs would allow greater access to RBC units that are more likely to result in partial or extended red cell antigen-matched or intraracial units for patients with SCD.

Through development of special blood products, better characterization of high-risk patients, sharing of red cell antigen profiles and transfusion-related histories, and expanded implementation of transfusion programs using primarily African-American donors, alloimmunization can be reduced in patients with SCD. Once alloimmunization risks are lowered and other complications such as iron overload are reduced, the broadening of transfusion indications should result in longer survival for patients with SCD.

References

1. Wayne AS, Kevy SV, Nathan DG. Transfusion management of sickle cell disease. Blood 1993;81:1109-23.
2. Cohen AR, Norris CF, Smith-Whitley K. Transfusion therapy for sickle cell disease. In: Capon SM, Chambers LA, eds. New directions in pediatric hematology. Bethesda, MD: American Association of Blood Banks, 1996: 39-88.
3. Ohene-Frempong K. Indications for red cell transfusion in sickle cell disease. Semin Hematol 2001;38:5-13.
4. Telen MJ. Principles and problems of transfusion in sickle cell disease. Semin Hematol 2001;38:315-23.
5. Emre U, Miller ST, Rao SP, Rao M. Alveolar-arterial oxygen gradient in acute chest syndrome of sickle cell disease. J Pediatr 1993;123:272-5.
6. Vichinsky EP, Styles LA, Colangelo LH, et al. Acute chest syndrome in sickle cell disease: Clinical presentation and course. Cooperative Study of Sickle Cell Disease. Blood 1997;89:1787-92.
7. Maitre B, Habibi A, Roudot-Thoraval F, et al. Acute chest syndrome in adults with sickle cell disease. Chest 2000;117:1386-92.
8. Serjeant GR, Serjeant BE, Thomas PW, et al. Human parvovirus infection in homozygous sickle cell disease. Lancet 1993;341:1237-40.
9. Rao S, Gooden S. Splenic sequestration in sickle cell disease: Role of transfusion therapy. Am J Pediatr Hematol Oncol 1985;7:298-301.
10. Ohene-Frempong K. Stroke in sickle cell disease: Demographic, clinical and therapeutic considerations. Semin Hematol 1991;28:213-19.
11. Vichinsky EP, Haberkern CM, Neumayr L, et al. A comparison of conservative and aggressive transfusion regimens in the perioperative management of sickle cell disease. The Preoperative Transfusion in Sickle Cell Disease Study Group. N Engl J Med 1995;333:206-13.
12. Morrison JC, Whybrew WD, Bucovaz ET. Use of partial exchange transfusion preoperatively in patients with sickle cell hemoglobinopathies. Am J Obstet Gynecol 1978;132:59-63.
13. Adams RJ, McKie VC, Hsu L, et al. Prevention of a first stroke by transfusions in children with sickle cell anemia and abnormal results on transcranial Doppler ultrasonography. N Engl J Med 1998;339:5-11.
14. Wilimas J, Goff JR, Anderson HR, Jr, et al. Efficacy of transfusion therapy for one to two years in patients with sickle cell disease and cerebrovascular accidents. J Pediatr 1980;96:205-8.
15. Wang WC, Kovnar EH, Tonkin IL, et al. High risk of recurrent stroke after discontinuance of five to twelve years of transfusion therapy in patients with sickle cell disease. J Pediatr 1991;118:377-82.
16. Russell MO, Goldberg HI, Hodson A, et al. Effect of transfusion therapy on arteriographic abnormalities and on recurrence of stroke in sickle cell disease. Blood 1984;63:162-9.

17. Sarnaik SA. Prevention of stroke by transfusions in children with sickle cell anemia. N Engl J Med 1998;339:1477-8.
18. Styles LA, Vichinsky E. Effects of a long-term transfusion regimen on sickle cell-related illnesses. J Pediatr 1994;125:909-11.
19. Miller ST, Wright E, Abboud M, et al. Impact of chronic transfusion on incidence of pain and acute chest syndrome during the Stroke Prevention Trial (STOP) in sickle-cell anemia. J Pediatr 2001;139:785-9.
20. Morrison JC, Schneider JM, Whybrew WD, et al. Prophylactic transfusions in pregnant patients with sickle hemoglobinopathies: benefit versus risk. Obstet Gynecol 1980;56:274-80.
21. Koshy M, Burd L, Wallace D, et al. Prophylactic red-cell transfusions in pregnant patients with sickle cell disease. A randomized cooperative study. N Engl J Med 1988;319:1447-52.
22. Rosse WF, Telen MJ, Ware RE. Transfusion support for patients with sickle cell disease. Bethesda, MD: AABB Press, 1998.
23. Rosse WF, Gallagher D, Kinney TR, et al. Transfusion and alloimmunization in sickle cell disease. The Cooperative Study of Sickle Cell Disease. Blood 1990;76:1431-7.
24. Vichinsky EP, Earles A, Johnson RA, et al. Alloimmunization in sickle cell anemia and transfusion of racially unmatched blood. N Engl J Med 1990;322:1617-21.
25. Sarnaik S, Schornack J, Lusher JM. The incidence of development of irregular red cell antibodies in patients with sickle cell anemia. Transfusion 1986;26:249-52.
26. Orlina AR, Unger PJ, Koshy M. Post-transfusion alloimmunization in patients with sickle cell disease. Am J Hematol 1978;5:101-6.
27. Cox JV, Steane E, Cunningham G, Frenkel EP. Risk of alloimmunization and delayed hemolytic transfusion reactions in patients with sickle cell disease. Arch Intern Med 1988;148:2485-9.
28. Davies SC, McWilliam AC, Hewitt PE, et al. Red cell alloimmunization in sickle cell disease. Br J Haematol 1986;63:241-5.
29. Ambruso DR, Githens JH, Alcorn R, et al. Experience with donors matched for minor blood group antigens in patients with sickle cell anemia who are receiving chronic transfusion therapy. Transfusion 1987;27:94-8.
30. Blumberg N, Ross K, Avila E, Peck K. Should chronic transfusions be matched for antigens other than ABO and Rho(D)? Vox Sang 1984;47:205-8.
31. Coles SM, Klein HG, Holland PV. Alloimmunization in two multitransfused patient populations. Transfusion 1981;21:462-6.
32. Aygun B, Padmanabhan S, Paley C, Chandrasekaran V. Clinical significance of RBC alloantibodies and autoantibodies in sickle cell patients who received transfusions. Transfusion 2002;42:37-43.

33. Olujohungbe A, Hambleton I, Stephens L, et al. Red cell antibodies in patients with homozygous sickle cell disease: A comparison of patients in Jamaica and the United Kingdom. Br J Haematol 2001;113:661-5.
34. Luban NL. Variability in rates of alloimmunization in different groups of children with sickle cell disease: Effect of ethnic background. Am J Pediatr Hematol Oncol 1989;11:314-19.
35. Moreira Jr G, Bordin JO, Kuroda A, Kerbauy J. Red blood cell alloimmunization in sickle cell disease: The influence of racial and antigenic pattern differences between donors and recipients in Brazil. Am J Hematol 1996;52:197-200.
36. Friedman DF, Lukas MB, Jawad A, et al. Alloimmunization to platelets in heavily transfused patients with sickle cell disease. Blood 1996;88: 3216-22.
37. Castro O, Sandler SG, Houston-Yu P, Rana S. Predicting the effect of transfusing only phenotype-matched RBCs to patients with sickle cell disease: Theoretical and practical implications. Transfusion 2002;42: 684-90.
38. Heddle NM, Blajchman MA. The leukodepletion of cellular blood products in the prevention of HLA-alloimmunization and refractoriness to allogeneic platelet transfusions. Blood 1995;85:603-6.
39. Heddle NM. A prospective study to determine the frequency and clinical significance of alloimmunization post-transfusion. Br J Haematol 1995; 91:1000-15.
40. Ness PM, Shirey RS, Thoman SK, Buck SA. The differentiation of delayed serologic and delayed hemolytic transfusion reactions: Incidence, long-term serologic findings, and clinical significance. Transfusion 1990;30: 688-93.
41. Pinkerton PH, Coovadia AS, Goldstein J. Frequency of delayed hemolytic transfusion reactions following antibody screening and immediate-spin crossmatching. Transfusion 1992;32:814-17.
42. Vamvakas EC, Pineda AA, Reisner R, et al. The differentiation of delayed hemolytic and delayed serologic transfusion reactions: Incidence and predictors of hemolysis. Transfusion 1995;35:26-32.
43. Reisner R, Butler G, Bundy K, Moore SB. Comparison of the polyethylene glycol antiglobulin test and the use of enzymes in antibody detection and identification. Transfusion 1996;36:487-9.
44. Alarif L, Castro O, Ofosu M, et al. HLA-B35 is associated with red cell alloimmunization in sickle cell disease. Clin Immunol Immunopathol 1986;38:178-83.
45. Garratty G. Severe reactions associated with transfusion of patients with sickle cell disease. Transfusion 1997;37:357-61.
46. Reisner EG, Kostyu DD, Phillips G, et al. Alloantibody responses in multiply transfused sickle cell patients. Tissue Antigens 1987;30:161-6.
47. Spanos T, Karageorga M, Ladis V, et al. Red cell alloantibodies in patients with thalassemia. Vox Sang 1990;58:50-5.

48. Singer ST, Wu V, Mignacca R, et al. Alloimmunization and erythrocyte autoimmunization in transfusion-dependent thalassemia patients of predominantly Asian descent. Blood 2000;96:3369-73.
49. Sandler SG, Mallory D, Wolfe JS, et al. Screening with monoclonal anti-Fy3 to provide blood for phenotype-matched transfusions for patients with sickle cell disease. Transfusion 1997;37:393-7.
50. Mallory D, Malamut D, Ginther A. Rare blood for patients with sickle cell anemia. Ann NY Acad Sci 1989;565:432-3.
51. Diamond WJ, Brown FL, Jr, Bitterman P, et al. Delayed hemolytic transfusion reaction presenting as sickle-cell crisis. Ann Intern Med 1980;93: 231-4.
52. Cummins D, Webb G, Shah N, Davies SC. Delayed haemolytic transfusion reactions in patients with sickle cell disease. Postgrad Med J 1991;67: 689-91.
53. Syed SK, Sears DA, Werch JB, et al. Case reports: Delayed hemolytic transfusion reaction in sickle cell disease. Am J Med Sci 1996;312: 175-81.
54. Anderson RR, Sosler SD, Kovach J, DeChristopher PJ. Delayed hemolytic transfusion reaction due to anti-Js(a) in an alloimmunized patient with a sickle cell syndrome. Am J Clin Pathol 1997;108:658-61.
55. Bowen DT, Devenish A, Dalton J, Hewitt PE. Delayed haemolytic transfusion reaction due to simultaneous appearance of anti-Fya and anti-Fy5. Vox Sang 1988;55:35-6.
56. Fabron A Jr, Moreira G Jr, Bordin JO. Delayed hemolytic transfusion reaction presenting as a painful crisis in a patient with sickle cell anemia. Rev Paul Med 1999;117:38-9.
57. Kalyanaraman M, Heidemann SM, Sarnaik AP, et al. Anti-s antibody-associated delayed hemolytic transfusion reaction in patients with sickle cell anemia. J Pediatr Hematol Oncol 1999;21:70-3.
58. King KE, Shirey RS, Lankiewicz MW, et al. Delayed hemolytic transfusion reactions in sickle cell disease: Simultaneous destruction of recipients' red cells. Transfusion 1997;37:376-81.
59. Larson PJ, Lukas MB, Friedman DF, Manno CS. Delayed hemolytic transfusion reaction due to anti-Go(a), an antibody against the low-prevalence Gonzales antigen. Am J Hematol 1996;53:248-50.
60. Milner PF, Squires JE, Larison PJ, et al. Posttransfusion crises in sickle cell anemia: Role of delayed hemolytic reactions to transfusion. South Med J 1985;78:1462-9.
61. Mintz PD, Williams ME. Cerebrovascular accident during a delayed hemolytic transfusion reaction in a patient with sickle cell anemia. Ann Clin Lab Sci 1986;16:214-18.
62. Rao KR, Patel AR. Delayed hemolytic transfusion reactions in sickle cell anemia. South Med J 1989;82:1034-6.
63. Solanki D MP. Delayed hemolytic transfusion reactions: An often-missed clinical entity. JAMA 1978;239:729-31.

64. Squires JE, Larison PJ, Charles WT, Milner PF. A delayed hemolytic transfusion reaction due to anti-Co[b]. Transfusion 1985;25:137-9.
65. Strupp A, Cash K, Uehlinger J. Difficulties in identifying antibodies in the Dombrock blood group system in multiply alloimmunized patients. Transfusion 1998;38:1022-5.
66. Petz LD, Calhoun L, Shulman IA, et al. The sickle cell hemolytic transfusion reaction syndrome. Transfusion 1997;37:382-92.
67. Le Pennec PY, Rouger P, Klein MT, et al. Study of anti-Fy[a] in five black Fy(a–b–) patients. Vox Sang 1987;52:246-9.
68. Orlina AR, Sosler SD, Koshy M. Problems of chronic transfusion in sickle cell disease. J Clin Apheresis 1991;6:234-40.
69. Campbell SA, Shirey RS, King KE, Ness PM. An acute hemolytic transfusion reaction due to anti-IH in a patient with sickle cell disease. Transfusion 2000;40:828-31.
70. Halverson G, Shanahan E, Santiago I, et al. The first reported case of anti-Do[b] causing an acute hemolytic transfusion reaction. Vox Sang 1994;66:206-9.
71. Castellino SM, Combs MR, Zimmerman SA, et al. Erythrocyte autoantibodies in paediatric patients with sickle cell disease receiving transfusion therapy: Frequency, characteristics and significance. Br J Haematol 1999;104:189-94.
72. Issitt PD, Combs MR, Bumgarner DJ, et al. Studies of antibodies in the sera of patients who have made red cell autoantibodies. Transfusion 1996;36:481-6.
73. Paglieroni TG, Ward J, Holland PV. Changes in peripheral blood CD5 (Bla) B-cell populations and autoantibodies following blood transfusion. Transfusion 1995;35:189-98.
74. Vichinsky EP, Luban NL, Wright E, et al. Prospective RBC phenotype matching in a stroke-prevention trial in sickle cell anemia: A multicenter transfusion trial. Transfusion 2001;41:1086-92.
75. Wenz B, Gurtlinger K, Wheaton D, Dugan EP. A mimicking red blood cell autoantibody accompanying transfusion and alloimmunization. Transfusion 1982;22:147-50.
76. Cullis JO, Win N, Dudley JM, Kaye T. Post-transfusion hyperhaemolysis in a patient with sickle cell disease: Use of steroids and intravenous immunoglobulin to prevent further red cell destruction. Vox Sang 1995; 69:355-7.
77. Chaplin HJ, Cassell M. The occasional fallibility of in vitro compatibility tests. Transfusion 1962;2:375-84.
78. Win N, Doughty H, Telfer P, et al. Hyperhemolytic transfusion reaction in sickle cell disease. Transfusion 2001;41:323-8.
79. Telen MJ, Combs MR. Management of massive delayed hemolytic transfusion reactions in patients with sickle cell disease (abstract). Transfusion 1999;39(Suppl):97S.

80. Charache S, Terrin ML, Moore RD, et al. Effect of hydroxyurea on the frequency of painful crises in sickle cell anemia. Investigators of the Multicenter Study of Hydroxyurea in Sickle Cell Anemia. N Engl J Med 1995;332:1317-22.
81. Ware RE, Zimmerman SA, Schultz WH. Hydroxyurea as an alternative to blood transfusions for the prevention of recurrent stroke in children with sickle cell disease. Blood 1999;94:3022-6.
82. Brown D. A rapid method for harvesting autologous red cells from patients with hemoglobin S disease. Transfusion 1988;28:21-3.
83. Castilho L, Rios M, Bianco C, et al. DNA-based typing of blood groups for the management of multiply-transfused sickle cell disease patients. Transfusion 2002;42:232-8.
84. Rios M, Hue-Roye K, Storry JR, Reiss RF. Cell typing the sensitized transfusion-dependent patient. Ann Clin Lab Sci 2000;30:379-86.
85. Pellegrino J Jr, Castilho L, Rios M, De Souza CA. Blood group genotyping in a population of highly diverse ancestry. J Clin Lab Anal 2001;15:8-13.
86. Tahhan HR, Holbrook CT, Braddy LR, et al. Antigen-matched donor blood in the transfusion management of patients with sickle cell disease. Transfusion 1994;34:562-9.
87. Issitt PD. Race-related red cell alloantibody problems. Br J Biomed Sci 1994;51:158-67.
88. Vichinsky E. Consensus document for transfusion-related iron overload. Semin Hematol 2001;38:2-4.
89. Ness PM. To match or not to match: The question for chronically transfused patients with sickle cell anemia. Transfusion 1994;34:558-60.
90. Charache S. Problems in transfusion therapy. N Engl J Med 1990;322:1666-8.
91. Castro O. Management of sickle cell disease: Recent advances and controversies. Br J Haematol 1999;107:2-11.
92. Reed W, Vichinsky EP. Transfusion therapy: A coming-of-age treatment for patients with sickle cell disease. Am J Pediatr Hematol Oncol 2001;23:197-202.
93. Kavitsky D, Nance S, Glackin K, et al. A novel method to obtain phenotypically similar blood for sickle cell disease patients and promote African-American donations (abstract). Transfusion 1998;38(Suppl):110S.
94. Squires JE. Artificial blood. Science 2002;295:1002-5.
95. Scott MD, Murad KL, Koumpouras F, et al. Chemical camouflage of antigenic determinants: Stealth erythrocytes. Proc Natl Acad Sci U S A 1997;94:7566-71.
96. Murad KL, Mahany KL, Brugnara C, et al. Structural and functional consequences of antigenic modulation of red blood cells with methoxypoly(ethylene glycol). Blood 1999;93:2121-7.

In: Herman JH, Manno CS, eds.
Pediatric Transfusion Therapy
Bethesda, MD: AABB Press, 2002

12

Transfusion Support in Pediatric Cardiac Surgery

CATHERINE S. MANNO, MD

FROM THE FIRST EFFORTS made by Blalock and Taussig in the 1940s,[1] cardiac surgery procedures for pediatric patients continued to improve and become more complex. As technology has permitted treatment of smaller and smaller patients, blood transfusion support for open-heart surgery in this patient group has become more challenging. Optimal transfusion support must address the key issues of 1) need for volumes exceeding 100 mL/kg, 2) underlying cardiac disease, 3) patient age and size, 4) hemostatic abnormalities, and 5) complex serologic techniques and procedures.

Catherine S. Manno, MD, Acting Chief, Division of Hematology, The Children's Hospital of Philadelphia, and Associate Professor of Pediatrics, School of Medicine, University of Pennsylvania, Philadelphia, Pennsylvania

In meeting the requirements for transfusion support in pediatric cardiac surgery, many approaches have been used, and practices vary widely. Some clinicians use hemoconcentration and bypass circuits modified for pediatric volumes to decrease the need for transfusion and thus exposure to multiple donors. Others turn to adjunctive pharmacologic therapies to achieve the same goal. This chapter discusses several different strategies currently in use to provide safe and effective transfusion support for this patient group.

Overview of Pediatric Cardiac Surgery

In addition to advances in technology that have resulted in the survival and treatment of smaller and smaller patients, other trends have surfaced. On one hand, blood transfusion support has increased as the surgical procedures themselves have become more complex.[2,3] For instance, infants may undergo palliative shunting procedures as a temporary measure, and return when they are older for definitive surgical repair. Often, the need for blood components is increased in repeat procedures[2] because of bleeding from the scar tissue. As can be expected, the more complex the surgical procedure, the greater the transfusion requirements. Types of cardiac surgery are listed in Table 12-1.

Yet, on the other hand, there are also trends toward decreased transfusion requirements. For example, transcatheter therapy is being used for a wide variety of procedures, thus limiting the need for component therapy to support congenital heart disease treatment.

In parallel with the trend toward smaller patients in cardiovascular surgery is a trend toward younger patients in pediatric cardiac transplantation. Infants now constitute 50% of pediatric cardiac surgical populations,[4] and over 50% of pediatric heart recipients are less than 5 years old.[5]

Achieving Hemostasis

Appropriate transfusion support to maintain perioperative hemostasis must be determined after consideration of several factors, including physiologic alterations in coagulation factor

Table 12-1. Comparative Complexity of Pediatric Cardiac Surgeries[3]

Complexity Level/Examples	Comments
Simple Aortic valvuloplasty Closure of ASD patch Blalock-Taussig shunt* Repair of partial anomalous pulmonary venous return Resection of subaortic membrane	Shortest time on CPB; shortest period of circulatory arrest; shortest suture lines; least need for transfusion support (avg 2.3 components)
Intermediate Closure of primum ASD with mitral valve replacement Repair of ASD with mitral valve replacement Repair of ASD/VSD patch Repair of incomplete AV canal Repair of complete AV canal Pulmonary valvotomy Repair of total anomalous pulmonary venous return Senning procedure† Closure of VSD patch Repair of VSD patch with resection of coarctation of aorta	
Complex Arterial switch Fontan procedure‡ Modified Glenn shunt§ Separation of aorta and pulmonary artery with repair of VSD patch Stage I palliation for hypoplastic left heart syndrome‖	Longest time on CPB; longest period of circulatory arrest; longest suture lines; most transfusion support (avg 6.3 components)

Modified from Manno et al.[3]

ASD = atrial septal defect; CPB = cardiopulmonary bypass; VSD = ventricular septal defect; AV = atrioventricular

*Subclavian to pulmonary artery anastomosis.

†An operation used in children with transposition of the great vessels that redirects the venous return using an intra-atrial baffle of autologous tissue.

‡An operation used in children with a single ventricle that separates the pulmonary from the systemic circulation.

§Superior vena cava to right pulmonary artery anastomosis.

‖Procedure consisting of 1) transection of the main pulmonary artery, 2) creation of a neoaorta, and 3) creation of a systemic to pulmonary artery shunt.

levels due to patient age, the hematologic abnormalities that have been described in children with congenital heart disease, and the severe bleeding that occurs as a result of cardiopulmonary bypass (CPB).

Impact of Patient Age

The human coagulation system is not fully developed at birth; rather, maturation occurs gradually until late childhood. Thus, neonates have low levels of Factors II, VII, IX, X, XI, XII, prekallikrein, and high-molecular-weight kininogen.[6] A slower rate of thrombin generation is evidenced by mildly prolonged prothrombin time and activated partial thromboplastin time. These differences are more pronounced in premature infants than in newborns.

Although these hemostatic derangements are physiologic in normal infants, they may become significant in those undergoing cardiac surgery. Underlying illness or dilution from CPB may exacerbate the hemostatic alterations. In addition to low coagulation factor levels, levels of coagulation inhibitors are also decreased in neonates. These altered inhibitor levels (protein C, protein S, antithrombin, and heparin cofactor II) as well as increase in a_2-macroglobulin, may result in difficulties in achieving adequate anticoagulation during CPB.

Impact of Underlying Disease

Children with congenital heart disease typically demonstrate one of several hemostatic abnormalities. Patient with cyanotic congenital heart disease may have shortened platelet survival.[7] Thrombocytopenia may be present.[8] Platelet dysfunction and impaired platelet aggregation have been reported.[9] Those who receive preoperative medications such as prostaglandins or amiodarone may experience decreased platelet function. Some patients have demonstrated an acquired reduction of very large von Willebrand factor multimers.[10] Underlying disease often results in reduced coagulation factor levels,[11] as well as the possibility of chronic DIC.[12,13]

Factors Associated with Cardiopulmonary Bypass

CPB causes hemostatic alterations through several mechanisms.[14] First, the hemodilution caused by large volumes of non-blood solutions used to prime the pump results in significantly reduced coagulation factor levels.[11,15,16] In pediatric patients, the prime volume may be two or three times larger than their blood volume. Second, when the blood is exposed to the surface of the extracorporeal circuit, the contact system is activated and consumption of coagulation factors is increased.[11,17] The area of exposure is proportionately greater for pediatric patients than for adults.

Third, agonists associated with CPB, such as epinephrine and adenosine diphosphate,[18] can cause impaired platelet aggregation. Too much or too little protamine (used to reverse heparinization) can also cause platelet dysfunction. A fourth mechanism, the loss of platelet surface antigens such as glycoprotein IIb/IIIa, fibrinogen receptors,[19] and platelet a_2-adrenergic receptors,[18] has been debated.[20]

Finally, the hypothermia induced during many cardiac procedures (to lower the metabolic demands) alters both platelet function and coagulation parameters.[21]

Selection of Blood Components

Many different approaches to component selection are used successfully in pediatric cardiac surgery, and there are no widely accepted practice standards. Factors that affect the choice of components include the experience and skill of the surgical team, and the type of surgery. All surgical blood ordering protocols should limit donor exposures and support good patient outcomes by maximizing oxygenation during CPB and minimizing bleeding.

Whole Blood

The hemostatic defects noted above can be addressed through the transfusion of "fresh" Whole Blood. The use of Whole Blood may also result in decreased donor exposures. However, Whole Blood is not widely available. In addition to meeting the patient's transfusion needs, Whole Blood is also used by some as the priming mixture for CPB pumps.[2] Others prime with a combination of Whole Blood and a balanced electrolyte solution such as Plasma-Lyte A (Baxter Hyland Healthcare, Glendale, CA).

In certain groups of patients, postsurgical blood requirements have been met through transfusion of recently collected or "fresh" Whole Blood. A study of 161 pediatric open-heart surgery patients compared the use of fresh Whole Blood and stored blood components that were reconstituted as Whole Blood.[3] Children less than 2 years old undergoing complex procedures who received blood less than 48 hours old experienced significantly less blood loss. In children over 2 years of age, postoperative blood loss was not affected by the freshness of the blood. Blood less than 6 hours old was no more effective than blood that was 24 to 48 hours old.

The hemostatic advantage of blood transfused 24 to 48 hours after collection is likely the result of better platelet function. In Whole Blood stored at 4 C for more than 48 hours, platelet function deteriorates and coagulation factor levels decrease. Furthermore, platelet function in fresh Whole blood is preserved because the unit does not undergo centrifugation. Platelet aggregation studies were more normal in children who received fresh Whole Blood compared with those who received Whole Blood reconstituted with stored components.[3] Similarly, in adults, a single unit of fresh whole blood has been shown to increase platelet counts equivalent to the increase achieved through 6 units of platelets.[22]

An important issue in the use of Whole Blood is the amount of time required for testing. The use of very fresh Whole Blood (less than 6 hours old) does not allow time for pretransfusion testing. While use of 24- to 48-hour Whole Blood does permit time for some pretransfusion testing, other testing such as nucleic acid amplification testing (NAT) requires more time. Thus, the hemostatic benefits of using Whole Blood within 24 to 48 hours of collection must be weighed against the (very small) viral safety advantage of using blood that has undergone NAT.

Another concern involves leukocyte reduction of Whole Blood. Because currently available leukocyte reduction filters also remove platelets, the use of Whole Blood is incompatible with leukocyte reduction.

Blood Components

As with Whole Blood, component therapy varies widely and no uniform criteria have been established. For example, some clinicians use red cell transfusion to maintain a hemoglobin level of greater than 10 g/dL[2,23] or higher (12 to 13 g/dL in neonates[24] and patients with cyanosis and residual shunts[23,24]). Others find 8 g/dL an acceptable hemoglobin level.[25]

Another concern is transfusion of large amounts of additive solutions, which may cause electrolyte disturbances in particularly small infants. In some facilities, RBC units are centrifuged to remove additive solutions, although the practice has not been studied extensively. Table 12-2 compares some advantages and disadvantages of RBCs and Whole Blood.

The use of platelet concentrates to maintain a platelet count of greater than 100,000/µL is recommended by some as a routine practice in the presence of bleeding or on the first postoperative day.[2] Platelet concentrates are also transfused in cases of severe bleeding when the platelet count is normal, in an effort to treat the platelet dysfunction induced by CPB. Postoperative hemorrhage in the presence of abnormal coagulation test results is often treated with Fresh Frozen Plasma (FFP).[2,23] Some clinicians have suggested the use of Cryoprecipitated AHF instead of FFP in neonates, who are likely to have low fibrinogen levels.[11]

Blood Testing and Modification

Blood intended for transfusion to pediatric patients scheduled to undergo cardiac surgery should undergo complete routine testing for infectious diseases; blood typing and antibody screening should also be performed. As with adults, pediatric patients with cold-reacting antibodies may experience hemolysis during deep hypothermia if antigen-positive blood has been transfused. Although this situation has not been studied extensively, some fa-

Table 12-2. Comparison of Fresh Whole Blood and Red Blood Cells in Pediatric Cardiac Surgery

Blood Component	Advantages	Disadvantages
Fresh Whole Blood (used 24 to 48 hours after collection)	Addresses hemodilution Better platelet formation Limits donor exposures Associated with reduced postoperative blood loss in very young patients undergoing complex procedures Can be used for CPB prime	Limited availability Cannot be leukocyte-reduced Does not permit time for NAT
Red Blood Cells	Readily available Can undergo NAT Can be leukocyte-reduced Can be used for CPB prime	Presence of additive solutions No platelets Increased donor exposures

cilities provide M-negative blood to patients with anti-M, to prevent potential hemolysis.

Several indications exist for the use of irradiated components in pediatric cardiac surgery. Chapter 7 discusses irradiation in detail. It should be noted that an additional indication for irradiation is for heart transplant recipients, because they will continue to receive immunosuppressive therapy. Other patients who should receive irradiated blood include those with the DiGeorge anomaly and those with cardiac lesions in whom the DiGeorge anomaly has not been definitively excluded.[17,26]

Blood Conservation

The importance of limiting donor exposure in pediatric patients is discussed in detail in Chapter 9. The use of aliquots and other technologies is reviewed in Chapter 10. In the setting of cardiac surgery, pediatric patients can benefit from newer surgical and CPB techniques that limit blood loss, the use of autologous blood, and the use of adjuctive pharmacologic therapy.

Modified CPB Technology

Although the hemodilution during CPB normally increases blood usage in pediatric patients, modifications can be made to reverse this trend. For instance, a reduction in the size of the oxygenator compartment in the CPB circuit can substantially reduce the priming volume—in comes cases, to as low as 80 mL.[4]

Another approach is to counteract the hemodilution itself through ultrafiltration. Water, electrolytes, and low-molecular-weight substances are removed as blood passes through the filter, resulting in hemoconcentration, rather than hemodilution. Although conventional ultrafiltration occurs during CPB, newer techniques of modified ultrafiltration are performed after CPB. The use of modified ultrafiltration results in significantly less blood loss and fewer postoperative transfusions,[27-30] and the technique is used routinely in many facilities.

Autologous Blood

The feasibility of preoperative autologous blood donation may be limited in pediatric patients because of their small blood volume. Some may not be candidates because of their poor venous access, anemia, hypoxemia, or cardiovascular instability. Nevertheless, the technique has proved to be beneficial in many pediatric patients. One study of autologous blood transfusion in pediatric cardiac surgery[31] demonstrated that patients had few adverse reactions to sequential phlebotomy, and used significantly less allogeneic blood. Decreased exposure to allogeneic blood has also been reported in pediatric patients who underwent preoperative autologous donation before other types of surgery.[32]

Autologous blood may also be recovered from the CPB circuit and used for postoperative transfusion. It has been demonstrated[33] that such intraoperative blood recovery does not result in increased bleeding, when compared with the use of allogeneic blood for postoperative transfusion. However, the risk of bacterial contamination in recovered blood stored for up to 18 hours at room temperature as well as increased free hemoglobin levels must be taken into consideration.

Pharmacologic Therapy

Pharmacologic agents have been demonstrated to decrease transfusion requirements in adult cardiac patients.[34-36] Aprotinin, a nonspecific protease inhibitor that preserves platelet function, has been extensively studied, but the results in pediatric cardiac surgery are conflicting. Some reports[37-39] have shown decreased blood loss and postoperative transfusion requirements, while others[34] show no improvement with aprotinin. Pediatric patients with complex cardiac malformations[37] or who are undergoing a repeat cardiac procedure[39] appear to benefit most from the use of aprotinin. This is likely due to the higher incidence of bleeding in these patients.

Because aprotinin is derived from a bovine source, there may be a risk of allergic reaction with re-exposure (as high as 6%[40]). The incidence of allergic reactions appears to be highest when the re-exposure occurs within 200 days of the initial exposure.[41] Therefore, repeat surgical procedures should be delayed if possible. Also recommended is administration of a test dose of aprotinin followed by monitoring for anaphylaxis for all repeat exposures.[41] Premedication with antihistamines or steroids has been used to decrease the risk of an allergic reaction to aprotinin. It is important to determine the individual patient's risk of allergic reaction and prevent its occurrence, because patients needing repeat procedures are the ones who can benefit most from aprotinin.

Tranexamic acid, which inhibits fibrinolysis, is another pharmacologic agent that has been shown to decrease blood loss and transfusion requirements in adult cardiac patients.[35,36] However, for the pediatric population, study results are not as clear, partly because few studies have been conducted and partly because the donors and methods of administration are not comparable.

One study of tranexamic acid given as a single 50 mg/kg dose showed decreased postoperative bleeding only in children with cyanotic heart defects.[42] Another study using a larger initial dose followed by continuous infusion of tranexamic acid showed decreased blood loss and transfusion requirements in children undergoing different types of repeat procudres.[43] Further research is needed to determine if pediatric patients truly derive benefit from this therapy.

Conclusion

Although great strides have been made in reducing blood loss in pediatric patients undergoing cardiac surgery, the majority of these tiny patients still need blood transfusion. Thus, the careful selection of blood components, the modification of CPB techniques, the use of autologous blood, and the potential use of adjuctive therapy remain key considerations. More studies are needed to determine whether successful approaches in adult patient populations are beneficial in the pediatric setting, and whether a consensus on practice standards can be formed.

References

1. Blalock A, Taussig HE. The surgical treatment of malformations of the heart in which there is pulmonary stenosis of pulmonary atresia. JAMA 1945;128:189-202.
2. Chambers LA, Cohen DM, Davis JT. Transfusion patterns in pediatric open heart surgery. Transfusion 1996;36:150-4.
3. Manno CS, Hedberg KW, Kim HC, et al. Comparison of the hemostatic effects of fresh whole blood, stored whole blood, and components after open heart surgery in children. Blood 1991;77:930-6.
4. Groom RC, Akl BF, Albus R, Lefrak EA. Pediatric pulmonary bypass: A review of current practice. Int Anesthesiol Clin 1996;34:141-63.

5. Addonizio LJ. Current status of cardiac transplantation in children. Curr Opin Pediatr 1996;8:520-6.
6. Andrew M, Paes B, Johnston M. Development of the hemostatic system in the neonate and young infant. Am J Pediatr Hematol Oncol 1990; 12:95-104.
7. Waldman JD, Czapek EE, Paul MH, et al. Shortened platelet survival in cyanotic congenital heart disease. J Pediatr 1975; 87:77-9.
8. Gross S, Keefer V, Liebman J. The platelets in cyanotic congenital heart disease. Pediatrics 1968;42:651-8.
9. Mauer HM, McCue CM, Caul J, Still WJ. Impairment in platelet aggregation in congenital cardiac disease. Blood 1972;40:207-15.
10. Gill JC, Wilson AD, Endres-Brooks J, Montgomery RR. Loss of the largest von Willebrand factor multimers from the plasma of patients with congenital heart defects. Blood 1996;67:758-61.
11. Kern FH, Morana NJ, Sears JJ, Hickey PR. Coagulation defects in neonates during cardiopulmonary bypass. Ann Thorac Surg 1992;54:541-6.
12. Komp DM, Sparrow AW. Polycythemia in cyanotic heart disease—a study of altered coagulation. J Pediatr 1970;76:231-6.
13. Ihenacho HN, Fletcher DJ, Breeze GR, Stuart J. Consumption coagulopathy in congenital heart disease. Lancet 1973;i:231-4.
14. Bevan DH. Cardiac bypass haemostasis: Putting blood through the mill. Br J Haematol 1999;104:208-19.
15. Mammen EF, Koets MH, Washington BC, et al. Hemostasis changes during cardiopulmonary bypass surgery. Semin Thromb Hemost 1985;11:281-92.
16. Chan AK, Leaker M, Burrows FA, et al. Coagulation and fibrinolytic profile of paediatric patients undergoing cardiopulmonary bypass. Thromb Haemost 1997;77:270-7.
17. Lin AE. Congenital heart defects in chromosome abnormality syndromes. In: Emmanoulides GC, Riemenschneider TA, Allen HD, Gutgesell HP, eds. Heart disease in infants, children, and adolescents including the fetus and young adult. Baltimore, MD: Williams & Wilkins, 1995:633-43.
18. Woodman RC, Harker LA. Bleeding complications associated with cardiopulmonary bypass. Blood 1990;76:1680-97.
19. Musial J, Niewiarowski S, Hershock D, et al. Loss of fibrinogen receptors from the platelet surface during simulated extracorporeal circulation. J Lab Clin Med 1985;105:514-22.
20. Kestin AS, Valeri CS, Khuri SF, et al. The platelet function defect of cardiopulmonary bypass. Blood 1993;82:107-17.
21. Milam JD. Blood transfusion in heart surgery. Surg Clin North Am 1982;63:1127-47.
22. Lavee J, Martinowitz U, Mohr R, et al. The effect of transfusion of fresh whole blood versus platelet concentrates after cardiac operations. J Thorac Cardiovasc Surg 1989;97:204-12.

23. Guay J, Rivard G. Mediastinal bleeding after cardiopulmonary bypass in pediatric patients. Ann Thorac Surg 1996;62:1955-60.
24. Bando K, Turrentine MW, Vijay P, et al. Effect of modified ultrafiltration in high-risk patients undergoing operations for congenital heart disease. Ann Thorac Surg 1998;66:821-8.
25. Cooley DA. Conservation of blood during cardiovascular surgery. Am J Surg 1995;170(Suppl):53-9.
26. Towbin JA, Greenberg F. Genetic syndromes and clinical molecular genetics. In: Garson A, Bricker JT, Fisher DJ, Neish SR, eds. The science and practice of pediatric cardiology, 2nd ed. Baltimore, MD: Williams & Wilkins, 1998:2627-700.
27. Koutlas TC, Gaynor W, Nicolson SC, et al. Modified ultrafiltration reduces postoperative morbidity after cavopulmonary connection. Ann Thorac Surg 1997;64:37-43.
28. Naik SK, Knight A, Elliot M. A prospective randomized study of a modified technique of ultrafiltration during pediatric open-heart surgery. Circulation 1991;84(Suppl III):422-31.
29. Ad N, Snir E, Katz J, et al. Use of the modified technique of ultrafiltration in pediatric open-heart surgery: A prospective study. Isr J Med Sci 1996;32:1326-31.
30. Draaisma AM, Hazekamp MG, Frank M, et al. Modified ultrafiltration after cardiopulmonary bypass in pediatric cardiac surgery. Ann Thorac Surg 1997;64:521-5.
31. Masuda M, Kawachi Y, Inaba S, et al. Preoperative autologous blood donations in pediatric cardiac surgery. Ann Thorac Surg 1995;60:1694-7.
32. Novak RW. Autologous blood transfusion in a pediatric population: Safety and efficacy. Clin Pediatr 1988;27:184-7.
33. Hishon ML, Ryan A, Lithgow P, Butt W. An evaluation of changes in composition and contamination of salvaged blood from the cardiopulmonary bypass circuit of pediatric patients. Heart Lung 1995;24:307-11.
34. Davies MJ, Allen A, Kort H, et al. Prospective, randomized, double-blind study of high-dose aprotinin in pediatric cardiac operations. Ann Thorac Surg 1997;63:497-503.
35. Coffey A, Pittmam J, Halbrook H, et al. The use of tranexamic acid to reduce postoperative bleeding following cardiac surgery: A double-blind randomized trial. Am Surg 1995;61:566-8.
36. Horrow JC, Hlavacek J, Strong MD, et al. Prophylactic tranexamic acid decreases bleeding after cardiac operations. J Thorac Cardiovasc Surg 1990;99:70-4.
37. Carrel TP, Schwanda M, Vogt PR, Turina MI. Aprotinin in pediatric cardiac operations: A benefit in complex malformations and with high-dose regimen only. Ann Thorac Surg 1998;66:153-8.
38. Penkoske PA, Entwistle LM, Marchak BE, et al. Aprotinin in children undergoing repair of congenital heart defects. Ann Thorac Surg 1995; 60(Suppl):529-32.

39. Miller BE, Tosone SR, Tam VK, et al. Hematologic and economic impact of aprotinin in reoperative pediatric cardiac operations. Ann Thorac Surg 1998;66:535-41.
40. Diefenbach C, Abel M, Limpers B, et al. Fatal anaphylactic shock after aprotinin reexposure in cardiac surgery. Anesth Analg 1995;80:830-1.
41. Dietrich W. Incidence of hypersensitivity reactions. Ann Thorac Surg 1998;65(Suppl):60-4.
42. Zonis Z, Seear M, Reichert C, et al. The effect of preoperative tranexamic acid on blood loss after cardiac operations in children. J Thorac Cardiovasc Surg 1996;111:982-7.
43. Reid RW, Zimmerman A, Laussen PC, et al. The efficacy of tranexamic acid versus placebo effect in decreasing blood loss in pediatric patients undergoing repeat cardiac surgery. Anesth Analg 1997;84:990-6.

In: Herman JH, Manno CS, eds.
Pediatric Transfusion Therapy
Bethesda, MD: AABB Press, 2002

13

Transfusion Support in Pediatric Surgery, Trauma, and the Intensive Care Unit

CHRISTOPHER J. FESTA, MD; ANDREW K. FENG, MD; AND DAVID BIGOS, MD

PEDIATRIC CRITICAL CARE medicine encompasses significant age ranges, physiologic variations, and medical and surgical pathologic conditions. A detailed discussion of the various aspects of transfusion therapy within the context of specific medical and surgical diagnoses is beyond the scope of this chapter. Rather, this discussion focuses on some general aspects of the application of trans-

Christopher J. Festa, MD, Assistant Professor of Pediatrics, Section of Critical Care, Temple University Children's Medical Center, Philadelphia, Pennsylvania; Andrew K. Feng, MD, Assistant Professor of Pediatrics, Floating Hospital for Children, Boston, Massachusetts; and David Bigos, MD, Associate Professor of Pediatrics and Director, Section of Critical Care, Temple University Children's Medical Center, Philadelphia, Pennsylvania

fusion therapy in the areas of pediatric surgery, trauma, and the intensive care unit (ICU).

Transfusion Triggers

Red Blood Cells

For many decades, transfusions were given as needed to maintain the hemoglobin above 10 g/dL and the hematocrit above 30%. This was primarily based on the recommendations of Adams and Lundy.[1]

Throughout the years, various investigators attempted to define the "optimal hematocrit" through a variety of studies. This optimal hematocrit was generally felt to maximize oxygen delivery. The equation for oxygen delivery is as follows:

$$DO_2 = CaO_2 \times CO$$

where DO_2 represents oxygen delivery, CaO_2 represents arterial oxygen content, and CO represents cardiac output. Proceeding further,

$$CaO_2 = (Hb \times 1.34) \times SaO_2 + (PaO_2 \times 0.0031)$$

where Hb represents hemoglobin, SaO_2 represents arterial oxygen saturation, and PaO_2 represents the arterial oxygen pressure. Thus,

$$DO_2 = [(Hb \times 1.34) \times SaO_2 + (PaO_2 \times 0.0031)] \times CO$$

There would be an almost linear relationship between hemoglobin and oxygen delivery if the increased viscosity from a higher hematocrit did not negatively affect the cardiac output. Thus, DO_2 increases with increasing hematocrit to a certain point at which the viscosity effects predominate and the DO_2 decreases. This point at which maximal DO_2 occurs is referred to as the optimal hematocrit.

Studies in animals have suggested that the maximal oxygen transport occurs at a hematocrit between 30 and 40%.[2-4] In the critically ill patient, clinicians may cite a transfusion target of a hematocrit ≥30% based on these models. In keeping with this general premise, volume resuscitation in the patient with unremitting shock and anemia should include blood. Crystalloid resuscitation alone would cause hemodilution, further lowering the hematocrit.

There is no agreement regarding a target value for hemoglobin and hematocrit transfusion triggers that apply to all patients and situations. Therefore, investigators have looked at signs and symptoms and multiple physiologic variables to determine if they could better represent an indication for the need for transfusion.

In children, however, signs and symptoms of anemia do not develop until the hemoglobin is extremely low. The physiologic values analyzed include such measures as mixed venous PO_2 or saturation, oxygen consumption, and oxygen extraction ratio. Whereas there are some data supporting the use of these variables in certain clinical situations, there is no widespread acceptance for the use of these types of data to determine the indication for transfusion. The issue of the red cell transfusion trigger for patients on mechanical ventilatory support is addressed later in this chapter.

Platelets

There are no established values for "safe" platelet counts for children who undergo the invasive procedures that occur in the area of critical care medicine. In fact, there are many instances in which resuscitative efforts involving invasive procedures are performed emergently in critically ill children before it is known that the patient is thrombocytopenic (platelet count <100,000/μL). It is generally accepted that a platelet count greater than 50,000/μL is adequate for hemostasis. Unlike extracorporeal membrane oxygenation (ECMO) and cardiopulmonary bypass (CPB), which are discussed later in this chapter, there are no studies that specifically address the risk of bleeding for critically ill children undergoing these invasive procedures.

The decision really is a matter of clinical judgment, in which the practitioner must balance the risk of morbidity and mortality associated with bleeding complications from the procedure(s) in question with the consequences of delaying the procedure until a platelet transfusion is completed. As a general rule, if the procedure is not emergent, platelets are given to patients whose platelet counts are less than 40-50,000/μL before most invasive procedures. The exceptions would be lumbar puncture and placement of an intracranial pressure monitor in which the desired goal would be a platelet count greater than 100,000/μL.

The practitioner must also factor in the specific disease or injury process into the decision. The classic example is the patient with idiopathic thrombocytopenic purpura (ITP). Many of these patients can be profoundly thrombocytopenic (platelet count <10,000/μL). In this case, platelet transfusion would be of little value, because transfused platelets would be rapidly bound to circulating antibodies and removed from the circulation.

Fresh Frozen Plasma

As with platelets, there are no established values for prothrombin time (PT) and activated partial thromboplastin time (aPTT) for critically ill children undergoing invasive procedures. Many critically ill children can have disseminated intravascular coagulation (DIC) associated with a variety of medical and surgical diagnoses. As is the case with thrombocytopenia, the critically ill child may require emergent invasive procedures in the resuscitative phase before the presence of a coagulopathy is known. In fact, bleeding from puncture or incision sites during or after the procedure may be the first sign to suggest the diagnosis. Again, the practitioner must balance the risk of morbidity and/or mortality associated with bleeding complications from the procedure(s) with the consequences of delaying the procedure. As a general rule, if the procedure is not emergent, fresh frozen plasma (FFP) is given to patients whose PT and aPTT are greater than 1.5 times normal before an invasive procedure.

Effect on Ventilator Response

Another group of patients for whom red cell transfusions are often given is those who require either high levels of or prolonged duration of mechanical ventilatory support. The rationale given is that the increased red cell mass and oxygen-carrying capacity will contribute to an improvement in patient status, thus facilitating the process of weaning the patient's level of support.

With respect to patients with high levels of mechanical ventilatory support, Asmundson and Kilburn[5] noted an improvement in survival rates for acute respiratory distress syndrome (ARDS) with red cell transfusion. As a general rule, if the level of mechanical ventilatory support or oxygen requirement (FiO_2 ≥0.6) is high, the patient should receive a red cell transfusion. For ARDS patients with high requirements for support, a hematocrit of 40 to 45% would be the goal. For patients with a moderate FiO_2 requirement (0.5-0.6) coupled with high positive end-expiratory pressure or poor compliance, red cell transfusion would be considered to maintain a hematocrit of 30 to 35% if the weaning process is likely to be protracted.

Schonhofer et al[6,7] demonstrated the value of transfusions given to anemic adult patients with chronic obstructive pulmonary disease who could not be weaned from mechanical ventilatory support. They demonstrated a significant reduction in minute ventilation and the work of breathing with a resultant unloading of the respiratory muscles. In addition, they showed an ability to be weaned more quickly from mechanical ventilation after transfusion. Similar benefits would appear to be potentially applicable to pediatric patients of a similar population.

Massive Transfusion

Massive transfusion in adults is defined as the replacement of a patient's entire blood volume in 24 hours or the transfusion of more than 10 RBC units over the same period. Translation of this definition into pediatric practice requires age and weight standardization.

Massive transfusions within the pediatric population, like those in the adult population, are frequent in trauma, CPB, and ECMO and when substantial blood loss occurs in complex nontraumatic surgical cases. Unlike the adult population, neonates with severe hyperbilirubinemia and others who receive exchange transfusion therapy may also qualify as massive transfusion recipients.

With advancing age, a child's circulating blood volume referenced to body weight decreases. Table 13-1 lists the average volume per kg of body weight for specific age groups within the pediatric population. This variance in circulating blood volume must be accounted for when formulating exchange volumes or attempting to define a population at risk for complications of massive transfusion therapy.

Aside from the well-recognized infectious complications associated with blood component exposure, a host of well-recognized acute metabolic complications are associated with massive blood transfusions. The complications of massive transfusion therapy can be categorized as either volume-related or rate-related.[8]

Table 13-1. Approximate Blood Volume for Age

Age	Blood Volume (mL/kg)
Preterm infant	90-105
Term newborn	78-86
1-12 months	73-78
1-3 years	74-82
4-6 years	80-86
7-18 years	83-90
Adults	68-88

Reproduced with permission from Barone MA. Harriet Lane handbook, 14th ed. St. Louis, MO: CV Mosby, 1996:285.

Volume-Related Complications

Volume-related complications occur when large replacement volumes are administered to a patient who requires volume resuscitation for treatment of an acute hemorrhage. In addition to third space accumulation with edema formation, several dilutional complications are encountered by the bedside clinician.

Thrombocytopenia

Dilutional thrombocytopenia is defined as a platelet count of less than 50,000/μL in the setting of massive transfusion. This dilutional effect is secondary to the transfusion of platelet-reduced RBC concentrates. Hippala et al[9] reported that, in adult patients undergoing surgery, approximately 230% of the patient's blood volume needed replacement before the platelet count dropped to below 50,000/μL. Unless clinical indications (ie, intracranial hemorrhage) that necessitate aggressive correction of thrombocytopenia exist, prophylactic transfusion of platelet concentrates is not indicated. Clearly, if a bleeding diathesis exists and can be attributed to thrombocytopenia or platelet dysfunction, correction should be considered.

Dilution of Coagulation Factors

Like that of platelets, the transfusion of large volumes of plasma-reduced RBC concentrates results in the dilution of circulating concentrations of coagulation factors. The use of whole blood appears to protect against this complication, but its lack of availability outside of elective surgical procedures limits its use. Of the clotting factors, fibrinogen appears to be the most susceptible.[9]

Clinical bleeding secondary to an overt dilutional coagulopathy is well recognized in the setting of massive transfusion therapy. The question presented to the bedside clinician is whether or not to administer FFP to replace clotting factors. Prophylactic administration of FFP is currently not recommended. It is recommended, however, that factor replacement therapy begin with evidence of a clinical bleeding diathesis. The decision algorithm for the bedside clinician confronted with an overt coagulopathy is challenging.

In the clinical setting, prophylactic transfusions to replace clotting factors are indicated only when the hemorrhage (by volume or location) is serious in its location or extent or for reversal of an underlying inherited or acquired coagulopathy (eg, warfarin intoxication). Although coagulation function studies (PT, aPTT) are used to guide factor replacement, there are questions as to their applicability in the acute-care setting. Delays in obtaining laboratory data may result in a delay in definitive therapy (factor replacement) for the patient. It is recommended that laboratory studies be used as a confirmatory test and that therapy, if clinically indicated in an urgent scenario, not be withheld.

Traditionally, the coagulopathy that develops in the setting of massive transfusion therapy is thought to be a result of dilution of procoagulants. The relative decrease in procoagulants leads to overt clinical bleeding. The dilution of anticoagulant factors such as protein C, protein S, and antithrombin that occurs with massive transfusion, however, leads to a hypercoagulable state. Data are lacking to support correction of these factors in the massive transfusion patient. However, with sepsis, activated protein C administration has been correlated with an improved outcome. There is also an increased risk of bleeding.[10]

Rate-Related Complications

In the setting of massive transfusion therapy, many major metabolic effects are related to the rate of blood component administration. (The more rapid the rate of infusion, the more profound the metabolic effects.) The vast majority of rate-related complications are the result of the manner in which RBC concentrates are stored. Each of the metabolic complications will be discussed briefly below.

A single unit of RBCs has a volume of approximately 250 mL and a hematocrit of approximately 70 to 80%. RBC concentrates are stored between 2 and 6 C for up to 35 days with the addition of specific solutions to the basic storage medium, CPDA. Storage of red cells results in specific biochemical alterations as a direct result of ongoing metabolism of the red cell. These biochemical changes are referred to as "storage lesions."

During storage, glycolytic and hexose-monophosphate (anaerobic) metabolic pathways continue to produce lactate. As lactate accumulates, the pH of the local environment falls, further inhibiting enzymatic activity. This decrease in enzymatic activity in turn decreases adenosine triphosphate (ATP) and 2,3-diphosphoglycerate (2,3-DPG) production. The lack of energy-rich substrate (ATP) results in alterations in the red cell membrane and ATPase-dependent osmotic channels (Na-K). The net effect is a decrease in membrane stability, resulting in rigid spherical cells that have a greater tendency to lyse. The decrease in 2,3-DPG increases the affinity of hemoglobin for oxygen that results in poor offloading of oxygen to the peripheral tissues, which further augments the acidosis. Other biochemical alterations noted in storage lesions include an elevation of lactate dehydrogenase and ammonia.

Electrolyte Disturbances

Several electrolyte disturbances are associated with the transfusion of stored blood. The sections below briefly describe these alterations, their physiologic effects, and treatment.

Hyperkalemia (Elevated Serum Potassium)

Extracellular potassium (K^+) accumulation in stored red cells is a result of the acidic environment that promotes K^+ flux out of the cell. In addition, altered energy-dependent ion-transport mechanisms and red cell lysis release intracellular K^+ into the external environment. With large-volume transfusions, significant K^+ loads are delivered to the patient. Although children tend to be more resistant to alterations in their serum K^+ than adults, a high burden promotes alterations in the myocardial resting membrane potential and decreases the rate of depolarization. This results in the classic electrocardiographic changes seen with hyperkalemia (peaked T waves, widened QRS, asystole). In addition to the electrocardiogram effects, the increased K^+ load decreases cardiac output. The rate of K^+ delivery plays a major role in its arrhythmogenic potential. Table 13-2 lists the standard therapy for hyperkalemia-induced arrhythmias.

Hypocalcemia (Low Ionized Serum Calcium)

As the ionized component of calcium is that which is physiologically active, the measurement of the ionized or active fraction of calcium provides a more precise picture of calcium activity than does total calcium (calcium bound to albumin). Hypocalcemia is best defined as a low serum ionized fraction and not a low total fraction that is affected by clinical conditions such as hypoalbuminemia. Although an equation exists (total calcium falls 0.8 mg/dL for every 1 g/dL decline in serum albumin from "normal") to correct for serum albumin, the measurement of the ionized form should be used when available.

With the rapid infusion of stored RBCs, citrate (an anticoagulant component of the storage solution) binds serum calcium. If citrate is infused rapidly, a dramatic decrease in serum calcium may occur. Citrate intoxication can occur when one RBC unit is infused over 5 to 10 minutes.[11] Citrate metabolism is decreased in hepatic disease, hypothermia, and poor perfusion states, all of which are potentially present in the patient who requires massive transfusion therapy. The rapid infusion of citrate with stored blood, along with the aforementioned physiologic states, is responsible for the development of hypocalcemia. The cardiovascular effects of hypocalcemia include hypotension, a narrowed pulse pressure, and prolonged QT intervals. Despite the serious implications of hypocalcemia, most normothermic adults withstand the effects of up to one RBC unit every 5 minutes.[12] In the infant and neonate population, the ability to withstand citrate infusion is limited by the immature hepatic function along with the inability to regulate body temperature. This makes such patients prone to the development of clinically significant hypocalcemia.

Table 13-2 lists the standard therapy for hypocalcemia. Frequent assessment of serum ionized calcium levels is crucial, es-

Table 13-2. Treatment of Biochemical Alterations Associated with Massive Transfusions

Abnormality	Physical Findings	Therapy
Hyperkalemia	ECG: Peaked T waves • Serum level 7.5 Loss of P wave Widened QRS complex • Serum level 8 ST depression • Serum level 9 Bradycardia/asystole • Serum level >9	Calcium Chloride 10-20 mg/kg • IV through central venous catheter • Preferential therapy for ECG changes secondary to hyperkalemia Calcium gluconate 100 mg/kd • Requires first pass to become biologically active • May be given through peripheral IV Sodium bicarbonate 1-2 mEq/kg • Creates alkalosis that drives K^+ intracellular Insulin 0.1 unit regular/kg with glucose 0.5 g/kg • Given in conjunction they promote K^+ cellular uptake • May also be continually infused Kayexalate Resin 1 g/kg/dose every 2-6 hours • May also be administered orally • Resin exchanges 2 Na^+ for 1 K^+ • Not intended for acute therapy Non-pharmacologic therapies • Hyperventilation (if mechanically ventilated) – Promotes alkalosis and drives K^+ intracellular – An easy acute intervention but may not produce substantial ECG changes • Inhaled Beta agonists – An acute intervention that promotes K+ uptake by muscle cells – Not a definitive therapy

(continued)

Table 13-2. Treatment of Biochemical Alterations Associated with Massive Transfusions (continued)

Abnormality	Physical Findings	Therapy
Hypocalcemia	Increased QT interval Hypotension	Calcium chloride 10-20 mg/kg via central line
Hypomag-nesemia	Prolonged PR interval Increased QT interval Torsades de pointes	Magnesium sulfate 25-50 mg/kg • 2 g maximum • Administer slowly (125 mg/kg/hour) • May cause hypotension
Hypoglycemia	Hypothermia Hypotension Acute CNS dysfunction Seizures Coma	Dextrose 0.5 - 1 g/kg IV • May be given IV push • D10-D12.5 may be administered through peripheral IV • Concentrations greater than D12.5 should be administered through central line if possible

pecially in infants and neonates. Calcium correction through intravenous infusion has been associated with death.[13]

Hypomagnesemia (Low Serum Magnesium)

The cardiac effects of hypomagnesemia (prolonged QT interval, torsades de pointes) are described in association with massive transfusion therapy.[14] Magnesium serves as a cofactor for parathormone to promote calcium release from bone (decreased Mg^+ promotes decreased Ca^+) and in addition serves as a cofactor in the function of the Na-K ATPase-dependent channels in the myocardium. This later effect predisposes the myocardium to the development of arrhythmias. The extent to which the development of hypomagnesemia is transfusion rate-related is unclear. Unlike the ionized fraction of calcium, magnesium is more frequently reported as a total level (bound to albumin). As with calcium, a correction formula exists for hypoalbuminemia (true magnesium = measured Mg + 0.05 (40 – albumin in g/L). Table 13-2 lists the standard treatment for hypomagnesemia.

Acidosis

Anaerobic metabolism promotes the development of an acidic pH in stored RBC units. Despite this, in the setting of massive transfusion, the patient's pH may become paradoxically alkalotic. The alkalemia that develops is secondary to the conversion of sodium citrate to sodium bicarbonate. In the setting of acute trauma or poor cardiac output, poor perfusion may result in a metabolic acidosis. Depending on this metabolic balance, the pH may be acidotic, alkalotic, or neutral. Without confirmation of the serum pH, prophylactic infusion of sodium bicarbonate may worsen the metabolic state of the patient. Serum pH should be assessed frequently as the therapy is given only if a severe alteration in pH is present.

Hypothermia

Profound hypothermia can occur with the infusion of large volumes of cold fluids. Because the survival of stored red cells is dependent upon a cold environment, the patient undergoing a massive transfusion is at risk for the development of hypothermia (<35 C). The rate at which the thermal load is delivered to the patient plays a crucial role in the development of hypothermia. Unlike the adult or older child, small infants and neonates have poor temperature-regulatory mechanisms and thus are extremely prone to the development of hypothermia.

A core body temperature less than 35 C impairs coagulation through its effect on platelets that are already reduced in number by the dilutional effect of a massive transfusion. It also impairs the metabolism of citrate and shifts the hemoglobin oxygen dissociation curve to the left, which impairs oxygen delivery at the tissue level.

In addition to these effects, hypothermia is associated with systemic hypotension through myocardial depression, and, if severe (≤33 C), it may result in ventricular arrhythmias. If possible, blood should be warmed in an appropriate warming device and to a neutral temperature before infusion. This is particularly true when it is to be transfused to young infants.

Postoperative Transfusion

RBCs

As previously stated, the "10/30" trigger for RBC transfusion is not a valid indication for transfusion. Instead, the focus has turned more toward oxygen delivery (DO_2) and consumption (VO_2). In other words, there is no preset hemoglobin and/or hematocrit level that is considered optimal or necessary for good management and outcome. Several researchers[15,16] have recommended against using a single criterion as the sole indication for transfusion. In 1996, the American Society of Anesthesiologists (ASA) Task Force on Blood Component Therapy added to their recommendations for RBC transfusion the statement, "Transfusion is rarely indicated when the hemoglobin concentration is greater than 10 g/dL and is almost always indicated when it is less than 6 g/dL, especially when the anemia is acute...."[17]

In addition, the Task Force specified that the indications for transfusion of autologous red cells may be more liberal than those for allogeneic red cells because of the lower (but still significant) risks associated with the former. When evaluating these recommendations, one must keep in mind that, even though an age range is often not specified, most of these guidelines are written for adults. Therefore, translation of issues such as prophylactic protection of an ischemic myocardium is usually irrelevant in the pediatric population.

Platelets

In the postoperative surgical patient, risk factors for the development of thrombocytopenia include sepsis, an extensive surgical wound, and the volume of blood transfused.[18] Because thrombocytopenia is commonly encountered in patients with these conditions, the question of the need for platelet transfusions occurs fairly often. Postoperative patients may have additional problems that potentially lower the threshold for platelet transfusion. One factor favoring a more aggressive approach is the potential for "microvascular" bleeding, such as bleeding at the surgical wound. Bleeding seen with standard incisions may be compounded by effects from massive transfusion. Although most authorities[17] recommend prophylactic platelet transfusions for platelet counts ranging from ≤5000 to 30,000/μL, these guidelines may be more pertinent to the nonsurgical patient. One group,[19] however, recommended prophylactic preoperative platelet transfusion for patients with associated risk factors for bleeding when the platelet count reaches 10,000 to 20,000/μL. The ASA Task Force suggests that the threshold for transfusion should be lower (ie, transfusing at a higher platelet count) for surgical patients because of the increased risk of complications from bleeding.[17] In addition, it states that, in the setting of a massive transfusion or when a patient exhibits microvascular bleeding secondary to suspected thrombocytopenia and/or platelet dysfunction, empiric platelet transfusion may prove beneficial. Despite this caveat, the Task Force recommends that patients receive transfusions for platelet counts below 50,000/μL and that transfusions be considered for platelet counts between 50,000 and 100,000/μL in conjunction with increased clinical consequences of bleeding from the surgical site.

FFP

For the general postoperative patient, deficiency of clotting factors tends to derive more from complications of massive transfusion than from the surgery itself. Conversely, patients who have an abnormal PT and aPTT preoperatively, and yet have no history of bleeding, do not appear to have any significant postoperative surgical bleeding.[20,21] Furthermore, preoperative testing of PT and aPTT has failed to predict postoperative chest tube drainage in children after cardiopulmonary bypass (CPB).[22] For patients undergoing CPB, clotting factor deficiency secondary to hemodilution is a well-recognized entity that usually normalizes spontaneously within 1 to 2 hours after discontinuation of bypass.[23]

Trauma patients who undergo surgical intervention may develop a postoperative coagulopathy through different mechanisms. This patient population may require aggressive transfusion therapy. In addition to the dilutional effect of massive transfusion, clotting factors may become depleted by a number of factors stemming from the trauma itself. One trigger is the presence of tissue destruction that causes the release of tissue thromboplastins that activate the clotting cascade. Burn victims with extensive tissue injury are a subgroup of patients with DIC related to their injury. In addition, trauma patients are prone to complications associated with prolonged environmental exposure that further augments the coagulopathic effects of the trauma itself. These patients typically present with significant hypothermia. When the core body temperature drops below 34 C, certain enzyme activity, such as serine proteases, may be inhibited. This leads to a prolongation of the PT and aPTT.[24]

Coagulopathy is also associated with traumatic brain injury. As with other organ systems, brain tissue, when injured, can potentially release thromboplastin and plasminogen activators that promote a coagulopathy. A retrospective study of 265 pediatric patients with abusive head trauma (shaken baby syndrome) found that prolongation of the PT is a common complication of parenchymal injury rather than vice versa. There was an insufficient number of patients for evaluation of aPTT and fibrinogen.[25]

In general, the NIH, the American College of Physicians, and the ASA Task Force agree on the following indicators to guide FFP transfusion: 1) massive transfusion with active bleeding; 2) urgent reversal of warfarin (Coumadin) therapy; and 3) active bleeding with a history or clinical course suggestive of an inherited or acquired coagulopathy.[16,17,26] The Task Force further recommends that FFP be given when microvascular bleeding is evident in combination with an elevated PT and aPTT (>1.5 times normal), when there is blood loss in excess of one blood volume, or when clotting times cannot be obtained in a timely fashion.[26] All groups also agree that the use of FFP as a volume expander is contraindicated. Some authors, however, recommend that certain component therapy be given empirically for trauma patients with active bleeding.[27] Other blood components contain a certain amount of clotting factors (see Table 13-3).

Cryoprecipitate

As with thrombocytopenia and clotting factor deficiencies, hypofibrinogenemia is a well-recognized dilutional effect in the postoperative period in the context of massive transfusion, in addition to its association with DIC. Recommendations from the American College of Physicians and the ASA Task Force with re-

Table 13-3. Clotting Factor Level Equivalents

Amount/Unit Value	Blood Component
1 U	Fresh Frozen Plasma
4-5 U	Platelets
1 U	Platelets Pheresis
1 U	Whole Blood*

*Whole Blood contains relatively decreased concentrations of Factors V and VIII, but the levels are still considered to be hemostatic.

gard to cryoprecipitate therapy are limited to patients with active or microvascular bleeding in conjunction with hypofibrinogenemia (<80-100 mg/dL), von Willebrand disease, and hemophilia A when Factor VIII concentrate is not available.[16,17] The Task Force also recommends prophylactic cryoprecipitate therapy for patients with von Willebrand disease refractory to desmopressin.[17] Furthermore, in the context of trauma, the ASA Task Force and other authorities recommend that cryoprecipitate be given empirically for active bleeding in massively transfused patients whose fibrinogen levels cannot be obtained in a timely fashion.[17,27]

Extracorporeal Membrane Oxygenation

ECMO or extracorporeal life support is a means of artificially providing oxygenation and/or perfusion through a mechanical pump to which the patient is attached. Briefly, the system consists of a cannula that drains systemic venous blood into the bypass circuitry (right atrial venous cannula), a roller pump, a membrane oxygenator, and a return cannula that may be either venous or arterial. The pump moves the blood forward in a nonpulsatile manner to the membrane oxygenator where gas exchange occurs through a semipermeable membrane using a countercurrent mechanism (blood in one direction, gas in the other). The blood is rewarmed and returned to the patient through either an arterial cannula (VA ECMO) or a venous cannula (VV ECMO).

Although ECMO is used in pediatric and adult patients, the predominant use and experience continue to be in the neonatal population with isolated pulmonary disease (persistent pulmonary hypertension and respiratory distress syndrome).

Transfusion practices in the ECMO patient center around two priorities. One is optimizing oxygen delivery, and the second is providing a precise balance between anticoagulation (to prevent clotting within the circuit) and coagulation (to avoid catastrophic hemorrhagic complications). With the initiation of ECMO, the patient is given a heparin bolus and a maintenance infusion is begun. The rate of heparin infusion is adjusted on the basis of a bedside activated clotting time (ACT) assay. An ACT between 180 and 220 seconds is the accepted therapeutic target. On average, the neonate receiving ECMO support has a mean daily blood usage of 250 mL of RBCs, 80 mL of FFP, and 2 units of platelets.[28] Frequent assessments of clinical status (perfusion, urine output), arterial blood gases, serum chemistries, complete blood counts, platelet counts, and clotting indices are standard.

Priming the Circuit

Before ECMO initiation, the circuit is primed with stored blood. With stored blood, as with massive transfusion, the effects of storage lesions, discussed previously, come into play. The priming blood is acidic in pH and may be low in calcium and high in potassium, all of which have detrimental effects on the native myocardium. Acidosis may be corrected with the administration of sodium bicarbonate or tromethamine. Electrolytes of the priming blood should be measured before the initiation of ECMO. The hypocalcemia and hyperkalemia (if excessive) should be corrected in standard fashion. Alternative priming solutions such as albumin have been studied in bypass as a means of decreasing the adverse effects seen with stored blood.

RBC Administration

During a standard ECMO course, multiple RBC transfusions are required to maintain adequate blood volume and to increase oxygen-carrying capacity and oxygen delivery in these critically ill patients. The target hematocrit varies, depending on the underlying pathologic process (patients with cyanotic congenital heart disease may tolerate a hematocrit well above that of the neonate with persistent pulmonary hypertension).

Platelet Administration

Platelet consumption by the ECMO circuit results in the need for frequent monitoring of the platelet count. Multiple platelet transfusions may be necessary during a routine ECMO course. In addition to this consumptive coagulopathy, the administration of heparin adds the risk of heparin-induced thrombocytopenia to the mix. These, along with the dilutional effect of massive transfusion, contribute to the development of thrombocytopenia. In addition to the above effects, platelet activation through contact with foreign surfaces decreases the absolute quantity of "functional" platelets. Platelets, when activated, release a multitude of mediators from alpha granules. These mediators have a wide array of physiologic effects, including activation of the coagulation cascade. The abnormal platelet function associated with platelet activation, as measured by the bleeding time, reverses rapidly when ECMO is discontinued.

Approximately 10 to 35% of neonates receiving ECMO support suffer a hemorrhagic complication. In the child receiving ECMO support, frequent platelet transfusions are often required to maintain the platelet count at above or equal to 80,000 to 100,000/µL. If invasive procedures are needed, much more aggressive replacement may be necessary.

Techniques by which the hemostatic mechanism can be tightly controlled assume major importance. Newer techniques involve the use of less thrombogenic circuits, newer anticoagulants, and protease inhibitors.

Clotting Factor Administration

The administration of clotting factors to a patient receiving anticoagulant therapy, in an effort to prevent clotting, seems counterproductive. Yet the precise balance of hemostasis favoring anticoagulation must exist to prevent the thrombotic complications associated with ECMO. Because ECMO results in a consumptive coagulopathy[29] and because it is apparent that alterations in coagulation are a predictor of intracranial hemorrhage in ECMO patients,[30] clotting factor replacement therapy is important. FFP and cryoprecipitate are administered to correct these deficiencies and prevent the balance of anticoagulation-coagulation from favoring excessive anticoagulation.

Cardiothoracic Surgery Transfusion

Cyanotic Heart Disease

Postoperative patients with persistent right-to-left intracardiac shunts (from palliative surgery or residual patent foramen ovale) benefit from an elevated hemoglobin level. Hemoglobin concentrations above 15 mg/dL have been shown to improve blood oxygen-carrying capacity and systemic oxygen transport.[31] The desaturation of systemic blood triggers red cell production to augment DO_2 and provide essential oxygen to the tissues. Often, red cell production exceeds that which provides optimal DO_2 and results in polycythemia. When red cell mass and polycythemia predominate over the effects of increased oxygen-carrying capacity, DO_2 is negatively affected and the tissues are deprived of oxygen by the stasis within the system. Under these circumstances, therapeutic blood letting to reduce red cell mass may be beneficial. On the other hand, anemia superimposed on baseline cyanosis can be harmful. It is essential, therefore, that the balance between increased oxygen-carrying capacity and microcirculatory stasis be carefully maintained.

Cardiopulmonary Bypass

CPB has significant effects on the coagulation system that are analogous to those seen with ECMO. The effects are predominantly limited to platelets and clotting factors. Platelets are affected in terms of both function and quantity. During CPB, platelets become activated and release alpha granules as well as other mediators, leaving a depleted pool of functional platelets. Subsequent worsening of platelet function, as seen in prolonged bleeding time, can be seen within minutes after the initiation of CPB. Reversal of prolonged bleeding time, however, begins spontaneously within 15 minutes after CPB is discontinued and becomes normal within 2 to 4 hours.[23] Platelet number is also reduced through hemodilution, although it will generally stay above 100,000/µL throughout the procedure.[23] In addition, hypothermia (a means of brain protection) is often induced during

CPB and the reduced core body temperature also affects platelets negatively.

With CPB, clotting factors become depleted primarily by hemodilution. Some specific issues regarding clotting factors and CPB in children are of note. First, infants up to 6 months of age do not produce "adult" levels of clotting factors. This shortfall is balanced by the relative deficiency of protein S, protein C, and antithrombin. Second, infants with cyanotic heart defects typically have 30% to 40% of normal factor levels. The reason for this is not completely clear, but it may be the compromised liver perfusion due to the cardiac defect.[32] Third, children with acyanotic cardiac lesions may be deficient in von Willebrand factor.[33] Although the etiology is unknown, the deficiency appears to resolve after repair of the defect. These deficiencies may explain the tendency for a more pronounced coagulopathy in younger patients undergoing CPB, which may be further compounded by the greater hemodilution effect associated with relatively larger priming volumes indexed to weight in smaller children. However, the coagulopathy induced during CPB may not have clinical significance, as abnormal clotting times tend to normalize within 12 hours after CPB.[23] In fact, in patients who have received FFP postoperatively or after CPB, clotting times have been observed to worsen with a concomitant increase in chest tube drainage.[22] Therefore, given the multitude of mechanisms favoring the development of a coagulopathy with CPB, platelet transfusions alone are advocated and appear to be the most efficacious means of effecting hemostasis in these patients.

The Maximum Surgical Blood Ordering Schedule

The maximum surgical blood ordering schedule (MSBOS) is a list of commonly performed surgical procedures and their usual blood requirements. The schedule is developed to cover the transfusion requirements in 80% to 90% of patients undergoing a specific procedure. The MSBOS is a tool by which an institution can audit its transfusion requirements for surgical procedures and develop a pattern of blood usage specific to each procedure.

While many transfusion guidelines for adults apply to pediatric patients as well, a separate pediatric MSBOS is recommended. (Appendix 13-1 gives an example of a MSBOS for pediatric patients.) This should be developed through the coordinated efforts of personnel representing transfusion service, surgery, anesthesiology, and neonatology.

Conclusion

Transfusion practices in pediatric surgery, trauma, and the intensive care unit encompass a spectrum of age, developmental physiology, and pathologic conditions. In the pediatric practice, transfusions vary from elective to increase oxygen-carrying capacity and oxygen delivery, through cardiothoracic surgery and ECMO in which DO_2 and hemostasis considerations predominate, to the emergent resuscitation of the trauma victim where volume resuscitation for hemodynamic support is added to the mix. An explicit understanding of the unique physiology of the developing child is essential to providing optimal transfusion support. The pediatric intensivist, anesthesiologist, or surgeon caring for the critically ill child understands the unique physiologic changes and is thus suited to work in concert with blood bank personnel to develop an optimal transfusion strategy for the pediatric patient.

References

1. Adams RC, Lundy JS. Anesthesia in cases of poor surgical risk: Some suggestions for decreasing the risk. Surg Gynecol Obstet 1942;74:1011.
2. Richardson TQ, Guyton AC. Effects of polycythemia and anemia on cardiac output and other circulatory factors. Am J Physiol 1959;197:1167-70.
3. Stehling L, Zaunder HL. Acute normovolemic hemodilution. Transfusion 1991;31:857-68.
4. Marini CP, Russo GC, Nathan IM, et al. Effect of hematocrit on regional oxygen delivery and extraction in an adult respiratory distress syndrome model. Am J Surg 2000;180:108-14.
5. Asmundson T, Kilburn KH. Survival of acute respiratory failure: A study of 239 episodes. Ann Intern Med 1969;70:471-85.

6. Schonofer B, Bohrer H, Kohler D. Importance of blood transfusion in anemic patients with COPD and unsuccessful weaning from respirator. Med Klin 1999;94:70-2.
7. Schonofer B, Wenzel M, Geibel M, Kohler D. Blood transfusion and lung function in chronically anemic patients with severe chronic obstructive pulmonary disease. Crit Care Med 1998;26:1824-8.
8. Goskowicz R. The complications of massive blood transfusion. Anesth Clin North Am 1999;17:960-78.
9. Hippala ST, Myllyla GJ, Vahtera EM. Hemostatic factors and replacement of major blood loss with plasma-poor red cell concentrates (abstract). Anesth Analg 1995;81:360.
10. Bernard GR, Vincet J, Laterre P, et al. Efficacy and safety of recombinant human activated protein C for severe sepsis. N Engl J Med 2001;344: 699-709.
11. Ludbrook J, Wynn W. Citrate intoxication: A clinical and experimental study. Br J Med 1985;2:523-8.
12. Denlinger JK, Nahrwood ML, Gibbs PS, et al. Hypocalcemia during rapid blood transfusion in anaesthesized man (abstract). Br J Anaesth 1976; 48:995.
13. Wolf PL, McCarty LJ, Hafleigh B. Extreme hypercalcemia following blood transfusion combined with intravenous calcium. Vox Sang 1970;19: 544-5.
14. Kulkaris P, Bhattacharya S, Petros AJ. Torsades de pointes and long QT syndrome following major blood transfusion. Anaesthesia 1992;47: 125-7.
15. Office of Medical Applications of Research, National Institutes of Health. Perioperative red blood cell transfusion. JAMA 1988;260:270-3.
16. American College of Physicians. Practice strategies for elective red blood cell transfusion. Ann Intern Med 1992;116:403-6.
17. Practice Guidelines for Blood Component Therapy. A report by the American Society of Anesthesiologists Task Force on Blood Component Therapy. Anesthesiology 1996;84:732-47.
18. Stephan F, Hollande J, Richard O, et al. Thrombocytopenia in a surgical ICU. Chest 1999;115:1363-70.
19. Office of Medical Applications of Research, National Institutes of Health: Platelet transfusion therapy. JAMA 1987;257:1777-80.
20. McVay PA, Toy PT. Lack of increased bleeding after paracentesis and thoracentesis in patients with mild coagulation abnormalities. Transfusion 1991;31:164-71.
21. Friedman EW, Sussman II. Safety of invasive procedures in patients with the coagulopathy of liver disease. Clin Lab Haematol 1989;11:119-204.
22. Miller BE, Mochizuki T, et al. Predicting and treating coagulopathies after cardiopulmonary bypass in children. Anesth Analg 1997;85:1196-202.

23. Woodman RC, Harker LA. Bleeding complications associated with cardiopulmonary bypass. Blood 1990;76:1680-97.
24. Spiess BD. Traumatic coagulopathies. Anesthesiol Clin North Am 1996; 14:29-38.
25. Hymel KP, Abshire TC, Luckey DW, Jenny C. Coagulopathy in pediatric abusive head trauma. Pediatrics 1997;99:371-5.
26. Office of Medical Applications of Research, National Institutes of Health. Fresh frozen plasma: Indications and risks. JAMA 1985;253:551-3.
27. Eddy VA, Morris JA, Cullinane DC. Hypothermia, coagulopathy and acidosis. Surg Clin North Am 2000;80:845-54.
28. McCoy-Paddington D, Judd WJ, Knafl P, et al. Blood use during extracorporeal membrane oxygenation. Transfusion 1990;30:307-9.
29. Urlesberger B, Zobel G, Zenz W, et al. Activation of the clotting system during extracorporeal membrane oxygenation in term newborn infants. J Pediatr 1996;29:264-8.
30. Hirthler MA, Blackwell E, Abbe D, et al. Coagulation parameter instability as an early predictor of intracranial hemorrhage during extracorporeal membrane oxygenation. J Pediatr Surg 1992;27:40-3.
31. Beekman RH, Tuuri DT. Acute hemodynamic effects of increasing hemoglobin concentration in children with a right to left shunt and relative anemia. J Am Coll Cardiol 1985;5:357-62.
32. Schulman SR, Kern FH, Greeley WJ. Coagulation disorders in congenital heart disease. In: Nichols DG, Cameron DE, Greeley WJ, et al, eds. Critical heart disease in infants and children. St. Louis: Mosby, 1995:401-13.
33. Gill JC, Wilson AD, Endres-Brooks J, Montgomery RR. Loss of largest von Willebrand factor multimers from the plasma of patients with congenital cardiac defects. Blood 1986;67:758-61.

Appendix 13-1. Example of a Surgical Blood Order Schedule (SBOS) for Pediatric Patients

Surgical Procedures	Units
Amputation (upper or lower extremity)	1
Anoplasty	1
Arthrodesis, hip	1-2
Arteriovenous fistula placement	T&S
Bladder tumor excision	1
Burn debridement	T&S-1
Cardiac surgery (including pump prime)	
Catheterization	1
Closed procedures	1-2
Open procedures	2-3
Patients >10 kg	4
Pacemaker insertion	T&S
Reoperations	2-4
Valve replacements	2-4
Cleft palate repair	T&S
Clitorectomy	1
Colectomy	1
Colostomy	T&S
Craniectomy	T&S-1
Craniofacial repair, complex	2-4
Craniosynostosis	1-3
Craniotomy for tumor	1-3
Cerebrospinal fluid shunts, replacement or revision	T&S
Cystectomy, ovarian	T&S
Extracorporeal membrane oxygenation	2-4
Encephalocoele repair	1
Endorectal pull-through	1
Enterostomy closure	T&S-1
Extrahepatic anastomosis (Kasai procedure)	2
Femoral neck repair	1-2
Fundoplication (Nissen procedure)	T&S
Gastroschisis repair	T&S-1
Hypospadias repair	T&S
Ileostomy	T&S
Intestinal resection	1
Knee and distal femur procedures	T&S-1
Laminectomy	
Limited	T&S-1
Fusion with instrumentation	2-4

Appendix 13-1. Example of a Surgical Blood Order Schedule (SBOS) for Pediatric Patients (continued)

Surgical Procedures	Units
Laparotomy	T&S-1
Limb salvage, with or without tumor resection	1
Liver biopsy	T&S
Liver resection	6
Liver transplant (equal number of units in reserve plus FFP and platelets)	6
Lobectomy, lung resection	1-2
Lung biopsy	T&S
Myelomeningocoele repair	T&S-1
Neck dissection	1-2
Nephrectomy	2
Neurofibroma excision	1
Nevus removal/scar revision	T&S
Osteotomy, long bones or joints	1-2
Pectus excavatum repair	T&S
Prosthesis (insertion/removal), long bones	1-2
Pyeloplasty	T&S
Pyelostomy	T&S
Renal transplant	
Donor	1
Recipient	2
Skin grafts, extensive	1-2
Splenectomy	
Complex (eg, Gaucher's disease)	2-3
Simple	T&S-1
Throacotomy	1-2
Thyroid, biopsy or resection	T&S
Tumor resection, long bones	2-4
Ureteroneocystostomy	T&S
Vascular malformation	1

T&S = type and screen. Used with permission from Hume HA. Role of the hospital transfusion service in assessing, ensuring, and improving the quality of pediatric transfusion therapy. In: Chambers LA, Issitt LA, eds. Supporting the pediatric transfusion recipient. Bethesda, MD: American Association of Blood Banks, 1994:151-8.

In: Herman JH, Manno CS, eds.
Pediatric Transfusion Therapy
Bethesda, MD: AABB Press, 2002

14

Pediatric Perioperative Blood Recovery

DAVID N. MOOLTEN, MD

THE "CELL SAVER" DEVICE HAS BEEN A FIXTURE in operative suites since the early 1980s. While devices capable of capturing and washing shed blood from the operative field or postoperative drainage were in routine use before that, it was concern over transfusion-transmitted infectious disease that made their use ubiquitous. Over the past decade, cost concerns and the implementation of operative techniques that reduce blood loss have winnowed the number and types of procedures in which recovery is customarily performed. Pediatric surgery has been no exception to these trends. The principles, methods, and technology used for pediatric blood recovery largely overlap those used for

David Moolten, MD, Medical Director, Penn-Jersey Regional Blood Services, American Red Cross, and Musser Blood Center, Philadelphia, Pennsylvania

recovery in adults. Nevertheless, the distinct physiology and surgical management of children create unique requirements for the appropriate practice of pediatric blood recovery.

Rationale for Blood Recovery

The rationale for blood recovery is fairly straightforward. Blood shed during surgery and/or during postoperative wound drainage contains intact functional red cells that may be collected, processed to eliminate deleterious cellular and/or noncellular material, and reinfused. Recovered blood is often touted for its freshness, immediate availability, compatibility, freedom from the risks associated with the transfusion of banked blood, and ability to reduce inventory requirements for banked blood.[1-3] Recovered red cells, if properly handled, are potentially of very high quality, according to several criteria, including red cell survival, the levels of 2,3-diphosphoglycerate (2,3-DPG), and concentration of cell-free hemoglobin.[4] In adults, parameters such as 2,3-DPG may be of questionable importance, except in the setting of massive transfusion.[5] In children, however, more controversy exists regarding the value of "fresh" blood.[6,7] However, despite its freshness, recovered blood may still have subtle defects when compared with patient blood.[8,9] Substances thought to play a potential role in posttransfusion complications include cytokines and eicosanoids.[10,11] Some have reported a low level of eicosanoids in washed recovered blood and no increase after transfusion—in contrast to reports of increased levels in banked blood and after transfusion.[12] However, others have reported finding no significant increase or difference in the concentration of eicosanoids among recovered, stored, or stored leukocyte-reduced blood.[13]

In general, the availability of banked allogeneic blood is not an issue for transfusion, but, in the setting of rapid, massive blood loss, blood recovery may be helpful.[14] In addition, autologous transfusion can appreciably lessen the need for allogeneic blood, which is of potential value, given the periodic occurrence of blood shortages.[15,16] On the other hand, blood recovery often contributes considerably less than preoperative autologous donation in this regard. As with adults, there may be children whose family's religious convictions prohibit the transfusion of allogeneic blood or even of banked autologous blood but whose convictions will, under certain circumstances, allow blood recovery.[17]

Types of Surgeries

Any surgical patient in whom bleeding is anticipated is a potential candidate for perioperative recovery. However, in practice, cost-effectiveness issues require that bleeding be routine and profuse enough to warrant recovery, which limits its use. In addition, the reinfusion of recovered blood is considered unsafe in certain surgical procedures and is contraindicated in those settings.

In adults, the most common surgical procedures in which blood recovery is performed are joint replacement, spinal surgery (noncongenital pathologic conditions), vascular repair of aneurysms or atherosclerotic disease in the peripheral vessels, and coronary artery bypass.[18] Conversely, in children, the most common indications are the correction of spine deformities associated with congenital disease and the correction of congenital heart defects. Much of the available literature regarding blood recovery is based on studies of surgical procedures in adults, which makes it difficult to reliably extrapolate to children conclusions drawn from that experience. Other conditions in which perioperative recovery has been reported in children include liver repair or transplantation, craniosynostosis surgery, the management of splenic injury, blunt abdominal trauma, and excisional burn surgery.[19-28]

Devices and Methods Used to Recover Blood

Semiautomated Cell Processors

Perioperative blood may be recovered and reinfused in two forms: washed or unwashed. The most commonly used and accepted strategy is for shed blood to be washed before reinfusion.[29] While it is possible to do this manually or even remotely using a standard blood bank cell washer (eg, COBE 2991, Gambro BCT, Lakewood CO), this is neither common nor practical. A dedicated semi-automated cell processor capable of rapid flow rates is typically used. Analogous to apheresis machines, these devices use an onboard centrifuge to separate blood according to sedimentation properties; an onboard computer to direct the flow of recovered blood, waste, and washed cells; peristalsis pumps; and a sterile disposable plasticware and tubing set to allow multi-patient use. Most devices rely on a discontinuous-flow circuit at whose heart is a centrifuge bowl of the Latham design (Fig 14-1), seminally developed during the 1940s for the purposes of blood fractionation. Variations of the design have been introduced, but the principal mechanics are ubiquitous.

Methods

In addition to a dedicated semi-automated cell processor and a disposable plasticware and tubing set, blood recovery procedures require several other supplies and pieces of equipment. A sterile, plastic reservoir (800 mL-4000 mL) in which to initially collect shed blood is required, typically filtered (either gross, 170 micron, or microaggregate 40 micron). Vacuum suction and a suction wand and tubing are needed (some cell-washing devices have the capability of generating an independent vacuum; otherwise, wall suction is adequate if excessive negative pressure is avoided). Anticoagulant is needed, and this can either be heparin or a citrate-based anticoagulant such as ACD or CPD. The preference is generally for heparin: should unwashed blood be requested for immediate reinfusion by the operative team, there would not be the potential for the complications associated with citrate toxicity (ie, chelation of divalent cations, particularly calcium and magnesium, with effects on neuromuscular function including cardiac arrhythmia and hypotension). Optional but generally recommended supplies include a transfer pack and a microaggregate filter (20-40 micron) for brief storage of the washed red cells after processing and transfusion of the patient by the staff of the operating theater or recovery room.

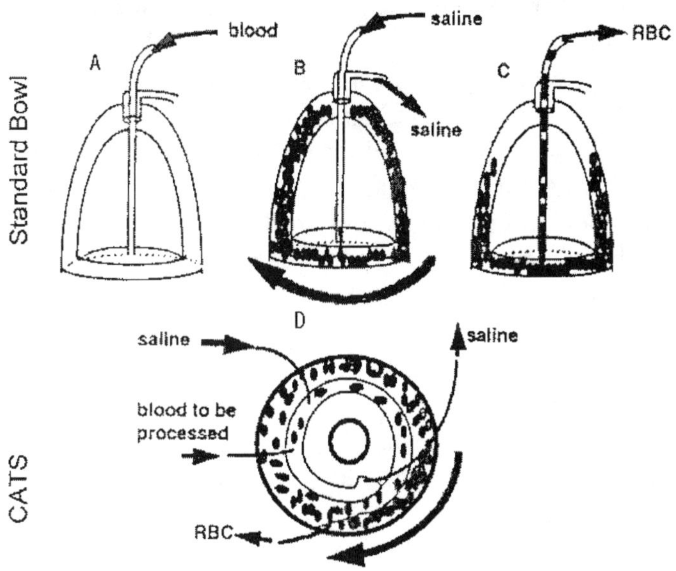

Figure 14-1. Schematic description of the blood processing procedure of a device using discontinuous operation (Standard Bowl) and the continuous autotransfusion system (CATS, Fresenius). With discontinuous operation, blood is pumped into the rotating separation chamber until it is filled with red cells (A). This blood is then washed with saline (B). After completion of this washing procedure, the centrifugation is stopped, and the washed red cells are pumped into the retransfusion bag (C). The entire procedure is repeated step-by-step if there is still blood to be processed. Thus, the blood is processed discontinuously in batches or units. In the CATS, blood is processed continuously. The separation chamber represents a blood channel in the shape of a double spiral (D). Blood is pumped into the inner spiral while the separation chamber is rotated. Because of centrifugal forces, red cells move to the outer spiral, and on their way, they are washed with saline added by an extra pump into the separation chamber. Substances of lighter density, such as debris and washing solution, leave the spiral at the innermost point. This is a continuous blood-processing procedure in which all steps (filling the chamber with blood, adding washing solution, pumping red cells into the retransfusion bag, and eliminating the waste) are performed in parallel, until all the blood is processed. Used with permission from Booke M, Fobker M, Fingerhut D, et al. Fat elimination during intraoperative autotransfusion: An in-vitro investigation. Anesth Analg 1997;85:959-62.

Aspiration from the operative site and/or postoperative drains is standard; blood may also be recovered from sponges.[30] When enough blood has been collected in the reservoir, the operator initiates the processing cycle. The amount of shed blood required to process a "full" bowl is dependent on the crude hematocrit of the unwashed reservoir contents, which is itself derivative of multiple factors including patient hematocrit, hemolysis in the operative field, irrigation fluid volume, and bowl size. Concerns over the quality of blood processed from partially packed bowls (see below) have led to commonly followed recommendations that such blood not be processed or transfused.[31-33] Certain manufacturers sanction the processing of partial bowls, but with stipulations such as the use of a greater volume of wash solution.[34] Bowls available for routine use range in volume from 55 mL to 375 mL. For smaller patients and/or procedures when lesser blood loss is anticipated, the 55-mL and 125-mL bowls might be superior, as they allow the processing of smaller volumes. For larger patients whose surgical procedures are likely to lead to substantial blood loss, a 225-mL bowl might be indicated.

The processing cycle consists of three phases: FILL (also known as PRIME), WASH, and EMPTY (also known as REINFUSE). The FILL phase transfers the reservoir contents to the bowl via a peristaltic pump. Because the bowl and tubing kits are not typically vacuum-packed, there is air in the bowl and tubing that is displaced by fluid during operation. The fluid forces air ahead of it (through the bowl and into the reinfusion bag). The contents are pumped into the bowl (the FILL stage) until the reservoir is empty. (Air may also enter the bowl at this stage. This air passes through the bowl and into the reinfusion bag.) Through centrifugal separation, cellular fluid entering the spinning bowl is separated into its components. A typical centrifuge speed might be 5000 to 6000 rpm with the transfer of shed blood from the reservoir to the bowl proceeding at a rate of between 300 to 400 mL/minute until red cells concentrated from the reservoir contents have filled the bowl and the upper level of the red cell layer is at the "shoulder" of the bowl.

At this time, the operator commences the WASH cycle, in which the contents of the spinning bowl are perfused with saline. The tubing from the reservoir is clamped, and the tubing from the saline bag is opened. The volume of saline may vary, but a volume at least four to six times the bowl volume is usually considered minimal from the standpoint of contaminant washout. The color of the effluent to the waste bag is also used as a subjective discriminant. Under normal operating procedures, it is common practice to allow the wash solution to enter the bowl at a slightly slower rate than that at which the shed blood was introduced. This tends to minimize the loss of RBCs to the waste bag, because of the change in the type of fluid entering the bowl, which may alter the separation dynamics. As an example, such a process might be used to recover a 125-mL component with a hematocrit of 50% to 65% from 300 to 400 mL of shed blood.

In some cases, it may be necessary to change the processing dynamics because of an urgent intraoperative requirement for transfusion. Under such circumstances, the processing speed can be increased to as much as 1000 mL/minute. This velocity of processing will result in the same recovered red cell mass, but in a much higher volume of diluent, primarily because of the increased pump speed and the resultant decreased dwell time in the centrifuge and looser packing. Conversely, if the pump speed is decreased, the red cell mass packs more tightly, and a product of the same volume but of higher red cell concentration is generated. This may be done for several reasons, particularly in a pediatric situation in which fluid overload may be a concern. Tighter packing is achieved by reducing inlet flow, which gives the red cells more time to sediment in the rapidly rotating bowl. Theoretically, there is a risk of "channeling" if the cells are packed too tightly. In such an instance, the wash solution may create channels in an overly packed product, resulting in a clear effluent line to visual inspection, but only as a result of the saline's having carved a path through the red cell layer. In such a case, the product should be reprocessed at a rate that does not allow such tight packing.

The operator now starts the EMPTY phase, in which the contents of the bowl are discharged into a reinfusion bag (also known as a holding bag). Reversing the rotation of the peristaltic pump draws the red cell mass out of the bowl, which forces the air in the tubing ahead of it into the holding bag. With later-model cell recovery devices, the pump action stops as soon as the air detector detects air. This detector is usually located close to the exit port of the bowl. At this point, there are red cells in the holding bag; however, there are viable red cells in the tubing between the bowl and the holding bag. Depending upon the manufacturer (and bowl size), there may be anywhere between 25 mL and 40 mL in this tubing. It is possible to manually purge this blood by initiating another EMPTY cycle until the tubing is full of air and the entire red cell volume has been transferred to the holding bag. Subsequently, the volume of red cells in the holding bag should approximate the advertised bowl capacity. When the emptying process is appropriately monitored, channeling may be detected, as an overly tight pack will not easily exit the bowl, and pockets of air will "burp" through the pack, triggering the air detector prematurely.

While it is possible to directly transfuse from the holding bag, allowing continuous processing and transfusion without intervention by the operative team, this is neither recommended nor generally done. The holding bag contains air and potentially fat, fibrin, platelet and/or white cell aggregates that may have escaped removal during washing; these have been implicated in perioperative coagulopathy.[31-33,35] Transfer of the holding bag contents to a properly labeled transfer pack from which the air is then physically removed helps avoid air embolism and allows recovered blood to be separated into discrete units for the purposes of inspection, transfusion, adverse reaction management, and tracking. Attachment of an inline microaggregate filter during the transfer-filling of each unit allows removal of residual contaminating material.

When the holding bag is empty and the contents have been drained by gravity into the transfer pack, the air in the transfer pack is manually aspirated by gently squeezing the air back up the tubing; this leaves a transfer pack with washed packed red cells suspended in saline, and no air. Although not a requirement, the presence of a dedicated operator facilitates the process and ensures that all steps are correctly performed in a timely manner. While some degree of automated operation is possible with many devices, experienced operators will frequently utilize the manual mode to optimize processing (eg, to fully empty the bowl and tubing during transfer to the holding bag, or to override machine switchover from fill to wash, as in the case of significant hemolysis, when the optical density sensor may be fooled into prematurely ending the fill cycle).

Other Types of Devices

A plethora of devices are available, differing primarily in the degree of automated operation possible and the availability of enhancements, such as on-board vacuum or optics for platelet-rich plasma sequestration. Dideco (Modena, Italy), Haemonetics (Braintree, MA), Gambro, and Fresenius (Hamburg, Germany) are the principal manufacturers.

The semiautomated cell processors used to wash red cells were primarily designed with adult patients in mind. Consequently, the extracorporeal volume (ECV) of the device circuit can be large relative to the blood volume of the smaller, pediatric patient. Unlike apheresis, in which the device directly draws blood from the patient, which creates the potential for hypovolemia, perioperative recovery occurs in a setting where blood loss in excess of physiologic tolerance is routinely corrected as part of operative management and recovered blood is simply one source of red cell mass and blood volume. Nonetheless, the practicality of recovery in patients when the device circuit volume is in excess of 10% to 20% of the child's red cell mass may be uncertain. For such device–patient pairings, operative management will require use of alternative red cell or blood volume sources before a quantity of blood has been shed sufficient to allow a full unit to be washed and returned.

Fortunately, for most devices, low ECV disposables are available, facilitating the use of recovery in smaller patients. A recent in-vitro study compared three devices (Haemonetics Cell Saver 5, Dideco Compact, and Fresenius CATS) for which lower ECV circuits are available, evaluating their ability to process small quantities of blood (100, 200, 300, and 400 mL of outdated RBC units reconstituted to 30% hematocrit with lactated Ringer's solution).[36] The investigators looked at recovery rate (fraction of starting red cell mass recovered), elimination rate (fraction of starting supernatant potassium removed), rate of processing, and the hematocrit in the processed unit. They recommended the Fresenius device, because of its rapid processing, ability to concentrate small quantities of blood (60%), and 100% recovery rate. The Dideco Compact (55-mL bowl) was also effective, generating a 50% hematocrit with 80% to 85% recovery. They could not recommend the Haemonetics device (125-mL bowl), because of its slow processing, low final hematocrit (25% for 100 mL, 34% for 300 mL), and intrinsic inefficiencies with respect to partially filled bowls. Out of concern for possible coagulopathies, they felt that partially filled bowls could not be processed. They point out that, while this shortcoming can be circumvented after the processing of an initial full bowl by using packed recovered cells to fill the bowl, such maneuvers will often result in unacceptable delays for transfusion. Partial bowls are still a potential concern with the Dideco device, but the small bowl size significantly mitigates the issue.

Other investigators have described a novel technique in which a standard autologous transfusion device (Dideco Stat) was used to process shed blood in patients 6 months to 10 years old who were undergoing surgery for hip dysplasia. The high ratio of ECV to total blood volume (TBV) was circumvented through the use of starch sedimentation to highly concentrate the large-volume, low-hematocrit recovered blood unit.[37] This method mitigates concerns about posttransfusion hypervolemia but still requires initial compensation for blood loss with acellular fluid, and it raises other issues, such as control of the manufacturing process in the operating room and the delayed availability of recovered red cells. Such issues make this approach unappealing, when more suitable devices and disposal are available.

Most devices employ a bowl design for the centrifugation chamber, but one significant variation uses a channel configured as a double spiral (Fresenius CATS). This approach affords continuous processing, which is intrinsically more efficient and whose circuits are typically of smaller volume (Fig 14-1). Cell processors that utilize continuous processing have special value in apheresis, where minimized ECV may be critical and where a bowl system predisposes to a much larger ECV, as a significant volume of the patient's plasma must spill before the bowl fills with packed red cells. In blood recovery, the advantage is smaller, as it is waste supernatant and not patient plasma that is spilled during red cell concentration. However, because excessive ECV and/or slower processing may necessitate the transfusion of alternative blood components, which may make blood recovery less effective, a continuous-flow device that offers an intrinsically lower ECV and faster processing may be of advantage in the smaller child. According to the manufacturer's claims, the CATS device is capable of processing as little as 15 mL of red cell mass; for a child with a hematocrit of 30%, this would mean blood loss of approximately 50 mL. Assuming a maximum allowable lost volume fraction of 15% of TBV at 70 mL/kg, the minimum mass of a child for whom such a device would ordinarily be practical would be approximately 5 kg. However, because as little as 50% of total operative blood loss may be aspirated and recovered, a more realistic figure may be 10 kg.[38]

The ECV of a bowl-based blood-recovery device is essentially the volume of the bowl and that of the tubing (30-70 mL) leading from the reservoir to the bowl, although, if manual mode is used, which allows purging of the tubing, then the ECV is simply the bowl volume. Therefore, the minimum ECV in a bowl-based system is 55 mL. Using the same assumptions as above, the minimum mass of a child for whom such a device would be practical would be around 10 kg if the bowl red cells were packed to the patient's hematocrit; a tighter pack would require a larger equivalent volume of patient blood loss and would increase the minimum mass.

It may be possible to perform blood recovery in smaller patients if the operative team chooses to delay red cell reinfusion and manage the initial loss of blood volume with other replacement fluids. A cell-washing machine that features low circuit volume and does not rely on centrifugation but on mixing and filtration as a means of isolating red cells is also available, but it has been associated with transient hematuria in pediatric orthopedic surgery patients.[39]

Immediate-Return Devices

Several devices are available that allow shed blood to be collected via suction into a reservoir and then simply filtered and reinfused without a washing step. Most of these devices consist of nothing more than a sterile container with a standard blood filter. An advantage of such devices is the ability to process and return small aliquots of blood, which is of potential value in pediatric perioperative recovery. Moreover, for small volumes of blood, an immediate-return strategy may be cheaper than one requiring washing, although even then not necessarily cost-effective.[40-42] However, there has been considerable controversy in the literature regarding the appropriate place for such techniques vis-á-vis standard cell washing.[43-45] Guidelines limiting the use of such devices that take into account the nature of the surgery and the presence in the wound of specific deleterious contaminants have generally been advised. For example, in cardiac surgery, there has been concern over coagulopathy occurring consequent to the reinfusion of fibrin degradation products, the release of inflammatory cytokines, and the presence of damaged platelets and/or white cells in shed mediastinal blood.[46-48]

Whereas the presence of supernormal levels of cytokines known to have potential deleterious effects can be documented in unwashed blood, a correlation between these supernormal levels and either a significant increase in in-vivo levels and/or clinical sequela unequivocally attributable to increased levels in the transfused blood has not been proven. In fact, some report the safe, effective use of such devices.[49] On the other hand, the clinical picture in patients who have complications is often confoundingly complex. Uncertainty exists as to which cytokines are involved in instigating or aggravating such complications. Moreover, it is unclear whether increased plasma levels are a prerequisite and, if so, which levels would represent thresholds.

Similarly, in adult orthopedic and vascular procedures, contamination of the wound and thus the recovery of blood with potentially toxic degradation materials, such as leukotrienes, C3a, lipase, and elastase, have raised concerns; washing appears ameliorative.[10,11,50,51] In orthopedic procedures, heavy contamination of the wound with debris and surgical materials such as bone cement may present risks, as might the potential for cytokine release.[43,52] Again, there is difference of opinion regarding the nature, degree, and danger of this contamination vis-á-vis unwashed blood.[53,54]

The use of immediate-return devices in pediatric surgery is less well evaluated. The risk of superfluous and potentially deleterious contaminants from unwashed blood is difficult to ascertain conclusively, and it may well vary with the specific nature of the surgical procedure. Nevertheless, limits on total blood processed and transfused through immediate-return devices during a given surgical procedure or over a set period have generally been advised, and some surgical departments and/or institutions have forbidden their use.

Medical Management of Pediatric Cell Recovery

In addition to the technical aspects of performing blood recovery, the supervening management of the activity is of importance to ensure its proper role in transfusion therapy with regard to efficacy, as well as the quality, safety, and cost-effectiveness of the overall process. Perhaps the single greatest issue confronting the physician in charge of a cell-recovery service is utilization. While the technology and practice of autologous transfusion has remained relatively constant over the past decade, a number of innovations have improved the safety of allogeneic transfusion and have reduced blood loss in complex procedures such as cardiac surgery.[55] Consequently, the efficacy of autologous transfusion has been challenged, and recent cost-benefit analysis for transfusion of preoperatively donated autologous blood suggested a lack of indication.[56] Others argue that such analysis cannot be validly extrapolated to children for at least two reasons: children live longer, which alters the value of avoiding complications through autologous transfusion; and complications specific to a pediatric population, such as alloimmunization of girls before they reach childbearing potential, were not included.[57] Perioperative recovery is not preoperative donation, but the relative costs of recovery are generally considered higher, and the relative contribution of recovered blood to transfusion was significantly less than that of banked autologous blood in studies where both were used.[58] Nevertheless, psychosocial factors play an enormous role in the use of autologous transfusion, and its use persists even when not cost-effective and where risk reduction vis-á-vis allogeneic transfusion is negligible. There are also legal considerations. Some states have codified a requirement that physicians offer autologous transfusion options to patients.[59] From a medicolegal standpoint, the use of autologous transfusion may be difficult to curtail in procedures for which it has been considered standard, even those that efficacy analysis alone might now proscribe.

A major drawback to cell recovery for some surgeries is poor cost-effectiveness. Overallocation is intrinsic to autologous transfusion, because there is a strong tendency to overpredict its need in the interests of ensuring that no allogeneic blood be used. Moreover, in the case of blood recovery, there is a high fixed cost generally associated with the availability of an operator and a device, coupled with a low overall rate of contribution to perioperative transfusion for many surgical procedures in which recovery has traditionally been used. One study analyzed breakeven points in the three principal categories of adult surgical procedures using recovery (cardiac, noncardiac vascular, and orthopedic); it reported that utilization for noncardiac vascular procedures was often cost-effective, that for cardiac procedures was sometimes cost-effective, and that for orthopedic procedures was never cost-effective.[60] Another study purported that, in abdominal aneurysm repair, a blood loss of 1000 mL and recovery volume of 750 mL or greater was required for cost-effectiveness.[61] On the other hand, the financial analyses used to ascertain cost-effectiveness in these studies did not take into account overhead expenses or the cost of complications of allogeneic transfusions and their management. In one of the largest analyses of blood recovery to date, investigators evaluated its efficacy and cost-effectiveness in 3022 patients undergoing cardiac surgery; they found blood recovery to be of economic benefit.[62] Similar analyses of pediatric procedures have not been reported as frequently. Blood losses in children may be lower in volume than those in adults, and thus they are lower relative to the volume of banked blood units and to the ECV of recovery device circuits; yet they still are high relative to the child's blood volume.[63] Whereas extrapolation from adult to pediatric surgical patients is untrustworthy because of myriad differences between the two populations, it would appear that, overall, a transfusion breakeven point of two standard red cell units might be attainable less often in children.[61]

On the other hand, there are certainly many pediatric surgical procedures in which substantial blood loss is routine or uniquely problematic.[64-67] For procedures in which blood loss is variable, it may be possible to use clinical criteria to anticipate which patients are more likely to have substantial bleeding.[67] The cost-effectiveness of blood recovery might be improved by limiting its use to such patients. Moreover, lower costs for blood recovery than for allogeneic transfusion in children have been reported in certain settings, such as intracranial neurosurgery.[64]

It is also possible to avoid some of the fixed costs associated with blood recovery through the use of alternative staffing and deployment strategies. These might include early dismissal of the blood recovery operator in cases when the operative team determined that blood loss would be insubstantial or, conversely, having the blood recovery operator on-call and summoned only when extensive blood loss is anticipated, with the operative team initiating aspiration of shed blood into the reservoir while the operator is en route.

The principal measure used to ascertain the efficacy of perioperative recovery has been the avoidance of donor exposure, with the optimal goal the performance of the surgical procedure without allogeneic transfusion. Subjective factors may influence the decision to transfuse, facilitating better results under study conditions than might otherwise be readily achievable. On the other hand, efforts to limit allogeneic exposure in children may be more concerted and comprehensive, may be facilitated by the parents, and may include alternative strategies such as designated-donor programs to reduce donor exposure.[68] Such increased effort may make autologous transfusion options more appealing and effective in pediatric populations.

Whereas many of the risks of allogeneic transfusion have been proven and quantified, others have not or remain controversial. One frequently cited example is the hypothesized risk of immunosuppression and resultant increased risk of infection and/or cancer relapse with associated costs, as measured by increased length of hospital stay.[69,70] However, even if immunosuppression were associated with allogeneic transfusion, it may not be uniquely associated; some investigators have suggested that the impact may be at least partially mediated by cytokines released from stored leukocytes. There is evidence that the release of such cytokines may occur in recovered blood as well.[12,13] Moreover, even where certain risks may be limited to allogeneic transfusion, because blood recovery does not by itself necessarily preclude the need for allogeneic transfusion, it is unclear whether simply reducing the number of allogeneic units for a given patient would have sufficient impact on transfusion risk to warrant the cost. Much of the available literature assumes a greater risk of allogeneic transfusion than of autologous transfusion and therefore considers the avoidance of donor exposure alone as sufficient evidence for efficacy. Such an approach may well have been intuitively if not rigorously compelling in the past, but the risk of allogeneic transfusion has dropped precipitously, and a fresh look at appropriate utilization criteria may be in order.

Evidence exists that autologous transfusion to adequately cover transfusion needs during major surgery is less likely in children than in adults; this is particularly due to the unavailability of preoperatively donated autologous blood, which compels greater reliance on blood recovery[69,71,72] and which may be dependent on the cutoff age considered safe and practical for pediatric autologous donation. Investigators using a minimum age of 3 years old [mean 8.6 (±3.9)] for preoperative donation reported that 75 (94%) of 80 children undergoing cardiac surgery avoided allogeneic blood transfusion by using preoperative donation alone.[73] On the other hand, standard preoperative donation may always be impossible in some surgeries, such as craniosynostosis correction, because of the child's age and size. The successful use of blood recovery in 18 patients undergoing this procedure has been reported, with 33% avoiding allogeneic blood transfusion and a 46.3% reduction in the volume of allogeneic blood transfused as compared to that in prospective nonrandomized controls.[74]

A number of studies have considered the ability of recovery to prevent allogeneic transfusion either alone or in combination with preoperative donation and/or hemodilution. In a recent evaluation of 142 patients undergoing scoliosis surgery, investigators found that blood recovery independently reduced average allogeneic transfusion requirements by more than 50% (5.1 vs 2.0 units) from the requirements of historical controls.[75] Conversely, others, evaluating 155 children (10-21 years old) undergoing spinal surgery—all of whom were able to donate autologous blood for themselves—reported that blood recovery contributed to avoiding allogeneic blood transfusion only in those with massive blood loss (2000 mL or greater).[76] In this group (12% of patients), 90% avoided allogeneic blood transfusion when blood recovery was performed, and 40% did so when it was not performed.

Another study analyzed the autologous transfusion experience in 82 patients (8-16 years old) undergoing spinal fusion.[71] Of these, 50% avoided allogeneic blood transfusion with preoperative autologous donation alone, 10% with blood recovery alone, and 77% with both. Of those undergoing blood recovery alone, 80% weighed less than 45 kg, which prohibited preoperative autologous donation. Others reported that the use of both sequestration (2 units) and recovery provided for 87% of the transfusion needs of 80 patients undergoing reconstructive spine surgery, while recovery alone provided for 49% of red cell transfusion needs in 302 patients.[77] In another series, 50 patients undergoing scoliosis surgery were supported with a combination of preoperative autologous donation and blood recovery, which, per case, contributed an average of 391 mL of washed red cells with an average hematocrit of 46%—approximately the red cell mass of one standard RBC unit.[78] The type of scoliosis surgery performed may significantly influence the adequacy and feasibility of preoperative autologous donation; one study found that patients with neuromuscular disorders were much less likely to successfully donate (25%) than those with idiopathic scoliosis (86%), of whom 97% did not receive allogeneic blood.[57] Recovery was not used in these patients, but the low availability of preoperative autologous donation in the former group would appear to make them more suitable candidates for recovery, and extraordinary bleeding in patients with such disorders has been reported.[65,66]

Complications of Transfusing Recovered Blood

Because autologous blood is not always "safer," utilization issues must be balanced with benefits on a case-by-case basis. This assumption seems intuitively sound, but it must be remembered that it is the quality of the process and not just the blood that must be comparatively evaluated. Early strategies for blood recovery were fraught with fatal complications including coagulopathy and air embolism, because of design flaws in the devices used.[35]

Currently, the potential complications of receiving recovered blood are primarily those caused by the infusion of damaged or hemolysed red cells, damaged or activated platelets, and/or white cells; activated coagulation and complement cascade components; and the infusion of operative wound contaminants or debris inadequately removed from shed blood. Damage to red cells may occur secondary to the trauma of surgery itself or to the presence of osmotically or chemically incompatible fluids in the wound, such as those used for cleansing or irrigation.[35,79] Damage may also occur during the recovery process, particularly during aspiration, and recommendations regarding suction vacuum pressure have been made.[80] The precise impact of reinfusing red cell debris remains controversial.[35]

Damage to platelets and white cells may also occur for similar reasons and has been associated with activation and/or the release of granules into recovered blood.[35] The potential for reperfusion injury caused by damaged and/or activated white cells has been hypothesized and the extensive leukocyte content of even washed recovered blood has been evaluated.[81] Cell recovery devices appear to remove white cells with various efficiencies.[81] Investigators using a dog model have reported that washed, recovered red cell suspensions may contain degradation products that had been released from white cells and/or platelets deposited on the centrifuge chamber during processing.[31] They further proposed that reinfusion of these toxic materials promulgated a "recovered blood syndrome" consisting of intravascular clotting and pulmonary damage, marked by intra-alveolar and perivascular hemorrhage, along with pulmonary edema. Leukocyte margination and occlusive thrombi in the pulmonary arterioles were also noted. Excessive saline dilution, high calcium concentration, and the aspiration of clotted blood were aggravating factors, and their avoidance has been recommended to enhance the safety of blood recovery.[31,32]

The levels of inflammatory and immunomodulatory substances such as leukotrienes and thromboxanes may be increased in shed blood, and a role for them in adverse effects of recovered blood transfusion has been suggested.[12] Cell washing will remove a substantial fraction of noncellular material, but the threshold at which any given undesirable substance can be considered "safe" is variable and arguable. Many substances are found or instilled in surgical wounds that have been shown to be deleterious to red cells or whose infusion is proscribed. A short list would include amniotic fluid, gastric fluid, bowel contents, clotting agents (eg, thrombin), irrigating solutions (eg, sterile water, betadyne), and topical antibiotics. Hence, the general practice is to wash and to process under conditions that minimize or forbid the presence of unwanted material in the wound and/or its aspiration into the reservoir and that favors its removal from processed units (adequate wash solution volume, no transfusion of partial bowls).

Contraindications to Cell Recovery

There are a number of general contraindications to cell recovery, most of which are applicable in pediatric surgery. These include those surgeries or operative maneuvers known to cause complications, as well as those in which potential complications have been hypothesized or modeled in vitro but not definitively shown in patients. The latter group, by far the larger, includes surgery in which there is bacterial contamination of the wound, such as abdominal trauma with bowel contents present, and contamination of the wound with amniotic fluid, such as during obstetric procedures, because of the potential risk of sepsis, coagulopathy, or amniotic fluid embolism.[35,82-84] Concerns about the use of blood recovery in neurosurgery, as brain tissue is highly provocative to the coagulation cascade, have led to a similar proscription.[25] On the other hand, some have questioned the absoluteness of these contraindications, suggesting that the risk is overstated and that cell washing adequately attenuates the risk.[25] In fact, the safe, successful use of blood recovery in pediatric neurosurgical procedures such as intracranial neurosurgery and craniosynostosis repair has been reported.[19,25,85] Similarly, some have claimed that the partial removal of a heavy bacterial load renders recovered blood safe enough to use in the setting of perforation.[74] The use of cell recovery in burn surgery, where bacterial contamination is a threat, has also been advocated.[26] There is evidence that blood recovery may be safely performed in the obstetric setting, although whether this would hold true when pregnant minors are involved is unknown.[86]

Blood recovery is contraindicated in patients with sickle cell disease, because of the risk for sickling and hemolysis consequent to aspiration and processing. However, some have reported successful use in sickle cell patients and have recommended precautions to reduce this risk.[87] Autologous transfusion can be helpful in alloimmunized patients, for whom finding compatible allogeneic blood can be difficult. Blood recovery is also contraindicated in the setting of malignancy when the purpose of the surgery is resection of a primary nonmetastatic tumor, because of the theoretical risk of disseminating aspirated tumor cells through transfusion, a risk substantiated by the clonogenicity in culture of tumor cells isolated from washed recovered blood.[88] Some have advocated processing techniques such as the use of filters or irradiation as a means of removing this risk.[89-93] Others base a willingness to recover blood on the nature of the tumor itself. In the adult population, the results of a few small studies in which no measurable increase in relapse rate or unusual sites or manifestations of relapse were reported have become the basis for the use of blood recovery in the resection of certain primary tumors, such as during radical prostatectomy, nephrectomy, and cystectomy.[35] Unfortunately, the small size of these studies and the short follow-up often preclude the drawing of definitive conclusions, as a rate of serious adverse effects comparable to the very low rate associated with allogeneic transfusion might well go undetected.[16,56,94] There is a danger in combining such potentially misleading results with a preconceived notion of the intrinsic superiority of autologous blood over allogeneic blood.

In fact, this is a general problem in the literature concerning blood recovery, as there is no large study or meta-analysis weighing the risk of recovery against its effectiveness as a means of directly avoiding the complications of allogeneic transfusion in either adult or pediatric patients. Especially in children, who have the greater fraction of their lives in front of them, potential unknown harm must be considered in any decision to use recovery, and certainly in a setting of relative contraindication. A similar statistical conundrum has plagued the proper safety analysis of preoperative autologous donation in adult patients; a number of studies "proving" the safety of bleeding higher-risk donors ultimately gave way to larger analyses that appeared to describe a quite different risk-benefit profile.[16,56,94]

Blood Recovery in Cardiothoracic Bypass Surgery and Ultrafiltration

Blood recovery is often performed in the context of a nondedicated extracorporeal circuit such as the perfusion pump utilized during bypass surgery.[95] Blood recovery procedures associated with perfusion may include direct reinfusion of shed blood through the perfusion pump or after standard cell washing. As an example, the recovery reservoir may be fitted with a Y-connector at the bottom, with one line leading to the processing kit and the other line to the pump. At various intervals, the recovery device operator might be asked by the perfusionist to transfer the contents of the reservoir to the pump in an effort to maintain volume and pressure within the extracorporeal circuit. Conversely, at the end of the procedure, the contents of the pump (≥2 L) might be transferred back to the reservoir and washed and concentrated in the recovery device.

Ultrafiltration has been used as means of recovering red cells from the bypass pump during or after pediatric cardiac surgery.[96] The authors report the procedure as safe, although significant, clinically manageable increases in plasma-free hemoglobin and activated clotting time were noted. In a study comparing immediate return, cell washing, and ultrafiltration as methods of red cell recovery in 60 patients during and after cardiopulmonary bypass in adults, no clinically significant difference among the three techniques was reported.[97]

Storage

As with adults, the routine storage of recovered blood, washed or unwashed, from children cannot be routinely recommended. While it is technically feasible to briefly store recovered blood units, that step raises issues regarding their quality, identification, labeling, handling, and documentation, as compared with other banked blood.[98,99] The potential for bacterial contamination and proliferation and the presence of uncertain quantities of superfluous materials contraindicate longer storage. The storage of shed, unwashed blood, with its greater risk for contamination, is similarly contraindicated.

Quality Assurance Issues

The need for quality systems in blood recovery has been proposed and explored by practitioners.[51] The AABB has established clearly defined standards for perioperative blood recovery.[99]

However, because recovery is performed in and controlled by the operating room, and because it is a service frequently outsourced to commercial providers, the blood banks of some institutions may choose not to be answerable for the quality of the activity.

The FDA has made recommendations in the area of perioperative transfusion, primarily regarding storage conditions of recovered blood, but it has otherwise largely avoided significant audit or enforcement activity.[98]

As mentioned above, recovered blood is potentially of very high quality. However, a number of technical and clinical factors may have detrimental effects on this quality. In essence, the preparation of any blood component is a kind of manufacturing, and the process controls that are in place directly affect the integrity of the component produced. Certainly, this is true of banked blood, whether allogeneic or autologous. One might question whether, if the same standard of current good manufacturing practice were applied to blood recovery, unvalidated procedures or techniques of uncertain efficacy such as using white cell filters to remove cancer cells would be considered acceptable, even in an autologous context. In contrast, preoperatively collected autologous banked blood can be an FDA-licensed product and subject to scrutiny similar to that for other manufactured products, with suitable provisos addressing its irreplaceability and allowing physician input regarding risk-benefit issues. Quality assurance includes quality control measures used to document that recovered blood meets standards for purity (absence of contaminating material) and potency (adequate hematocrit). Although the latter is straightforward, the former is less so. Some have advocated potassium as a surrogate marker.[100] In general, quality control is performed periodically to validate the process and its components (ie, operator practices and proficiency, device integrity).

Conclusion

Cell recovery has a definitive role in the perioperative transfusion management of children. However, this role is constrained by the technical capabilities of available devices and a lack of cost-effectiveness and even of efficacy in some surgeries. Measures to refine utilization to those cases more likely to have blood loss that justifies recovery may be indicated. Certainly, independent oversight of the recovery activity (such as through AABB accreditation) so as to ensure safe practice is essential to realize the advantages of autologous transfusion even in this group. The best use of blood recovery appears to be the supplementation of preoperative autologous donation and other strategies to limit donor exposure in pediatric surgical patients.

References

1. Khan RM, Bassett HF. Intraoperative autologous blood transfusion: Report of a technique. Thorax 1975;30:447-51.
2. Dorang LA, Klebanoff G, Kemmerer WT. Autotransfusion in long-segment spinal fusion. An experimental model to demonstrate the efficacy of salvaging blood contaminated with bone fragments and marrow. Am J Surg 1972;123:686-8.
3. Klebanoff G. Early clinical experience with a disposable unit for the intraoperative salvage and reinfusion of blood loss (intraoperative autotransfusion). Am J Surg 1970;120:718-22.
4. Stehling L, ed. Perioperative autologous transfusion. Arlington, VA: American Association of Blood Banks, 1991:92.
5. Mollison PL, Engelfriet CP, Contreras M. Blood transfusion in clinical medicine. 8th ed. London: Blackwell Scientific Publications, 1987: 136-7.
6. Petaja J, Lundstrom U, Leijala M, et al. Bleeding and use of blood products after heart operations in infants. J Thorac Cardiovasc Surg 1995; 109:524-9.
7. Manno CS, Hedberg KW, Kim HC, et al. Comparison of the hemostatic effects of fresh whole blood, stored whole blood, and components after open heart surgery in children. Blood 1991;77:930-6.
8. McShane AJ, Power C, Jackson JF, et al. Autotransfusion: Quality of blood prepared with a red cell processing device. Br J Anaesth 1987; 59:1035-9.
9. Kirkpatrick UJ, Adams RA, Lardi A, McCollum CN. Rheological properties and function of blood cells in stored bank blood and salvaged blood. Br J Haematol 1998;101:364-8.
10. Sieunarine K, Langton S, Lawrence-Brown MM, et al. Elastase levels in salvaged blood and the effect of cell washing. Aust N Z J Surg 1990;60: 613-6.

11. Sieunarine K, Lawrence-Brown MM, Goodman MA, et al. Plasma levels of lipid mediators, leukotriene B4 and lyso platelet-activating factor, in intraoperative recovered blood. Vox Sang 1992;63:168-71.
12. Jacobi K, Walther A, Lorler H, Neidhardt B. Plasma levels of eicosanoids after transfusion of intraoperatively salvaged blood. Vox Sang 2000; 78:31-6.
13. Jacobi KE, Wanke C, Jacobi A, et al. Determination of eicosanoid and cytokine production in salvaged blood, stored red blood cell concentrates, and whole blood. J Clin Anesthesiol 2000;12:94-9.
14. Klebanoff G, Dorang LA, Kemmerer WT, et al. Repair of surahepatic caval laceration employing autotransfusion: An experimental model to demonstrate the effectiveness of intraoperative blood salvage under conditions of massive hemorrhage. J Trauma 1972;12:422-4.
15. Valbonesi M, Frisoni R, Florio G, Ferrari M. Intraoperative blood salvage: A new artificial organ? Int J Artif Organs 1995;18:136-42.
16. Haugen RK, Hill GE. A large-scale autologous blood program in a community hospital. A contribution to the community's blood supply. JAMA 1987;257:1211-14.
17. Malan TP Jr, Whitemore J, Maddi R. Reoperative cardiac surgery in a Jehovah's Witness: Role of continuous cell salvage and in-line reinfusion. J Cardiothorac Anesthesiol 1989;3:211-14.
18. Williamson KR, Taswell HF. Indications for intraoperative blood salvage. J Clin Apheresis 1990;5:100-3.
19. Velardi F, Di Chirico A, Di Rocco C, et al. "No allogeneic blood transfusion" protocol for the surgical correction of craniosynostoses. II. Clinical application. Childs Nerv Syst 1998;14:732-9.
20. Velardi F, Di Chirico A, Di Rocco C, et al. "No allogeneic blood transfusion" protocol for the surgical correction of craniosynostoses. I. Rationale. Childs Nerv Syst 1998;14:722-31.
21. Estrin JA, Belani KG, Karnavas AG, et al. A new approach to massive blood transfusion during pediatric liver resection. Surgery 1986;99: 664-70.
22. Farrar RP, Hanto DW, Flye MW, Chaplin H. Blood component use in orthotopic liver transplantation. Transfusion 1988;28:474-8.
23. Dzik WH, Jenkins R. Use of intraoperative blood salvage during orthotopic liver transplantation. Arch Surg 1985;120:946-8.
24. Witte CL, Esser MJ, Rappaport WD. Updating the management of salvageable splenic injury. Ann Surg 1992;215:261-5.
25. Velardi F, DiChirico A, DiRocco C. Blood salvage in craniosynostosis surgery. Childs Nerv Syst 1999;15:695-710.
26. Jeng JC, Boyd TM, Jablonski KA, et al. Intraoperative blood salvage in excisional burn surgery: An analysis of yield, bacteriology, and inflammatory mediators. J Burn Care Rehabil 1998;19:305-11.

27. Smith RS, Meister RK, Tsoi EK, Bohman HR. Laparoscopically guided blood salvage and autotransfusion in splenic trauma: A case report. J Trauma 1993;34:313-14.
28. Wesson DE, Ein SH, Villamater J. Intraoperative autotransfusion in blunt abdominal trauma. J Pediatr Surg 1980;15:735-6.
29. Popovsky MA, Devine PA, Taswell HF. Intraoperative autologous transfusion. Mayo Clin Proc 1985;60:125-34.
30. Ronai AK, Glass JJ, Shapiro AS. Improving autologous blood harvest: Recovery of red cells from sponges and suction. Anaesth Intensive Care 1987;15:421-4.
31. Bull MH, Bull BS, Van Arsdell GS, Smith LL. Clinical implications of procoagulant and leukoattractant formation during intraoperative blood salvage. Arch Surg 1988;123:1073-8.
32. Bull BS, Bull MH. Enhancing the safety of intraoperative RBC salvage. J Trauma 1989;29:320-5.
33. Bull BS, Bull MH. The salvaged blood syndrome: A sequel to mechanochemical activation of platelets and leukocytes? Blood Cells 1990;16:15-20.
34. Cell salvage washout performance with partial bowls. Haemonetics Cell Saver 5, clinical performance summary. Braintree, MA: Haemonetics Corporation, August 1996.
35. Dzik WH, Sherburne B. Intraoperative blood salvage: Medical controversies. Transfus Med Rev 1990;4:208-35.
36. Booke M, Hagemann O, Van Aken H, et al. Intraoperative autotransfusion in small children: An in vitro investigation to study its feasibility. Anesth Analg 1999;88:763-5.
37. Michaelis G, Melzer C, Biscoping J, Hempelmann G. Mechanical autologous transfusion in orthopedic surgery in children. Is the use of mechanical autologous transfusion possible even in pediatric orthopedic surgical procedures? Anaesthetist 1995;44:501-7.
38. Ray JM, Flynn JC, Bierman AH. Erythrocyte survival following intraoperative autotransfusion in spinal surgery: An in vivo comparative study and 5-year update. Spine 1986;11:879-82.
39. Keverline JP, Sanders JO. Hematuria associated with low-volume cell saver in pediatric orthopedics. J Pediatr Orthop 1998;18:594-7.
40. Rollo VJ, Hozack WJ, Rothman RH, et al. Prospective randomized evaluation of blood salvage techniques for primary total hip arthroplasty. J Arthroplasty 1995;10:532-9.
41. Umlas J, Foster RR, Dalal SA, et al. Red cell loss following orthopedic surgery: The case against postoperative blood salvage. Transfusion 1994;34:402-6.
42. Marks RM, Vaccaro AR, Balderston RA, et al. Postoperative blood salvage in total knee arthroplasty using the Solcotrans autotransfusion system. J Arthroplasty 1995;10:433-7.

43. Rosolski T, Mauermann K, Frick U, Hergert M. Direct autotransfusion systems deliver blood of inadequate quality. Anasthesiol Intensivmed Notfallmed Schmerzther 2000;35:21-4.
44. Reents W, Babin-Ebell J, Misoph MR, et al. Influence of different autotransfusion devices on the quality of salvaged blood. Ann Thorac Surg 1999;68:58-62.
45. Tawes RL Jr, Sydorak GR, DuVall TB. Postoperative salvage: A technological advance in the 'washed' versus 'unwashed' blood controversy. Semin Vasc Surg 1994;7:98-103.
46. Schmidt H, Bendtzen K, Mortensen PE. The inflammatory cytokine response after autotransfusion of shed mediastinal blood. Acta Anaesthesiol Scand 1998;42:558-64.
47. Sloand E, Alyono D, Yu M, Klein H. Platelet membrane glycoproteins and microvesicles in blood from postoperative salvage: A study in cardiac bypass patients. Transfusion 1995;35:738-44.
48. Lawrence-Brown MM, Couch C, Halliday M, et al. D-dimer levels in blood salvage for autotransfusion. Aust N Z J Surg 1989;59:67-70.
49. Khan RM, Siddiqui AM, Natrajan KM. Blood conservation and autotransfusion in cardiac surgery. J Cardiac Surg 1993;8:25-31.
50. Sieunarine K, Wetherall J, Lawrence-Brown MM, et al. Levels of complement factor C3 and its activated product, C3a, in operatively salvaged blood. Aust N Z J Surg 1991;61:302-5.
51. Koehler LC, Williamson KR, Taswell HF. A comprehensive program to ensure quality in intraoperative blood salvage. J Intraven Nurs 1991; 14:193-7.
52. Avall A, Hyllner M, Bengtson JP, et al. Greater increase in cytokine concentration after salvage with filtered whole blood than with washed red cells, but no difference in postoperative hemoglobin recovery. Transfusion 1999;39:271-6.
53. Arnestad JP, Hyllner M, Bengston JP, et al. Removal of activated complement from shed blood: Comparison of high- and low-dilutional haemofiltration. Acta Anaesthesiol Scand 1998;42:811-15.
54. Dalen T, Brostrom LA, Engstrom KG. Cell quality of salvaged blood after total knee arthroplasty. Drain blood compared to venous blood in 32 patients. Acta Orthop Scand 1995;66:329-33.
55. Ferraris VA, Ferraris SP. Limiting excessive postoperative blood transfusion after cardiac procedures. A review. Tex Heart Inst J 1995;22: 216-30.
56. Etchason J, Petz L, Keeler E, et al. The cost effectiveness of preoperative autologous blood donations. N Engl J Med 1995;332:719-24.
57. Murray DJ, Forbes RB, Titone MB, et al. Transfusion management in pediatric and adolescent scoliosis surgery. Efficacy of autologous blood. Spine 1997;22:2735-40.

58. Thompson HW, Luban NL. Autologous blood transfusion in the pediatric patient. J Pediatr Surg 1995;30:1406-11.
59. Stehling L, Zauder HL. Autologous blood salvage procedures. Biotechnology 1991;19:47-73.
60. Solomon MD, Rutledge ML, Kane LE. Cost comparison of intraoperative autologous versus homologous transfusion. Transfusion 1988;28:379-82.
61. Goodnough LT, Monk TG, Sicard G. Intraoperative salvage in patients undergoing elective abdominal aortic aneurysm repair: An analysis of cost and benefit. J Vasc Surg 1996;24:213-18.
62. Ikeda S, Johnston MF, Yagi K, et al. Intraoperative autologous blood salvage with cardiac surgery: An analysis of five years' experience in more than 3,000 patients. J Clin Anesth 1992;4:359-66.
63. Williams GD, Bratton SL, Riley EC, et al. Association between age and blood loss in children undergoing open heart operations. Ann Thorac Surg 1998;66:870-5; discussion 875-6.
64. Cataldi S, Bruder N, Dufour H, et al. Intraoperative autologous blood transfusion in intracranial surgery. Neurosurgery 1997;40:765-71.
65. Forst J, Forst R, Leithe H, Maurin N. Platelet function deficiency in duchenne muscular dystrophy. Neuromuscul Disord 1998;8:46-9.
66. Katz K, Tamary H, Lahav J, et al. Increased operative bleeding during orthopedic surgery in patients with type I Gaucher disease and bone involvement. Bull Hosp Jt Dis 1999;58:188-90.
67. Ozier YM, Le Cam B, Chatellier G, et al. Intraoperative blood loss in pediatric liver transplantation: Analysis of preoperative risk factors. Anesth Analg 1995;81:1142-7.
68. Brecher ME, Taswell HF, Clare DE, et al. Minimal-exposure transfusion and the committed donor. Transfusion 1990;30:599-604.
69. Faenza A, Cunsolo A, Selleri S, et al. Correlation between plasma or blood transfusion and survival after curative surgery for colorectal cancer. Int Surg 1992;77:264-9.
70. Murphy PJ, Connery C, Hicks GL Jr, et al. Homologous blood transfusion as a risk factor for postoperative infection after coronary artery bypass graft operations. J Thorac Cardiovasc Surg 1992;104:1092-9.
71. Novak RW. Autologous blood transfusion in a pediatric population. Safety and efficacy. Clin Pediatr 1988;27:184-7.
72. Werner AL, Zarandy M, Lilliston E. Intraoperative cell salvage for pediatric orthopedic surgery—is it still needed? (abstract). Transfusion 2000;40(Suppl):100S.
73. Masuda M, Kawachi Y, Inaba S, et al. Preoperative autologous blood donations in pediatric cardiac surgery. Ann Thorac Surg 1995;60:1694-7.
74. Jimenez DF, Barone CM. Intraoperative autologous blood transfusion in the surgical correction of craniosynostosis. Neurosurgery 1995;37:1075-9.

75. Lennon RL, Hosking MP, Gray JR, et al. The effects of intraoperative blood salvage and induced hypotension on transfusion requirements during spinal surgical procedures. Mayo Clin Proc 1987;62:1090-4.
76. Simpson MB, Georgopoulos G, Eilert RE. Intraoperative blood salvage in children and young adults undergoing spinal surgery with pre-deposited autologous blood: Efficacy and cost effectiveness. J Pediatr Orthop 1993;13:777-80.
77. Shulman G, Solanki DR, Nicodemus CL, et al. Audit of autotransfusion in spine surgery. Int Orthop 1998;22:303-7.
78. Anand N, Idio FG Jr, Remer S, Hoppenfeld S. The effects of perioperative blood salvage and autologous blood donation on transfusion requirements in scoliosis surgery. J Spinal Disord 1998;11:532-4.
79. Orliaguet G, Dahmani S, Meyer P. [Acute hemolysis following perioperative blood salvage in children operated for the surgical correction of craniosynostosis]. Ann Fr Anesth Reanim 2001;20:28-31.
80. Gregoretti S. Suction-induced hemolysis at various vacuum pressures: Implications for intraoperative blood salvage. Transfusion 1996;36: 57-60.
81. Connall TP, Zhang J, Vaziri ND, et al. Leukocyte CD11b and CD18 expression are increased in blood salvaged for autotransfusion. Am Surg 1994;60:797-800.
82. Perttila J, Leino L, Poyhonen M, Salo M. Leukocyte content in blood processed by autotransfusion devices during open-heart surgery. Acta Anaesthesiol Scand 1995;39:445-8.
83. Horst HM, Dlugos S, Fath JJ, et al. Coagulopathy and intraoperative blood salvage (IBS). J Trauma 1992;32:646-52.
84. Waters JH, Biscotti C, Potter PS, et al. Amniotic fluid removal during cell salvage in the cesarean section patient. Anesthesiology 2000;92: 1531-6.
85. Rebarber A, Lonser R, Jackson S, et al. The safety of intraoperative autologous blood collection and autotransfusion during cesarean section. Am J Obstet Gynecol 1998;179:715-20.
86. Boudreaux JP, Bornside GH, Cohn I Jr. Emergency autotransfusion: Partial cleansing of bacteria-laden blood by cell washing. J Trauma 1983;23:31-5.
87. Rainaldi MP, Tazzari PL, Scagliarini G, et al. Blood salvage during cesarean section. Br J Anaesth 1998;80:195-8.
88. Fox JS, Amaranath L, Hoeltge GA, et al. Autologous blood transfusion and intraoperative cell salvage in a patient with homozygous sickle cell disease. Cleve Clin J Med 1994;61:137-40.
89. Hansen E, Wolff N, Knuechel R, et al. Tumor cells in blood shed from the surgical field. Arch Surg 1995;130:287-93.

90. Wiesel M, Gudemann C, Staehler G, et al. Separation of urologic tumor cells from Cell Saver blood using a membrane filter. A new method in autotransfusion? Urologe 1992;31:182-5.
91. Hansen E, Knuechel R, Altmeppen J, Taeger K. Blood irradiation for intraoperative autotransfusion in cancer surgery: Demonstration of efficient elimination of contaminating tumor cells. Transfusion 1999;39: 608-15.
92. Karczewski DM, Lema MJ, Glaves D. The efficiency of an autotransfusion system for tumor cell removal from blood salvaged during cancer surgery. Anesth Analg 1994;78:1131-5.
93. Hansen E, Schlosser S, Altmeppen J, et al. Irradiation of wound blood from tumor surgery for retransfusion. Beitr Infusionsther Transfusionsmed 1994;32:502-4.
94. Popovsky MA, Whitaker B, Arnold NL. Severe outcomes of allogeneic and autologous blood donation: Frequency and characterization (letter). Transfusion 1996;36:761.
95. Hishon ML, Ryan A, Lithgow P, Butt W. An evaluation of changes in composition and contamination of salvaged blood from the cardiopulmonary bypass circuit of pediatric patients. Heart Lung 1995;24: 307-11.
96. Friesen RH, Tornabene MA, Coleman SP. Blood conservation during pediatric cardiac surgery: Ultrafiltration of the extracorporeal circuit volume after cardiopulmonary bypass. Anesth Analg 1993;77:702-7.
97. Sutton RG, Kratz JM, Spinale FG, Crawford FA Jr. Comparison of three blood-processing techniques during and after cardiopulmonary bypass. Ann Thorac Surg 1993;56:938-43.
98. Food and Drug Administration. Memorandum: Guidance for autologous blood and blood components. (March 15, 1989) Rockville, MD: CBER Office of Communications, Training, and Manufacturers Assistance, 1989.
99. Santrach P, ed. Standards for perioperative autologous blood collection and administration, 1st ed. Bethesda, MD: American Association of Blood Banks, 2001.
100. Szpisjak DF, Edgell DS, Bissonnette B. Potassium as a surrogate marker of debris in cell-salvaged blood. Anesth Analg 2000;91:40-3.

In: Herman JH, Manno CS, eds.
Pediatric Transfusion Therapy
Bethesda, MD: AABB Press, 2002

15

Therapy for Hemophilia and von Willebrand Disease

JOSEPH G. PRESSEY, MD, AND
CATHERINE S. MANNO, MD

FOR MOST OF THE PAST CENTURY, the life expectancy and quality of life of hemophilia patients steadily climbed. According to Swedish death registries, the life expectancy of those with severe hemophilia in 1920 was merely 11 years. During the period from 1961 to 1980, the mean lifespan of persons with severe hemophilia in Sweden had reached 56 years due to the advent of more specific therapies for Factor VIII and Factor IX deficiency.[1] However, the detection of AIDS in hemophilia patients in 1983 har-

Joseph G. Pressey, MD, Clinical Instructor, Division of Oncology, The Children's Hospital of Philadelphia, and Catherine S. Manno, MD, Acting Chief, Division of Hematology, The Children's Hospital of Philadelphia, and Associate Professor of Pediatrics, School of Medicine, University of Pennsylvania, Philadelphia, Pennsylvania

kened an era of increasing morbidity and mortality in the hemophilia population.[2] The majority of patients with severe hemophilia treated in the early 1980s contracted human immunodeficiency virus (HIV) and many of those have since died of AIDS. Likewise, many hemophilia patients treated during the same era became infected with hepatitis C virus (HCV) as a result of contaminated factor concentrates.[3] The recognition that such deadly viruses were frequently transmitted in pooled-plasma concentrates prompted a revolution in product advances and safety during the last 15 years. The identification and characterization of the Factor VIII and Factor IX genes has led to the advent of recombinant clotting factors. Improved virus inactivation procedures in plasma-derived factor concentrates and the production of recombinant factor products have significantly decreased the risk of infectious transmission in hemophilia patients. Other advances include prophylactic strategies that allow affected children to lead more active lives with decreased incidence of chronic joint damage from hemorrhage. Despite these improvements, patients with hemophilia and severe von Willebrand disease (vWD) are at constant risk of life-threatening hemorrhage, necessitating limitations on athletic and recreational activities, a particularly difficult task in otherwise healthy, energetic children.

Hemophilia patients and their families should be followed closely in tertiary pediatric hospitals with designated centers for the diagnosis and treatment of hemophilia. Pediatric hematologists, orthopedic surgeons, physical therapists, nurses and social workers play integral roles in the management of these patients and their families. Patients and parents must be thoroughly educated on the signs and symptoms of bleeding complications, particularly intracranial hemorrhage (ICH). Access to rapid and appropriate treatment is paramount in preventing severe and chronic complications from bleeding.

Demographics and Etiology

Hemophilia is caused by a partial or complete absence of coagulation Factor VIII or coagulation Factor IX, resulting from mutations in the genes encoding each protein. About 1 in 5000 males is affected with hemophilia; 80% of patients have Factor VIII deficiency (hemophilia A) and 20% of patients have Factor IX deficiency (hemophilia B).[4] The genes encoding Factor VIII and Factor IX are each located on the long arm of the X chromosome. Thus, hemophilia A and B are inherited as X-linked diseases and most patients inherit the disease from their mothers. In approximately 30% of cases, mutations of Factors VIII or IX develop spontaneously with no family history of a bleeding disorder.[5] The incidence of hemophilia is spread evenly among ethnic, racial, and geographic groups. Rarely, heavily lyonized females with hemophilia trait may experience mild to moderate bleeding symptoms.

von Willebrand disease is the most common congenital bleeding disorder and is inherited in an autosomal fashion, affecting males and females equally. The majority of vWD patients have a mild quantitative deficiency of von Willebrand factor (vWF) and typically have only minor mucosal bleeding or menorrhagia, or prolonged bleeding after tooth extraction or surgery. Approximately 5% of vWD patients have severe disease with undetectable amounts of vWF and consequently a more serious bleeding diathesis.

Numerous forms of Factor VIII and Factor IX mutations have been described in hemophilia patients and carriers. Base-pair substitutions, including missense, nonsense, and splice site mutations are the most common alterations detected.[6] Genetic deletions of varying sizes are also implicated in Factor VIII and IX mutations. Approximately 40% to 50% of mutations of Factor VIII result from inversions of DNA sequence within intron 22.[7] Investigators have sought a correlation between the genetic alteration of the hemophilia genes and the clinical phenotype

Presentation and Diagnosis

Hemophilia patients without a family history may present in the neonatal period with prolonged bleeding after circumcision. Other presentations include recurrent unusual or severe bruising, persistent mucosal bleeding (commonly a torn frenulem during infancy), or hemarthrosis. Joint bleeds are rare during the first year of life due to the limited mobility in such young children. Approximately 1% to 4% of newborns with severe hemophilia suffer intracranial bleeding episodes, underlining the necessity for pediatric hematologists to be involved during the prenatal period, if possible.[8] If there is a family history of hemophilia, cord blood can be assayed for Factor VIII or Factor IX activity immediately after birth. In older children, an activated partial thromboplastin time (aPTT) may be used as a screen for Factor VIII or Factor IX deficiency, followed by assays for Factor VIII and Factor IX and vWD, depending on the clinical situation. While bleeding times are typically prolonged in patients with hemophilia, this test is typically of little use in diagnosis, particularly in newborns and infants.

von Willebrand disease includes numerous variants, such as quantitative and qualitative defects in the vWF protein, with most patients possessing mild quantitative deficiency of vWF (type 1 vWD). Such patients typically present with frequent mucosal bleeding, menorrhagia, or perioperative hemorrhage. Screening for vWD should include F:VIII activity, vWF, and ristocetin cofactor (R:Co) assays. Because these levels tend to fluctuate in an unpredictable way, the diagnostic testing may at times be normal in an affected individual. It is recommended that screening be performed on three separate occasions before ruling out vWD.

Clinical Characteristics

The activated form of Factor VIII is a cofactor required for activation of Factor IX; together they function to activate Factor X in the coagulation cascade; therefore, a deficiency of either factor translates into identical bleeding manifestations. The degree of factor deficiency dictates the severity of hemorrhagic manifestations. Hemophilia is conventionally divided into three clinical categories: severe, moderate, and mild. Severe hemophilia is defined as factor activity less than 1% of normal. Mild and moderate hemophilia are characterized by factor activities between 1% and 5% and between 5% and 20%, respectively. The rarity of spontaneous hemorrhage clinically differentiates mild and moderate from severe hemophilia patients. Patients with severe Factor VIII or Factor IX deficiency may experience spontaneous or traumatic joint and soft tissue bleeding. In the setting of hemarthrosis, patients note a sensation of warmth and fullness in the joint, followed by decreased mobility, pain, and edema. Prompt factor replacement and joint immobilization are integral to reducing the damage associated with acute and chronic joint bleeding. Recurrent hemarthrosis leads to debilitating hemophilic arthropathy, significantly hindering the quality of life of hemophilia patients. A more critical concern for hemophilia patients is the risk of life-threatening events such as intracranial hemorrhage. Head trauma, documented or suspected, must be evaluated by trained medical personnel immediately and factor replacement administered as quickly as possible, even before the completion of CT scans or complete physical examination. Other worrisome clinical situations include bleeding into closed body spaces that can accommodate large volumes of blood. The retroperitoneum and thighs are particularly susceptible to significant blood accumulation with few concomitant physical signs or symptoms appearing before a patient becomes severely anemic. Compartment syndrome is another complication associated with hemophilia, with bleeding into the closed compartment of the forearm causing potential compromise to neural and vascular structures. Bleeding of the tongue and airway also present potential emergencies, necessitating rapid treatment, airway monitoring, and protection of the airway.

Therapy for Hemophilia A and B

The introduction of highly purified plasma-derived and recombinant Factor VIII concentrates has revolutionized the treatment and prevention of bleeding complications in persons with hemophilia. Most patients in Western Europe and the United States, particularly newly diagnosed patients, now receive recombinant factor concentrates exclusively. However, plasma-derived factor concentrates are considered extremely safe and have the advantages of lower cost and typically more ample supply than recombinant factor concentrates.

Plasma-Derived Factors VIII and IX Concentrates

Numerous Factor VIII and Factor IX concentrates derived from pooled plasma (typically from about 60,000 donors) are available in the United States (see Table 15-1). While a potential risk of infection transmission with these products persists, the likelihood has been greatly reduced by the introduction of donor screening, as well as virus inactivation techniques such as pasteurization, solvent/detergent (S/D) treatment, and nanofiltration. Pasteurization of factor concentrates involves heating the product in aqueous solution to 60 C for 10 hours (Humate-P and Monoclate-P, Aventis Behring, King of Prussia, PA). The S/D technique is particularly useful in inactivating viruses with lipid envelopes, including HIV, HBV, and HCV. S/D treatment alone is not effective in removing nonenveloped viruses such as hepatitis A and parvovirus B19. Outbreaks of hepatitis A in hemophilia patients, particularly in Europe, are well documented.[9,10] These outbreaks have led manufacturers to utilize at least two methods of virus inactivation for plasma-derived factor concentrates. Likewise, parvovirus B19 may be transmitted in plasma-derived factor concentrates, as evidenced by active infection or seroconversion after administration of factor concentrate to hemophilia patients. Patients who have received pooled factor concentrates possess higher-than-average parvovirus B19 seropositivity.[11] Most often, parvovirus causes mild or no symptoms in infected patients; however, immunocompromised patients may suffer severe or persistent infection with reticulocytopenia and anemia. While parvovirus typically causes mild disease in the healthy patient, its ability to resist virus inactivation suggests that other robust blood-borne infectious agents might also be transmitted in plasma-derived products. Creutzfeldt-Jakob disease (CJD) is another potential transmissible agent, although no such cases have been documented in patients receiving blood components or factor concentrates.[12] Variant CJD is caused by a different prion with unique incubation characteristics. The pos-

Table 15-1. Plasma-Derived Factor VIII and Factor IX Products

Factor Purity	Virus Inactivation	Purification	Comments
Factor VIII Products			
Low Purity			
Cryoprecipitated AHF	None		Not recommended for known hemophiliacs
Intermediate Purity			
Humate-P (Aventis Behring)	Pasteurization		Licensed for vWD
High Purity			
Alphanate (Alpha)	Solvent/detergent, heat treated, filtered	Gel chromatography	Contains vWF
Koate-HP (Baxter)	Solvent/detergent		Human albumin
Ultra High Purity			
Hemofil-M (Baxter)	Solvent/detergent	Immunoaffinity chromatography	Trace mouse protein
Monoclate-P (Aventis Behring)	Pasteurization	Immunoaffinity chromatography	Human albumin
Factor IX Products			
Low Purity (Prothrombin complex concentrates)			
Konyne 80 (Bayer)	Heat treated		
Bebulin VH (Immuno)	Heat treated		
High Purity			
Alphanine SD (Alpha)	Solvent/detergent	Chromatography, filtered	

sibility of transmitting variant CJD in plasma-derived factor concentrates has caused great concern, particularly in Great Britain.[13]

All factor concentrates undergo chromatography steps to enhance product purity (the ratio of clotting protein/nonclotting product) of the final product. Purification techniques include immunoaffinity chromatography.

Some intermediate and high-purity plasma-derived Factor VIII concentrates contain high levels of vWF. These products, Humate-P (Aventis Behring) and Alphanate (Alpha Therapeutic Corporation, Los Angeles, CA) provide a therapeutic option for vWD patients who respond poorly to DDAVP, develop tachyphylaxis after repeated doses of DDAVP, or require treatment for serious bleeding. Otherwise, for hemophilia patients, particularly those who have not previously received factor products, recombinant factor products are often prescribed.

Recombinant Factor VIII and Factor IX

In 1984, the human Factor VIII gene was cloned and expressed by Genentech (San Francisco, CA) and Genetics Institute (Cambridge, MA). This finding led to the prelicensing trials of recombinant Factor VIII preparations (Recombinate, Healthcare Corp, Hyland Immuno, Glendale, CA and Kogenate, Bayer Biological Corp, West Haven, CT) in the early 1990s. Recombinant products have a theoretically minimal potential for viral transmission to patients who need factor concentrates (see Table 15-2). For production of recombinant factor, the Factor VIII gene is expressed in the Chinese hamster ovary (CHO) (Recombinate) or baby hamster kidney cell lines (Kogenate). The original formulations required the addition of pasteurized human albumin stabilization of the final protein product; however, newer versions of recombinant Factor VIII in development contain little or no foreign protein. Recombinant Factor IX has since been licensed for the treatment of patients with hemophilia B (Benefix, Genetics Institute/Wyeth, Collegeville, PA). The production of this recombinant Factor IX requires no human or animal protein for cell

Table 15-2. Recombinant Factor VIII and Factor IX Products

Products	Added Protein	Purification
Factor VIII		
Recombinate (Baxter)	Stabilized with human albumin	Immunoaffinity chromatography
Kogenate FS (Bayer)	None	Ion-exchange and MoAb chromatography
Helixate FS (Aventis Behring)	Stabilized with human albumin	Ion-exchange and MoAb chromatography
Bioclate (Aventis Behring)	Stabilized with human albumin	Immunoaffinity chromatography
ReFacto (Genetics Institute/Wyeth)	Human albumin in cell culture	Chromatography purification
Factor IX		
Benefix (Genetics Institute/Wyeth)	No animal or human protein added	Chromatography purification

culture or product stabilization, essentially eliminating the risk of known viral transmission.

Several so-called second-generation recombinant Factor VIII products have recently been licensed in the United States. One recombinant Factor VIII concentrate (ReFacto, Genetics Institute/Wyeth) has been made without the B-domain of the native Factor VIII molecule, resulting in the smallest active Factor VIII protein found in plasma-derived factor concentrates. The advantages of this modified protein include its enhanced resistance to degradation as well as no need for addition of human or animal protein for product stabilization. However, human albumin and recombinant insulin are required for culture of the transfected CHO cells. In initial studies, 32 of 101 previously untreated patients who received B-domain-depleted recombinant Factor VIII developed inhibitors.[14] Sixteen of these patients were classified as high responders (greater than or equal to 5 Bethesda units); these results are comparable to inhibitor development in previous recombinant Factor VIII reports. Kogenate FS (Bayer) is a second-generation recombinant Factor VIII that uses sucrose as a postproduction stabilizer, obviating the need for human albumin in the final product.[15,16]

DDAVP

Mild hemophilia A patients and symptomatic female carriers often respond well to DDAVP (desmopressin) in the setting of mild to moderate bleeding. DDAVP induces rapid release of vWF and Factor VIII from endothelial storage sites. Given parenterally (0.3 μg/kg) or intranasally, DDAVP (150 to 300 μg) may be repeated every 12 to 24 hours, as needed to control hemorrhage. For more serious bleeding or in the setting of tachyphylaxis to DDAVP, mild hemophilia patients should receive Factor VIII concentrate. After diagnosis, persons with mild hemophilia should be scheduled for a trial of DDAVP to assess each patient's response. Typically, a two- to threefold rise in Factor VIII levels will be observed. This response to DDAVP should be reproducible in future administrations.[17] DDAVP has proven to be a safe therapy. Side effects include facial flushing or warmth and a risk of syndrome of inappropriate antidiuretic hormone. Patients are recommended to limit their fluid intake to two-thirds of normal for 12 to 18 hours after administration to avoid hyponatremia. Especially close attention is necessary when administering DDAVP to patients with seizure disorders.

Dosage Considerations

The dose of therapeutic products and the duration of treatment can vary with the type of bleeding (see Table 15-3). One U/kg body weight of recombinant Factor VIII will raise the patient's plasma level by 0.02 units/mL (or 2%). One U/kg of plasma-derived Factor VIII will raise the factor level by 1%. The initial

Table 15-3. Sample Guidelines for Factor VIII and Factor IX Dosing in Treatment of Bleeding in Severe and Moderate Hemophilia*

Type of Bleeding	Factor Correction	Duration of Treatment	Ancillary Treatment/ Comments
Head trauma	100% for all head trauma in severe hemophilia	30% to 50% correction every 12 hours for one to two doses	Always treat before CT scan, even without bleeding or neurologic symptoms
Tongue or neck swelling	100% factor correction	As necessary for hemostasis	Patients must be evaluated by physician to rule out airway obstruction
Compartment syndrome	70% to 100% correction	30% to 50% dosing every 12 hours	Patients with nerve compression should be admitted and monitored
Flank or abdominal pain	Patients should receive 70% to 100% correction	Duration dependent on nature of bleeding	CT of abdomen/pelvis should be obtained to evaluate bleeding
Hemarthrosis (minor or early bleeding)	50% to 70% correction	30% correction in 12 hours, consider repeating at 24 to 36 hours	Splint joint for 48 to 72 hours

(continued)

Table 15-3. Sample Guidelines for Factor VIII and Factor IX Dosing in Treatment of Bleeding in Severe and Moderate Hemophilia* (continued)

Type of Bleeding	Factor Correction	Duration of Treatment	Ancillary Treatment/ Comments
Hemarthrosis (chronic, late, or target joint)	70% correction	30% correction at 12 and 24 hours	Factor IX patients should receive second dose at 4 to 8 hours and third at 24 hours
Muscle bleeding	30% correction	Follow up at 12 to 24 hours	Immobilize area
Thigh/ileopsoas bleeding	70% correction	Maintain factor level above 30% for 2 to 6 days	Monitor hemoglobin level to rule out significant blood loss; bedrest recommended
Fractures	70% correction	Maintain above 30% for 5 to 7 days	
Sutures	70% correction	30% correction during removal	Attempt steri-strips, if possible

*From the Children's Hospital of Philadelphia

half-life of Factor VIII is 6 to 8 hours. Subsequent half-life is 8 to 12 hours.

Recombinant Factor IX is dosed according to the following equation: % rise in factor level multiplied by patient's weight multiplied by 1.2. Plasma-derived Factor IX is dosed as follows: % rise in factor level multiplied by patient's weight. The initial half-life of Factor IX is 4 to 6 hours, with a subsequent half-life of 18 to 24 hours. Peak recovery and half-life of BeneFix (Genetics Institute/Wyeth) varies among hemophilia B patients; many clinicians recommend individual pharmacokinetic evaluation to optimize dosing of Benefix for an individual patient with hemophilia.

Mouth bleeding is common in hemophilia patients. Alpha-aminocaproic acid (Amicar, Amgen, Thousand Oaks, CA) (100 mg/kg every 6 hours for 5 days), an antifibrinolytic agent, or topical thrombin may be used to augment hemostasis if mucocutaneous bleeding is mild. Amicar is contraindicated in the setting of hematuria or within 12 hours of prothrombin complex concentrate (PCC) or activated prothrombin complex concentrate (aPCC) administration due to a risk of thrombosis. For more severe oral bleeding, 30% factor correction is recommended (every 12 hours for Factor VIII and 24 hours for Factor IX). Patients are encouraged to maintain a soft diet and avoid pacifiers to allow clot stabilization.

Dental procedures that require local infiltration or may cause minor bleeding should be proceeded with a 30% factor correction. Patients undergoing dental extractions should begin Amicar therapy the preceding night and continue for 5 days after the procedure. A 70% factor correction before the procedure should be given; follow-up treatments may be recommended if dental surgery is extensive.

Hematuria should be followed closely in hemophilia patients. If there is no history of trauma or pain, patients may be successfully managed with bed rest and aggressive hydration. A 30% factor correction may be used with bed rest if the bleeding continues. If hematuria is associated with trauma or pain, or is observed in those with mild hemophilia, aggressive factor replacement and radiographic (preferably ultrasonography) imaging should be utilized in order to define a site of bleeding.

Prophylactic Treatment of Severe Hemophilia

Episodic treatment of bleeding remains the way in which factor concentrate therapy is most often delivered to hemophilia patients. In the setting of acute hemarthrosis, rapid and accurate factor replacement is crucial in limiting the accumulation of blood in the joint space that results in pain and disability. Likewise, prompt concentrate infusion will help stop significant blood loss into body spaces with the potential to hold large volumes of blood, such as the retroperitoneum or thighs.

The development of chronic arthropathy in hemophilia patients stems from recurrent acute hemarthrosis. As blood enters the joint space and induces irritation of the synovial membrane, vascular proliferation in the synovium develops. Subsequently, with the presence of excess vasculature, even otherwise normal use of the joint can lead to further bleeding and irritation. With repeated bleeding and chronic inflammation, scar tissue in the joint cartilage forms, leading to debilitating joint disease.[18]

Prophylactic therapy is aimed primarily at preventing this chronic joint damage in those with severe hemophilia. First recommended by Professor I.M. Nilsson and others in Sweden in the late 1950s, the objective of prophylaxis was to modify the phenotype of persons with severe hemophilia to that of mild or moderate patients by keeping factor levels above 1% most of the time.[19] "Primary" prophylaxis is begun shortly after affected boys begin ambulating, typically at 1 or 2 years of age. "Secondary" prophylaxis, on the other hand, is started in severe hemophilia patients who have developed recurrent hemarthrosis in one or more "target" joints, defined as a joint with three bleeding episodes in a 6-month period. Primary prophylaxis may serve to prevent even early chronic arthropathy from developing in patients who may otherwise experience debilitating joint disease. Secondary prophylaxis may better address the heterogeneity among those with severe hemophilia, sparing some patients and families from the necessity of intravenous infusions, either through peripheral veins or indwelling central catheter, two or three times per week (see Table 15-4). Further, secondary prophylaxis avoids unnecessary expenditure of limited factor con-

Table 15-4. Typical Factor VIII and Factor IX Prophylaxis Regimens*

Factor	Dose
Factor VIII	25 to 30 U/kg on Monday and Wednesday and 40-50 U/kg on Friday
Factor IX	40 to 50 U/kg two days per week

*The goal of prophylaxis is to maintain factor levels >1%. The actual dose for each patient should be based upon individual factor recovery.

centrates and health-care resources. Prophylactic therapy requires that either 1) family members be trained in administering factor infusions or 2) a home nurse travel to the patient's home for therapy. Some patients, particularly younger boys with limited venous access, need indwelling catheter placement, which requires surgery and leads to a risk of bacterial sepsis and thrombosis.[20,21]

Inhibitors in Hemophilia Patients

The development of inhibitors, alloantibodies directed against Factor VIII or Factor IX, poses a challenging complication in the management of hemophilia patients. While inhibitors do not lead to more frequent bleeding, hemorrhages in affected patients are often more difficult to control. Inhibitor formation should be suspected in patients who are no longer responding to appropriate doses of factor concentrate or when the half-life of factor concentrated appears to be shortening in a particular patient. Inhibitors are detected using inhibitor assays (either the Bethesda assay or the Neimegen modification). In a German study as many as 51% of severe hemophilia A patients developed inhibitors.[22] However, an inhibitor incidence of 12% to 25% is more commonly reported in severe Factor VIII-deficient patients.[23] An analysis of patients with Factor VIII deficiency revealed that inhibitors were unlikely to develop in patients with missense mutations or small deletions (4% to 7%). In contrast, those with large deletions, nonsense mutations, or inversions involving intron 22 more frequently developed inhibitors to Factor VIII (34% to 38%).[24] Likewise, hemophilia B patients who develop inhibitors are more likely to have large deletions or nonsense mutations. An improved understanding of the structure and function of Factors VIII and IX will facilitate the development of less immunogenic factor replacement therapy and eventual gene therapy for hemophiliacs. Hemophilia B patients are less likely to develop inhibitors, with approximately 1% to 3% having high-titer inhibitor formation. During clinical trials of recombinant Factor VIII, 35% of previously untreated patients developed inhibitors, typically within 10 to 11 days of treatment. However, in one-third of the cases the inhibitor was found to be transient, resolving in weeks to months.[25] First- and second-degree relatives of high-titer inhibitor patients are four times more likely to develop inhibitors than other hemophilia patients, suggesting a familial predisposition. The greater likelihood of inhibitor development found in certain families may be a function of the particular gene mutation or other, yet undefined, shared inherited factors. Further, inhibitor formation has been demonstrated to be four times more likely in severe hemophilia patients than in mild hemophilia patients. This is particularly evident in patients whose factor mutations are the result of missense mutations, large deletions, or inversions resulting in the production of little or no structurally normal Factor VIII protein.[26]

Alloantibodies directed against Factor VIII or Factor IX are detected using in-vitro assays that measure the inhibitor's ability to block Factors VIII or IX procoagulant activity. In the commonly used Bethesda assay, patient plasma containing inhibitor is mixed and incubated at 37 C for 2 hours with a known quantity of Factor VIII derived from multidonor pooled plasma.[27] The reciprocal of the plasma dilution that neutralizes Factor VIII equals the number of inhibitor units per mL of plasma, or Bethesda units (BU). Low-titer inhibitors are conventionally defined as less than 10 BU. Patients with more than 10 BU are classified as having high-titer inhibitors; when re-exposed to Factor

VIII or Factor IX, they exhibit an increase in inhibitor titer (anamnestic response). These high-responder patients cannot be treated successfully with Factor VIII or Factor IX concentrates. Other means of measuring inhibitor levels include the in-vitro New Oxford method,[28] chromogenic assays, and nonfunctional immunoassays.[29]

Management of Bleeding in Patients with Inhibitors

Patients with low-titer inhibitors may achieve hemostasis when treated with higher doses of factor concentrates, are treated more frequently, or both. Often, low-titer inhibitors are transient and require no treatment for inhibitor eradication. On the other hand, patients with high-titer inhibitors typically present a more daunting challenge for hematologists.

Several medical treatments are available for the treatment of bleeding in hemophilia patients with high-titer inhibitors (see Table 15-5). In the past, prothrombin complex and activated prothrombin complex concentrates were the mainstay of therapy in affected patients. More recently, recombinant Factor VIIa (NovoSeven, NovoNordisk, Princeton, NJ) has found favor among hematologists as a safe and reliable treatment for bleeding in high-responder patients. Less common treatment modalities include porcine Factor VIII concentrate, immunosuppressives, immunoadsorption on protein A columns, and plasma exchange.

PCCs (Konyne-80, Bayer, and Proplex-T, Baxter), containing vitamin-K-dependent Factors II, VII, IX, and X, were developed and used in the early 1970s for treatment of hemophilia B and were found to be effective in some patients with high-titer inhibitors. These PCCs helped effect hemostasis by bypassing the need for Factor VIII or Factor IX in patients with high-titer inhibitors.[30] The aPCCs were developed to improve treatment for patients with inhibitors to Factors VIII or IX (Autoplex-T and FEIBA, Baxter) and were found to be more effective in controlled comparisons.[31] The recommended dose for PCCs and aPCCs is 50 to 75 U/kg per dose and may be repeated at 8-, 12-, or 24-hour intervals. Serious drawbacks to these concentrates include lack of a laboratory test to follow treatment efficacy and the risks of

Table 15-5. Comparison of Treatments for Bleeding Patients with High-Titer Inhibitors

Product	Dose	Advantages	Disadvantages
Recombinant Factor VIII	100 to 150 U/kg during ITT	Useful for ITT Measure with lab assay	No efficacy for acute bleeds Anamnestic response
Plasma-derived Factor VIII		Useful for ITT Measure with lab assay	Pooled plasma product Anamnestic response
PCCs (Konyne-80, Bayer and Proplex-T, Baxter) and aPCCs (Autoplex-T, Nabi and FEIBA VH, Bayer)	50-75 U/kg	Long half-life Activated form more efficacious	Pooled plasma products Risk of thrombosis Anamnesis Allergic response No lab assay available
Recombinant Factor VIIa (NovoSeven, NovoNordisk)	90 U/kg, repeat	No anamnesis No viral risk	Short half-life Expensive Risk of thrombosis(?)
Porcine Factor VIII (Hyate:C, Ipsen Biopharm)		No viral transmission Lab assay available	Cross-reactivity to Factor VIII antibodies Allergic reaction Porcine Factor VIII antibodies

ITT = immune tolerance therapy

venous thromboembolism, disseminated intravascular coagulation, and myocardial infarction, particularly in patients receiving therapy over an extended period of time.[32,33] In addition, these plasma-derived products carry a risk of viral transmission, although no reported cases of HIV or HCV seroconversion have been reported with the use of aPCCs.[34] FEIBA, with low levels of Factor VIII, has been associated with triggering anamnestic responses in as many as 31% of patients.[35]

Porcine Factor VIII (Hyate:C, Ipsen Biopharm, Wrexham, UK) is a less frequently used modality of therapy in hemophilia patients with inhibitors. Factor VIII derived from pig plasma will participate in the coagulation cascade. Patients with inhibitors possessing no cross-reactivity with porcine Factor VIII may be good candidates to receive Hyate:C. However, disadvantages of porcine Factor VIII include a risk of allergic reaction to animal product, thrombocytopenia, or the development of high-titer inhibitors specific for porcine Factor VIII.

Recombinant Factor VIIa (NovoSeven) is produced in CHO cells without the use of human or animal protein. Numerous reports have documented the efficacy of recombinant Factor IIa in high-titer inhibitor patients with both mild and serious bleeding.[36,37] Advantages of recombinant Factor VIIa include relative efficacy and no risk of viral transmission or anamnesis. Drawbacks to recombinant Factor VIIa include short half-life, expense, and lack of laboratory assay to follow efficacy.

Immune Tolerance Therapy in High-Titer Inhibitor Patients

Once a high-titer inhibitor has been diagnosed and confirmed in a hemophilia patient, immune tolerance therapy (ITT) should be initiated in a timely manner. ITT is regarded as the best means of eliminating high-titer inhibitors and is generally most successful if begun soon after diagnosis of a patient's high-responder status.[38] In general, ITT is most successful in patients with low inhibitor titers at initiation and those in whom the highest historical inhibitor titer <100 BU.[38]

Two widely cited ITT regimens for hemophilia A include the Bonn and Malmö protocols. Developed in the 1970s, the original Bonn protocol for patients with inhibitors >5 BU consisted of twice daily Factor VIII infusions (100 U/kg) to induce tolerance of Factor VIII and aPCC as prophylaxis against serious hemorrhage. Once the patient's inhibitor level falls below 1 BU, the Factor VIII dose is changed to 150 U/kg daily. While successful in most patients, the Bonn protocol may need to be continued for many years to achieve immune tolerance.[39] More recent modifications of the Bonn protocol include lower Factor VIII doses and the addition of corticosteroids.[40] Developed later, the Malmö regimen relies heavily on immunomodulation with cyclophosphamide, plasmapheresis with a sepharose and protein A column, and intravenous immunoglobulin. The immune suppression is targeted at preventing anamnestic responses and has proven to be highly successful, albeit, more toxic.[41]

Reports of ITT in hemophilia B patients are few, given that inhibitors rarely develop in such patients. In addition to an overall poorer response to ITT, hemophilia B patients have been found to experience a high rate of nephritic syndrome while undergoing immune tolerance.[42]

Diagnosis and Management of Newborn Hemophilia Patients

Several potential complications are unique to the newborn hemophilia patient. Ideally, women who are known carriers of hemophilia should be counseled regarding the risk of giving birth to a boy with hemophilia as well as about the implications of the disease including symptoms and treatment. Although not widely utilized, a number of techniques are available to diagnose hemophilia prenatally in pregnant women who are known or suspected carriers of the hemophilia trait. At 11 to 13 weeks of gestation chorionic villus sampling may be employed to determine the gender of the fetus and diagnose hemophilia by restriction fragment length polymorphism. In the second trimester, the diagnosis of hemophilia may be achieved using amniocentesis or sampling of umbilical cord blood. Likewise, ultrasonography in the second trimester may be used to determine the gender of the fetus and potentially rule out hemophilia.

All newborn males delivered to hemophilia trait carriers should have cord blood drawn for Factors VIII or IX assays. Neither Factors VIII nor IX cross the placenta; hence, the mother's factor levels will not affect the infant's plasma levels. Factor VIII production in the neonate is at adult levels (50% to 150%), allowing accurate diagnosis of hemophilia A in the newborn. Because vitamin-K-dependent clotting factors do not reach normal adult levels until postnatal day 90, the accurate diagnosis of hemophilia B may not be made easily in the neonatal period. Infants with very low Factor IX levels in the severely affected range may have moderate to mild levels by 6 months of age.

The delivery of infants with known or suspected hemophilia should be performed with the utmost caution. The risk of ICH in newborns with hemophilia appears to be increased in vacuum extraction and forceps deliveries, but is not eliminated by caesarean section. In a series of 117 hemophilia patients, Ljung reported the incidence of bleeding in 9 of 87 vaginal deliveries, 11 of 17 vaginal extractions, and 3 of 13 caesarean sections.[43]

A recent review of reported cases of bleeding in newborns with Factor VIII or IX deficiency revealed a variety of bleeding presentations. Intracranial hemorrhage was detected in 27% of patients, 13% had subgaleal or cephalohematoma, 16% had persistent puncture site bleeding, and 30% demonstrated bleeding at circumcision.[44]

Suspected or documented ICH should be treated with 100% correction of factor concentrate. If a diagnosis of hemophilia has been confirmed, recombinant factor or highly purified plasma-derived factor is the treatment of choice. In patients without a specific diagnosis, Fresh Frozen Plasma may be used because it contains both Factor VIII and Factor IX. Such patients with ICH are typically treated for a 2-week period. Other precautions for patients born to hemophilia carriers or who are otherwise suspected of Factors VIII or IX deficiency include avoidance of circumcision in the neonatal period and perhaps altogether. However, many patients are not suspected of having hemophilia until after prolonged postoperative bleeding. Fibrin sealant has reduced hospitalization and the need for factor concentrates following certain procedures.[45] General recommendations for preventing hemorrhage in newborns with hemophilia include avoiding venipuncture and intramuscular injections, if possible. Accordingly, hepatitis B vaccinations may be given subcutaneously and oral formulations of vitamin K may also be used in lieu of intramuscular injections. If venipuncture or intramuscular injections are required, firm pressure should be applied to the site for 5 minutes following the procedure.

von Willebrand Disease

von Willebrand disease typically manifests with mucocutaneous bleeding, menorrhagia, and perioperative or posttraumatic hemorrhage. One to two percent of the general population is affected by quantitative or qualitative vWF protein defects. vWF is a large multimeric protein that is produced by endothelial cells and megakaryocytes and is stored in Weibel-Palade bodies in endothelial cells and α-granules in platelets. vWF protein functions by binding platelets to the surface of damaged vascular endothelium. vWD may result from a variety of genetic defects caused by decreased or absent vWF or production of defective vWF protein. The protein also binds and stabilizes Factor VIII from proteolytic degradation. vWF circulates in the blood as multimers that are as large as 20 million daltons. Such large multimers are particularly adept at hemostasis as a result of numerous binding sites and the volume of the molecule.

von Willebrand Disease Variants

The most common form of vWD, the type 1 variant, affects 80% of all vWF patients (see Table 15-6). Such patients possess a heterozygous deficiency of vWF, producing vWF:Ag and R:Co between 20 and 40 units/dL. Type 1 vWD patients manifest bleeding symptoms such as epistaxis or menorrhagia, or bleed after trauma, surgery, or dental extractions. DDAVP is the best mode of therapy for most such situations, once a patient is documented to be a responder. Patients should have a three- to sixfold rise in R:Co after DDAVP administration, either intravenous

Table 15-6. Variants of von Willebrand Disease

Type (incidence)	Defect	Diagnosis	Treatment
1 (80%)	Decreased production of vWF	Decreased vWF:Ag, R:Co, Factor VIII; normal multimers	DDAVP or plasma-derived Factor VIII/vWF
2A (10-12%)	Abnormally small multimers	Decreased vWF:Ag and R:Co; small multimers; decreased RIPA	Plasma-derived Factor VIII/vWF
2B (3-5%)	vWF spontaneously agglutinates platelets	Increased RIPA-LD, possible decrease in vWF:Ag and R:Co; abnormal multimers	Plasma-derived Factor VIII/vWF
2N (1-2%)	Abnormal Factor VIII binding site	Decreased vWF:Ag, R:Co, and Factor VIII	Plasma-derived Factor VIII/vWF
2M (1-2%)	Abnormal binding site for GPIb	Decreased vWF:Ag and R:Co	Plasma-derived Factor VIII/vWF
Platelet-type (pseudo) von Willebrand disease	Absence of platelet GPIb receptor	Decreased vWF:Ag and R:Co; abnormal multimers	Platelet transfusion
3 (1-3%)	Absence of vWF	Low or absent vWF:Ag, R:Co, and Factor VIII	Plasma-derived Factor VIII/vWF

(0.3 μg/kg) or nasal (2 puffs, 300 μg). In addition, patients may benefit from α-aminocaproic acid or tranexamic acid (antifibrinolytic therapies to stabilize clot formation). For major surgery, plasma-derived Factor VIII containing vWF (Humate-P and Alphanate) may be advised, particularly in patients in whom DDAVP gives only a marginal response.

Type 3 vWD (severe vWD) is marked by low or unmeasurable levels of vWF and Factor VIII. Such patients typically respond poorly to DDAVP therapy and require plasma-derived Factor VIII/vWF to control bleeding. The disease may result from homozygous (autosomal recessive) mutations or compound heterozygous defects. Homozygous patients may experience severe bleeding, even spontaneous hemarthrosis.

Type 2A vWD is marked by abnormally small vWF multimers that are degraded rapidly. Patients typically respond poorly or only transiently to DDAVP, necessitating the use of plasma-derived Factor VIII/vWF for bleeding episodes. On the other hand, type 2B vWD results from abnormal multimers that spontaneously bind to platelets, leading to clearance of the largest high molecular weight multimers and mild thrombocytopenia. The diagnosis of type 2B vWD is aided by the finding of increased ristocetin-induced platelet aggregation to low doses of ristocetin (RIPA-LD). Although some reports suggest that DDAVP may be helpful in patients with type 2B disease, plasma-derived Factor VIII/vWF is generally the treatment of choice. While varying degrees of thrombocytopenia may coexist with type 2B vWD, therapy should focus upon raising vWF levels to the normal range. Type 2N vWD stems from the inability of vWF to bind and stabilize Factor VIII. This diagnosis should be considered when a deficiency of Factor VIII is out of proportion with the low level of vWF or when Factor VIII half-life is unexpectedly short after the administration of Factor VIII concentrate. Type 2M vWD results from lack of glycoprotein (GP) Ib binding sites on the vWF, leading to a decreased agglutination in response to ristocetin in vitro. The diagnosis of type 2M disease should be suspected in the setting of disproportionately low R:Co and vWF:Ag.

Platelet-type pseudo von Willebrand disease results from a defect in the platelet GPIb receptor, resulting in loss of high-molecular-weight multimers and low vWF levels. While this variant resembles type 2B, from both a phenotypic and laboratory perspective, the treatment for platelet-type pseudo von Willebrand disease is platelet transfusion rather than infusion of plasma-derived vWF.

Treatment of Bleeding in vWD Patients

Type 1 vWD patients (and selected type 2 patients) who have demonstrated a therapeutic increase in Factor VIII and vWF levels in response to DDAVP may receive a dose of 0.3 μg/kg intravenously over 20 to 30 minutes in response to (or to prevent) mild clinical bleeding. The Stimate formulation (Aventis Behring, King of Prussia, PA) of intranasal DDAVP may also be used, one spray (150 μg) in one nostril if the patient weighs <50 kg or one spray in each nostril (300 μg) if the patient weighs >50 kg. Patients with type 3 disease or those who are unresponsive to DDAVP should receive either Humate-P or Alphanate. Dosing recommendations are different for these products and are available on the package insert.

References

1. Cahill MR, Colvin BT. Haemophilia. Postgrad Med J 1997;73:201-6.
2. Lederman MM, Scillian JJ, Jones PK, Schacter B. Impaired cell-mediated immunity in patients with classic hemophilia. N Engl J Med 1983;308: 79-83.
3. Troisi CL, Hollinger FB, Hoots WK, et al. A multicenter study of viral hepatitis in a United States hemophilic population. Blood 1993;81:412-18.
4. Montgomery RR, Gill JC, Scott JP. Hemophilia and von Willebrand disease. In: Nathan DG, Orkin SH, Oski FA, Ginsburg D, eds. Nathan and Oski's hematology of infancy and childhood, 5th ed. Philadelphia, PA: WB Saunders, 1998:1631-59.
5. Giannelli F, Green PM. The molecular basis of haemophilia A and B. Baillieres Clin Haematol 1996;9:211-28.
6. Mannucci PM, Tuddenham EG. The hemophilias—from royal genes to gene therapy. N Engl J Med 2001;344(23):1773-9.
7. Lakich D, Kazazian HH Jr, Antonarakis SE, Gitschier J. Inversions disrupting the factor VIII gene are a common cause of severe haemophilia A. Nat Genet 1993;5:236-41.
8. Baehner RL. Hemophilia in the first year of life. N Engl J Med 1966; 275:424-528.

9. Centers for Disease Control and Prevention. Hepatitis A among persons with hemophilia who received clotting factor concentrate—United States, September-December 1995. MMWR Morb Mortal Wkly Rep 1996; 45(2):29-32.
10. Chudy M, Budek I, Keller-Stanislawski B, et al. A new cluster of hepatitis A infection in hemophiliacs traced to a contaminated plasma pool. J Med Virol 1999;57:91-9.
11. Gaboulaud V, Parquet A, Tahiri C, et al. Prevalence of IgG antibodies to human parvovirus B19 in haemophilia children treated with recombinant factor (F)VIII only or with at least one plasma-derived FVIII or FIX concentrate: Results from the French haemophilia cohort. Br J Haematol 2002;116:383-9.
12. Klein R, Dumble LJ. Transmission of Creutzfeldt-Jakob disease by blood transfusion. Lancet 1993;341:768.
13. Ludlam CA. New-variant Creutzfeldt-Jakob disease and treatment of haemophilia. Executive Committee of the UKHCDO. United Kingdom Haemophilia Centre Directors' Organisation (letter). Lancet 1997;350: 1704.
14. Courter SG, Bedrosian CL. Clinical evaluation of B-domain deleted recombinant factor VIII in previously untreated patients. Semin Hematol 2001;38:52-9.
15. Abshire TC, Brackmann HH, Scharrer I, et al. Sucrose formulated recombinant human antihemophilic factor VIII is safe and efficacious for treatment of hemophilia A in home therapy—International Kogenate-FS Study Group. Thromb Haemost 2000;83:811-16.
16. Yoshioka A, Shima M, Fukutake K, et al. Safety and efficacy of a new recombinant FVIII formulated with sucrose (rFVIII-FS) in patients with haemophilia A: A long-term, multicentre clinical study in Japan. Haemophilia 2001;7:242-9.
17. Rodeghiero F, Castaman G, Di Bona E, Ruggeri M. Consistency of responses to repeated DDAVP infusions in patients with von Willebrand's disease and hemophilia A. Blood 1989;74:1997-2000.
18. Lusher J. Treatment of congenital coagulopathies. In: Mintz P, ed. Transfusion therapy: Clinical principles and practice. AABB Press, Bethesda, MD: 1999:97-128.
19. Nilsson IM, Berntorp E, Lofqvist T, Pettersson H. Twenty-five years' experience of prophylactic treatment in severe haemophilia A and B. J Intern Med 1992;232:25-32.
20. Journeycake JM, Quinn CT, Miller KL, et al. Catheter-related deep venous thrombosis in children with hemophilia. Blood 2001;98:1727-31.
21. Vidler V, Richards M, Vora A. Central venous catheter-associated thrombosis in severe haemophilia. Br J Haematol 1999;104:461-4.
22. Ehrenforth S, Kreuz W, Scharrer I, et al. Incidence of development of factor VIII and factor IX inhibitors in haemophiliacs. Lancet 1992;339: 594-8.

23. Addiego J, Kasper C, Abildgaard C, et al. Frequency of inhibitor development in haemophiliacs treated with low-purity factor VIII. Lancet 1993;342:462-4.
24. Schwaab R, Brackmann HH, Meyer C, et al. Haemophilia A: Mutation type determines risk of inhibitor formation. Thromb Haemost 1995;74: 1402-6.
25. Lusher JM, Arkin S, Abildgaard CF, Schwartz RS. Recombinant factor VIII for the treatment of previously untreated patients with hemophilia A. Safety, efficacy, and development of inhibitors. Kogenate Previously Untreated Patient Study Group. N Engl J Med 1993;328:453-9.
26. Antonarakis SE, Rossiter JP, Young M, et al. Factor VIII gene inversions in severe hemophilia A: Results of an international consortium study. Blood 1995;86:2206-12.
27. Kasper CK, Aronson D, Counts R, et al. Proceedings: A more uniform measurement of factor VIII inhibitors. Thromb Diath Haemorrh 1975;34:612.
28. Rizza CR, Biggs R. The treatment of patients who have factor VIII antibodies. Br J Haematol 1973;24:65-82.
29. Scandella D, Mattingly M, de Graaf S, Fulcher CA. Localization of epitopes for human factor VIII inhibitor antibodies by immunoblotting and antibody neutralization. Blood 1989;74:1618-26.
30. Kelly P, Penner JA. Antihemophilic factor inhibitors. Management with prothrombin complex concentrates. JAMA 1976;236:2061-4.
31. Sjamsoedin LH, Mauser-Bunschoten L, van Geijlswijk EP, et al. The effect of activated prothrombin-complex concentrate (FEIBA) on joint and muscle bleeding in patients with hemophilia A and antibodies to factor VIII. A double-blind clinical trial. N Engl J Med 1981;305:717-21.
32. Chavin SI, Siegel DM, Rocco TA Jr, Olson JP. Acute myocardial infarction during treatment with an activated prothrombin complex concentrate in a patient with factor VIII deficiency and a factor VIII inhibitor. Am J Med 1988;85:245-9.
33. Lusher JM. Use of prothrombin complex concentrates in management of bleeding in hemophiliacs with inhibitors—benefits and limitations. Semin Hematol 1994;31:49-52.
34. Kulkarni R, Aledort LM, Berntorp E, et al. Therapeutic choices for patients with hemophilia and high-titer inhibitors. Am J Hematol 2001;67: 240-6.
35. Negrier C, Goudemand J, Sultan Y, et al. Multicenter retrospective study on the utilization of FEIBA in France in patients with factor VIII and factor IX inhibitors. French FEIBA Study Group. Factor Eight Bypassing Activity. Thromb Haemost 1997;77:1113-19.
36. Lusher J, Ingerslev J, Roberts H, Hedner U. Clinical experience with recombinant factor VIIa. Blood Coagul Fibrinolysis 1998;9:119-28.
37. Santagostino E, Gringeri A, Mannucci PM. Home treatment with recombinant activated factor VII in patients with factor VIII inhibitors: The advantages of early intervention. Br J Haematol 1999;104:22-6.

38. Mariani G, Scheibel E, Nogao T, et al. Immune tolerance as treatment of alloantibodies to factor VIII in hemophilia. The International Registry of Immune Tolerance Protocols. Semin Hematol 1994;31(Suppl 4):62-4.
39. Brackmann H, Oldenburg J, Schwaab R. Immune tolerance for the treatment of factor VIII inhibitors—20 years [of] Bonn protocol. Vox Sang 1996;70(Suppl 1):30-5.
40. Ewing NP, Sanders NL, Dietrich SL, Kasper CK. Induction of immune tolerance to factor VIII in hemophiliacs with inhibitors. JAMA 1988;259:65-8.
41. Nilsson IM, Berntorp E, Zettervall O. Induction of immune tolerance in patients with hemophilia and antibodies to factor VIII by combined treatment with intravenous IgG, cyclophosphamide, and factor VIII. N Engl J Med 1988;318:947-50.
42. Warrier I. Management of haemophilia B patients with inhibitors and anaphylaxis. Haemophilia 1998;4:574-6.
43. Ljung R. Genetic diagnosis of hemophilia A. Pediatr Hematol Oncol 1994;11:9-11.
44. Kulkarni R, Lusher J. Perinatal management of newborns with haemophilia. Br J Haematol 2001;112:264-74.
45. Kavakli K. Fibrin glue and clinical impact on haemophilia care. Haemophilia 1999;5:392-6.

In: Herman JH, Manno CS, eds.
Pediatric Transfusion Therapy
Bethesda, MD: AABB Press, 2002

16

Childhood Idiopathic Thrombocytopenic Purpura

NORMA B. LERNER, MD

PEDIATRIC IDIOPATHIC OR immune thrombocytopenic purpura (ITP) is a common, usually self-limited, hemorrhagic disorder characterized by isolated thrombocytopenia in an otherwise healthy child, most often between the ages of 2 and 10 years.[1,2] The incidence is approximately 4 per 100,000 children per year and the onset often follows a viral infection or, rarely, a live-virus immunization.[1-3] Most children have a relatively uncomplicated clinical presentation, characterized by petechiae, bruising, and, less commonly, mucosal bleeding.[4] The thrombocytopenia usually resolves within 6 months; however, a minority of patients

Norma B. Lerner, MD, Clinical Associate Professor of Pediatrics, Pediatric Hematology/Oncology, University of Rochester School of Medicine and Dentistry, Galisano Children's Hospital at Strong, Rochester, New York

may go on to have a chronic course.[1] There has been and continues to be a great deal of controversy regarding the appropriate evaluation and management of this disorder.

Pathophysiology

ITP results from platelet antigen-specific autoantibodies. Antibody of primarily the immunoglobulin G (IgG) class, and more rarely the IgM class, coats the platelet, permitting macrophage Fc-receptor binding and ultimately causing the platelet's demise.[5] Van Leeuwen et al[6] were the first investigators to specifically identify platelet membrane glycoprotein IIb/IIIa (GPIIb/IIIa) as the target antigen in adult chronic ITP. A later study revealed that IgG-F(ab')$_2$ fragments (purified from sera derived from patients with chronic and acute ITP) bound to normal platelet membranes. The fragments did not bind to platelet membranes derived from patients with Glanzmann's thrombasthenia, a disorder characterized by the absence of GPIIb/IIIa.[7] Autoantibodies to platelet antigens have been identified in ITP patients' sera and platelet eluates by immunoblot, immunobead, and MAIPA techniques.[8-10] Autoantibodies are most often identified against GPIIb/IIIa (also known as $\alpha II_b \beta_3$ integrin or CD41/CD61), although other platelet epitopes have been targeted.[11-13] Platelet-specific antibodies have been detected in 27% to 68% of children and with less frequency in the acute, as opposed to the chronic, cases.[11]

Few investigations have been directed at elucidating the cellular immune mechanisms that are responsible for autoantibody production.[12] It is thought that autoreactive B lymphocytes secrete platelet antibodies in ITP. The production of antibody is felt to be regulated by cellular and soluble mechanisms primarily involving T lymphocytes.[13] A number of T helper lymphocyte immunoregulatory defects have been described, including abnormal responses to mitogens and platelets, depressed autologous mixed lymphocyte reactions, and abnormal T-cell subpopulations.[13-15] It has been found that GPIIb/IIIa is one of the major target antigens recognized by platelet reactive CD4+ T cells in patients with ITP. These GPIIb/IIIa-reactive CD4+ T cells appear to provide helper activity to promote the production of platelet-binding GPIIb/IIIa antibodies, implying that these autoreactive T cells are involved in the production of platelet autoantibodies in patients with ITP.[16,17] The serum cytokine pattern identified in patients with ITP (increased levels of Interleukin (IL)-2 and IL-11 and interferon-gamma, decreased levels of IL-4, and normal levels of thrombopoietin) is compatible with a Th 1 kind of T-helper cell cytokine response and a down-regulated type Th 2 response.[18]

Diagnosis

Clinical Presentation

Children with acute ITP typically present with an abrupt onset of bruising and petechiae often in an atomic locations not exposed to trauma. Mucosal bleeding is observed in approximately one third of cases.[19] Patients have otherwise normal physical findings. In particular, there is no evidence of hepatosplenomegaly, lymphadenopathy, jaundice, or pallor.[1,19] Children with chronic ITP often have a more insidious onset of symptoms and tend to be older than those with acute ITP.[1,19]

Laboratory Studies

The complete blood count (CBC) and peripheral blood smear frequently reveal a platelet count that is less than 20,000/μL.[3] Children who have a more subtle presentation and often go on to have a more chronic course may have somewhat higher platelet counts (>30,000/μL).[1] The hemoglobin will be normal except in circumstances where substantial bleeding has occurred or there is an associated immune hemolytic anemia (Evans syndrome). The red cell indices, white cell count, and differential will also be normal. A review of the peripheral smear often shows that the few platelets present are large in size. The erythrocyte and leukocyte morphologies are normal and there is no evidence of microangiopathy. The prothrombin time and partial thromboplastin time are also normal in ITP and, as would be expected, the bleeding time is generally prolonged. When suspected, tests for associated infections such as Epstein-Barr virus should be pursued.

Platelet-associated antibody studies, while highly sensitive (90%), are of limited diagnostic benefit because of their lack of specificity (30%).[20] Reticulated platelets, representing the youngest platelets in the circulation, can be measured by analyzing RNA content.[21] Increased numbers of reticulated platelets are detected in ITP and the test has been found to have a strong positive predictive value.[21,22] The maximum peak of the platelet volume distribution curve, as measured by the Coulter Counter Max M (Beckman-Coulter, Fullerton, CA) has also proved useful when there is a need to distinguish ITP from other thrombocytopenic disorders.[23]

There is much difference of opinion among pediatric hematologists regarding whether it is necessary to perform a marrow aspiration when a diagnosis of ITP is being considered. Most hematologists will agree that if there is diagnostic doubt or if lymphadenopathy, hepatosplenomegaly, or another CBC abnormality is noted, a marrow examination is in order.[1,2] Some investigators see no reason to perform a marrow aspiration in the setting of typical ITP, no matter what the planned therapy. However, both an audit in the United Kingdom and a survey in the United States revealed that most practitioners will order a marrow examination prior to giving corticosteroids.[24-26] This approach is likely a result of the doctor's concern that he or she might otherwise jeopardize a child's long-term survival should that child indeed have leukemia. The risk of missing the diagnosis of leukemia in children with typical hematologic features of ITP has been calculated to be less than 1%.[27] Nonetheless, respondents to a national audit reported that they had seen children ultimately diagnosed with acute leukemia who had received steroids for presumed ITP.[25]

Children with ITP of more than 6 months' duration often have an associated autoimmune disease or immunodeficient state. A more extensive workup should be pursued in this setting. The patient should be evaluated for immunoglobulin deficiency and human immunodeficiency virus (HIV). Tests for antiphospholipid syndrome, systemic lupus erythematosus (SLE), and, where indicated, autoimmune thyroid disease, should also be obtained.

Differential Diagnosis

As noted previously, ITP is characterized by isolated thrombocytopenia with bruising and perhaps mucosal bleeding as the only clinical manifestations. With the possible exception of drug-induced thrombocytopenia, disorders considered in the differential diagnosis would be associated with additional clinical or laboratory abnormalities. In these circumstances, the physician should consider immune platelet destruction secondary to medications or HIV infection as well as non-immune destruction as a result of hemolytic uremic syndrome, thrombotic thrombocytopenic purpura, disseminated intravascular coagulation, or type II von Willebrand disease. Decreased platelet production can be seen in the setting of medication use, congenital abnormalities such as Fanconi anemia or thrombocytopenia absent radii syndrome, or acquired states such as leukemia, aplastic anemia, and nutritional deficiencies of B12 or folate. Certain qualitative platelet disorders are sometimes associated with thrombocytopenia as well. Hypersplenism and Kasabach-Merritt syndrome should also be considered. Pseudothrombocytopenia, or an artifactually low platelet count secondary to platelet clumping in tubes containing EDTA, should also be kept in mind, particularly when a low platelet count is incidentally noted and is not associated with a clinical history of bruising.

Treatment

There are strong differences of opinion regarding treatment for children with ITP who do not have significant hemorrhage.[1] ITP-associated intracranial hemorrhage (ICH) is an extremely rare event, but a life-threatening one. The avoidance of ICH appears to be the main reason why some hematologists have advocated prophylactic treatment for clinically well children with severe thrombocytopenia. The incidence of ICH in the first week is about 0.1% to 0.2% but rises to about 1% in those with platelet counts less than 20,000/μL, 6 to 12 months after diagnosis.[2] ICH is thus so rare that about 10,000 children would need to be prospectively treated to prove or disprove a treatment's preventive efficacy.[3,25] Lilleyman[3] reviewed all cases of ICH in children with ITP and found 14 cases over 20 years. Thirteen of 14 children had <10,000/µL platelets and eight children had additional risks. Only 1 of 14 children had definitely not received treatment, in five the treatment history was unclear, and eight had been treated with corticosteroids or IVIG.[3] In addition to the lack of evidence that treatment has an impact upon the development of ICH, there are also no data to suggest that treatment protects against any major bleeding or ultimately affects the evolution to chronic ITP.[28]

There are currently two sets of guidelines in the English literature regarding the management of acute ITP in childhood. The British Haematology Group[4] suggests that for children presenting with bruising only and no mucosal bleeding, no treatment is perfectly reasonable, regardless of the platelet count. When treatment is pursued, the authors recommend low doses of prednisolone, not to exceed 2 mg/kg/day, in view of "troublesome side effects." IVIG is recommended only 1) for emergency treatment of patients who are refractory to steroids or 2) to cover essential surgeries.[4] The report of the American Society of Hematology[29] recommends that all children with platelet counts <20,000/µL and significant mucous membrane bleeding, and those with counts <10,000/µL and minor purpura, should be treated with regimens of IVIG or glucocorticoids.[29] Not only are there discrepancies between the two sets of guidelines, but audits performed subsequent to their creation reveal that practitioners often fail to follow the guidelines.[25,26] The American recommendations in particular, although they "rely largely on opinion" that was later described as "polarized," may have put pressure on physicians to treat their patients.[29-31]

Patients Without Serious Bleeding

Current approaches to patients with ITP who do not have major hemorrhage include observation or therapy with corticosteroids, IVIG, or anti-D immune globulin.

Observation

Over the years, several investigators have strongly advocated approaching acute childhood ITP with observation only.[32] This tactic includes education about the nature of the disease as well as reassurance regarding its usual course. The child's activities, as well as the use of medications such as nonsteroidal anti-inflammatories or aspirin-containing compounds, are limited. The children make regularly scheduled visits to their pediatrician, CBCs are regularly performed, and parents are advised to contact medical personnel with any bleeding episodes, head trauma, or headache. A recent retrospective study of children with acute ITP examined outcomes in 55 patients for whom this management approach was predominantly used. Only those children with bleeding from the entire gingiva or with epistaxis requiring tamponade were treated with prednisone at 2 mg/kg/day for 3 days. Despite the fact that 37 of 55 patients had initial platelet counts of <10,000/μL and 10 of these had active mucosal bleeding, no life-threatening bleeding occurred and there were no deaths.[31]

Corticosteroids

Corticosteroids interfere with macrophage binding and clearance of antibody-coated platelets. They also decrease the production of platelet antibodies and may increase capillary endothelial stability.[33-35] Over the years, a number of regimens have been tested in children with ITP, but these approaches have never been submitted to a comparative randomized trial. Table 16-1 summarizes regimens of prednisone, prednisolone, or methylprednisolone that have been used in a variety of published studies.[33,36-46] In practice, prednisone is often given in a dose of 1-2 mg/kg/day for up to 2 weeks and then tapered. A pilot study revealed that a shorter course at higher dose (4 mg/kg/day × 4 days) may raise the count as quickly as IVIG. While inexpensive, particularly when compared with other treatment modalities, corticosteroids are associated with a number of side effects including

Table 16-1. Corticosteroid Doses in Childhood ITP

Study	Corticosteroid	Dosage
Bellucci et al[36]	Prednisone/prednisolone (given orally)	0.25 mg/kg/day or 1 mg/kg/day × 3 weeks then taper over 4th week
Buchanan and Holtkamp[33] Ozsoylu et al[37]	Prednisone (given orally)	2 mg/kg/day × 2 weeks ± taper over 3rd week
Suarez et al[38]	Prednisone (given orally)	4-8 mg/kg/day × 3 days then taper
Carcao et al[39] Blanchette et al[40,41]	Prednisone (given orally)	4 mg/kg/day × 4 days; 4 mg/kg/day × 7 days then taper over 2 weeks
Imbach et al[42] Sartorius et al[43]	Prednisone/prednisolone (given orally)	60 mg/m^2/day × 21 days
Albayrak et al[44]	Methylprednisolone (given orally)	30 mg/kg/day or 50 mg/kg/day × 7 days
Rosthoj et al[45] Van Hoff and Ritchy[46] Ozsoylu et al[37]	Methylprednisolone (given intravenously)	30 mg/kg/day × 2 days; 30 mg/kg/day × 3 days; 30 mg/kg/day × 3 days, then 20 mg/kg/day × 4 days, then 10 mg, 5 mg, 2 mg, and 1 mg/kg/day × 1 week each

weight gain, mood swings, sleep disturbance, hypertension, and hyperglycemia.

Intravenous Immunoglobulin

IVIG competitively inhibits Fc receptors on mononuclear phagocytes and reduces their number and affinity.[47-50] These effects serve to protect antibody-coated platelets from being destroyed.[42,51] Depressed haptoglobin levels during IVIG therapy have suggested a role for preferential sequestration of immunoglobulin-coated red cells, producing competitive inhibition of the macrophage binding of platelets.[52] IVIG also modulates platelet antibody production and alters T-cell subsets, T-cell proliferation, and B-cell function.[53-56]

Various regimens appear to be comparably effective (Table 16-2); however, lower doses are associated with fewer side effects and are obviously less expensive.[40-42,44,45,47,57-60] When compared to observation, standard dose prednisone, and anti-D immune globulin, IVIG produces the most rapid rise in platelet count.[40-42] Prednisone at 4 mg/kg/day for 4 days may, however, be comparable in this regard.[39]

IVIG has been associated with complications such as headache, vomiting, and fever in up to 75% of children.[2] Less commonly, IVIG has precipitated aseptic meningitis and transient

Table 16-2. IVIG Doses in Childhood ITP

Study	Dose of IVIG
Imbach et al[42,47,57]	0.4 g/kg/day × 5 days
Albayrak et al[44]	0.5 g/kg/day × 5 days
Blanchette et al[40,41] Rosthoj et al[45]	1 g/kg/day × 2 days
Blanchette et al[41]	0.8 g/kg × 1 day
Rosthoj et al[45,58] Tarantino et al[59]	0.8-1 g/kg × 1-2 days
Warrier et al[60]	250 mg, 400 mg, 500 mg, or 1 g/kg/day × 2 days

hemiplegia.[61-63] Symptoms associated with these side effects are of particular concern in patients with very low platelet counts and often initiate the pursuit of expensive studies.[61] Neurologic complications can be diminished by treating with prednisone at 2 mg/kg/day for 5 days.[64] This approach, however, may add corticosteroid side effects and raise issues regarding the need for marrow aspiration. It must always be kept in mind that while carefully prepared, IVIG is a pooled blood product and viral infection is always a risk. To date there have been no reports of HIV transmission; however, hepatitis C was found to be transmitted in Gammagard preparations (Baxter Healthcare Corporation, Deerfield, IL) given during 1993-1994.[65]

Anti-D Immune Globulin

Anti-D is a polyclonal antiserum that is directed against the D antigen on erythrocytes. It is believed that the preparation coats the patient's D-positive erythrocytes and, by diverting the reticuloendothelial system to these cells, diminishes platelet destruction.[59] Anti-D has been found to have no demonstrable effect upon lymphocyte numbers or function.[51]

Table 16-3 presents a summary of studies regarding anti-D dosing.[41,59,66,67] One manufacturer (Cangene Corporation, Winnepeg, Canada) currently recommends 50 μg/kg. Anti-D is effective only in those patients who are D-positive and have a functioning spleen.[1] In the only prospective, comparative study, anti-D was associated with a somewhat slower initial platelet re-

Table 16-3. Anti-D Doses in Childhood ITP

Study	Dose of Anti-D
Blanchette et al[41]	25 μg/kg/day × 2 days
Bussel et al[66]	10 μg/kg/day × 1 day then 20 μg/kg/day; 25 μg/kg/day × 1 day, repeat day 3 and day 4 as needed
Tarantino et al[59]	About 45-50 μg/kg/day × 1 day
Frieberg and Mauger[67]	16-127 μg/kg (median = 61 μg/kg)

sponse than was IVIG or prednisone.[41] The preparation is given as a rapid single infusion which is an advantage over other treatment modalities.[59] While anti-D was initially felt to have few side effects, recent reports of significant hemolysis necessitating transfusion are of obvious concern.[68,69] Furthermore, the risk of viral transmission must also be considered with this preparation.

Treatment Comparisons

Table 16-4 presents six investigations that compared particular ITP treatments.[40-42,44,45,59] All but one were randomized prospective studies. The platelet count was used as the measure of efficacy. Treatment doses varied from study to study and firm conclusions regarding relative efficacy are difficult to make with assurance. Overall, the studies suggested that IVIG and higher doses of prednisone produced faster platelet responses than anti-D at 20 µg/kg/day for 2 days. Another investigation, however, found comparably fast responses with a 45-50 µg/kg/day anti-D regimen. The comparative incidence of chronic ITP or ICH was not studied.

Patients With Serious Bleeding

For the small minority of patients with ITP who experience major hemorrhage, local interventions to control bleeding as well as therapies aimed at quickly increasing the platelet count are recommended. Intravenous corticosteroids (methylprednisolone 30 mg/kg/day for 3 days) and IVIG have been advised, as has the possible use of concomitant platelet transfusion in larger than normal doses.[2,4,28,29] Notably, because ITP is a consumptive platelet disorder, platelet transfusion is recommended only in the context of life-threatening bleeding and is not to be used in other instances of ITP.[2] If these approaches fail, emergency splenectomy may be attempted.

Chronic ITP

While chronic disease tends to be the norm in adults, thrombocytopenia persists for more than 6 months in only 15% to 20% of children with ITP.[70] These children are usually older,

Table 16-4. Comparative Studies of ITP Treatment in Children

Study*	Corticosteroid	IVIG	Anti-D	Results
Imbach et al[42]	Prednisone 60 mg/m^2 × 21 days (given orally)	0.4 g/kg/day × 5 days		Comparable for rapid responders; others responded better if given IVIG
Blanchette et al[40]	Prednisone 4 mg/kg/day × 7 days then taper over 2 weeks (given orally)	1.0 g/kg/day × 2 days		No difference in time to achieve platelet count of >20,000/µL
Albayrak et al[44]	Methylprednisolone 30 mg or 50 mg/kg/day (given orally)	0.5 g/kg/day × 5 days		No difference in platelet response
Blanchette et al[41]	Prednisone 4 mg/kg/day × 7 days then taper over 2 weeks (given orally)	1.0 g/kg/day × 2 days; 0.8 mg/kg/day × 1 day	25 µg/kg/day × 2 days	IVIG and prednisone were significantly faster than anti-D in time to achieve platelet count of >20,000/µL
Rosthoj et al[45]	Methylprednisolone 30 mg/kg × 2 days (given intravenously)	1.0 g/kg/day × 2 days		IVIG induced higher platelet counts after 72 hours
Tarantino et al[59]		0.8-1.0 g/kg/days × 1-2 days	45-50 µg/kg/day × 1 day (1 patient treated × 2 days)	No difference in time to achieve platelet count >20,000/µL

*All studies were randomized and prospective except for Tarantino et al,[59] which was a retrospective study.

and their problem is often associated with an underlying disease such as SLE. For those children without significant bleeding, careful observation and reasonable restriction of activities may well be the most rational approach, given the potentially toxic and/or unproven therapies currently available.[2] Clearly, where observation is used, treatment should be pursued in the context of surgery or accidents. Therapeutic modalities described for acute disease may also be given on a chronic basis. Both corticosteroids and IVIG generally fail to alter the course of the disease once it becomes chronic or refractory to therapy and side effects may become more burdensome over time.[71,72] Pulsed high-dose dexamethasone in particular was tested in children after it was found to be remarkably effective in 10 adult patients with chronic ITP.[73] Unfortunately, only a minority of patients with childhood ITP achieved durable remission with this regimen.[74-77] While also not curative, repeated doses of anti-D may maintain reasonable platelet counts. Its long-term use, however, is compromised by its cost as well as by the potential for hemolysis.[70]

Adults with chronic, refractory ITP are often treated with splenectomy. This approach, even for symptomatic children, is not as readily pursued in pediatric populations. The risk of postsplenectomy sepsis has historically been of paramount concern; however, regular penicillin prophylaxis as well as appropriate immunizations appear to have largely prevented this complication. Splenectomy is also less popular in pediatric populations because of this group's greater likelihood of late remission. A predicted spontaneous remission rate of 61% has been documented after 15 years.[78] Finally, it has been suggested that those patients who respond poorly to corticosteroids or IVIG may be the least likely to respond to splenectomy.[79,80] Unfortunately, these are frequently the very children for whom therapy is sought. A recent retrospective review of 38 evaluable children who underwent elective splenectomy for ITP found laparoscopic or open procedures to be safe and effective for most children. There were no cases of postsplenectomy sepsis and a median 2.1 year follow-up revealed normal platelet counts in 76.3% of patients, a percentage consistent with many previous reports.[70]

These earlier reports also included rather short follow-up periods.[81-84] The one study that followed patients for at least 4 years reported a lower response rate compared with that after 1 year, raising questions regarding the durability of remission.[81]

Small trials employing danazol, interferon, or chemotherapeutic agents, alone or in combination, have produced variable success and substantial side effects.[85,86] Cyclosporine, an immunosuppressive agent known to interfere with T-cell activation, has been tried in small studies of pediatric patients with the intent of suppressing autoreactive T cells. These studies have also produced only mixed success.[87,88] Rituximab, a genetically engineered anti-CD20 monoclonal antibody that is known to deplete B cells, was recently tested and proved to have some limited efficacy in a group of adult patients with chronic ITP.[89] This therapy has not as yet been studied in pediatric ITP patients.

Conclusion

Controversy abounds regarding the appropriate evaluation and therapy for pediatric ITP. At present, most recommendations are not evidence-based. Many investigators have noted the need for well-designed clinical trials. The intent of such studies would be to: 1) shed light on the natural history of ITP and the associated incidence of ICH and major hemorrhage, 2) define predictors of chronic, refractory disease and the likelihood of serious bleeding, and 3) make therapeutic comparisons using measures of bleeding, morbidity, and mortality, rather than platelet count, as outcome variables. These objectives are beginning to be addressed, as evidenced by the establishment of an intercontinental registry for childhood ITP (www.unibas.ch/itpbasel). The registry's goal is to "gain key data about childhood ITP" and to ultimately provide a database that would justify randomized trials. Finally, in addition to clinical studies, there is also a need for further basic investigations to better define the immune dysregulation indicative of pediatric ITP. In this way, rational, effective therapies can be developed and utilized when they are needed.

References

1. Medeiros D, Buchanan GR. Idiopathic thrombocytopenic purpura: Beyond consensus. Curr Opin Pediatr 2000;12:4-9.
2. Bolton-Maggs PH. Idiopathic thrombocytopenic purpura. Arch Dis Child 2000;83:220-2.
3. Lilleyman JS. Intracranial haemorrhage in idiopathic thrombocytopenic purpura. Arch Dis Child 1994;71:251-3.
4. Eden OB, Lilleyman JS. Guidelines for management of idiopathic thrombocytopenic purpura. Arch Dis Child 1992;67:1056-8.
5. Winiarski J. Mechanisms in childhood idiopathic thrombocytopenic purpura (ITP). Acta Paediatr 1998;424(Suppl):54-6.
6. van Leeuwen EF, van der Ven JT, Engelfriet CP, von dem Borne AE. Specificities of autoantibodies in autoimmune thrombocytopenia. Blood 1982;59:23-6.
7. Winiarski J, Ekeland E. Antibody binding to platelet antigens in acute and chronic idiopathic thrombocytopenic purpura: A platelet membrane ELISA for the detection of antiplatelet antibodies in serum. Clin Exp Immunol 1986;63:459-65.
8. Winiarski J. IgG and IgM antibodies to platelet membrane glycoprotein antigens in acute childhood idiopathic thrombocytopenic purpura. Br J Haematol 1989;73:88-92.
9. Berchtold P, McMillan R, Tani P, et al. Autoantibodies against platelet membrane glycoproteins in children with acute and chronic immune thrombocytopenic purpura. Blood 1989;74:1600-2.
10. Taub J, Warrier I, Holtkamp C, et al. Characterization of autoantibodies against the platelet glycoprotein antigens IIb/IIIa in childhood idiopathic thrombocytopenic purpura. Am J Hematol 1995;48:104-7.
11. Wadenvik H, Stockelberg D, Hou M. Platelet proteins as autoantibody targets in idiopathic thrombocytopenic purpura. Acta Paediatr 1998; 424(Suppl):26-36.
12. Semple JW. Immunobiology of T helper cells and antigen-presenting cells in autoimmune thrombocytopenic purpura (ITP). Acta Paediatr 1998;424(Suppl):41-5.
13. Hedlund-Treutiger I, Wahlström J, Elinder G. Role of the T cell receptor in idiopathic thrombocytopenic purpura (ITP). Acta Paediatr 1998; 424(Suppl):46-50.
14. Semple JW, Freedman J. Increased anti-platelet T helper lymphocyte reactivity in patients with autoimmune thrombocytopenia. Blood 1991; 78:2619-25.
15. Semple JW, Milev Y, Cosgrave D, et al. Differences in serum cytokine levels in acute and chronic autoimmune thrombocytopenic purpura: Relationship to platelet phenotype and antiplatelet T-cell reactivity. Blood 1996;87:4245-54.

16. Kiwana M, Kaburaki J, Ikeda Y. Autoreactive T cells to platelet GPIIb-IIIa in immune thrombocytopenic purpura. J Clin Invest 1998;102:1393-402.
17. Kiwana M, Kaburaki J, Kitasato H, et al. Immunodominant epitopes on glycoprotein IIb-IIIa recognized by autoreactive T cells in patients with immune thrombocytopenic purpura. Blood 2001;98:130-9.
18. Anderson J. Cytokines in idiopathic thrombocytopenic purpura (ITP). Acta Paediatr 1998;424(Suppl):61-4.
19. Chu Y, Korb J, Sakamoto K. Idiopathic thrombocytopenic purpura. Pediatr Rev 2000;21(3):95-103.
20. Kelton JG. The measurement of platelet-bound immunoglobulins: An overview of the methods and the biological relevance of platelet-associated IgG. Prog Hematol 1983;13:163-99.
21. Saxon BR, Mody M, Blanchette VS, Freedman J. Reticulated platelet counts in the assessment of thrombocytopenic disorders. Acta Paediatr 1998;424(Suppl):65-70.
22. Saxon BR, Blanchette VS, Butchart S, et al. Reticulated platelet counts in the diagnosis of acute immune thrombocytopenic purpura. J Pediatr Hematol Oncol 1998;20:44-8.
23. Niethammer AG, Forman EN. Use of the platelet histogram maximum in evaluating thrombocytopenia. Am J Hematol 1999;60:19-23.
24. Buchanan GR. Childhood acute idiopathic thrombocytopenic purpura: How many tests and how much treatment required? (editorial). J Pediatr 1985;106:928-9.
25. Bolton-Maggs PHB, Moon I. Assessment of UK practice for management of acute childhood idiopathic thrombocytopenic purpura against published guidelines. Lancet 1997;350:620-3.
26. Vesely S, Buchanan GR, Cohen A, et al. Self-reported diagnostic and management strategies in childhood idiopathic thrombocytopenic purpura: Results of a survey of practicing pediatric hematology/oncology specialists. J Pediatr Hematol Oncol 2000;22:55-61.
27. Calpin C, Dick P, Poon A, Freedman W. Is bone marrow aspiration needed in acute childhood idiopathic thrombocytopenic purpura to rule out leukemia? Arch Pediatr Adolesc Med 1998;152:345-7.
28. Medeiros D, Buchanan GR. Major hemorrhage in children with idiopathic thrombocytopenic purpura: Immediate response to therapy and long-term outcome. J Pediatr 1998;133:334-9.
29. George JN, Woolf SH, Raskob GE, et al. Idiopathic thrombocytopenic purpura: A practice guideline developed by explicit methods for the American Society of Hematology. Blood 1996;88:3-40.
30. George JN. Initial management of immune thrombocytopenic purpura in children: Is supportive counseling without therapeutic intervention sufficient? (editorial). J Pediatr 2000;137:598-600.
31. Dickerhoff R, von Ruecker A. The clinical course of immune thrombocytopenic purpura in children who did not receive intravenous immuno-

globulins or sustained prednisone treatment. J Pediatr 2000;137: 629-32.
32. Buchanan GR, de Alarcon PA, Feig SA, et al. Acute idiopathic thrombocytopenic purpura—management in childhood (letter). Blood 1997;89: 1464-5.
33. Buchanan GR, Holtkamp CA. Prednisone therapy for children with newly diagnosed idiopathic thrombocytopenic purpura. A randomized clinical trial. Am J Pediatr Hematol Oncol 1984;6:355-61.
34. Kitchens CS. Amelioration of endothelial abnormalities by prednisone in experimental thrombocytopenia in the rabbit. J Clin Invest 1977;60: 1129-34.
35. Kitchens CS, Pendergast JF. Human thrombocytopenia is associated with structural abnormalities of the endothelium that are ameliorated by glucocorticosteroid administration. Blood 1986;67:203-6.
36. Bellucci S, Charpak C, Chastang G, Tobelem G. Low doses *v* conventional doses of corticoids in immune thrombocytopenic purpura (ITP): Results of a randomized clinical trial in 160 children, 223 adults. Blood 1988;71: 1165-9.
37. Ozsoylu S, Irken G, Karabent A. High-dose intravenous methylprednisolone for acute childhood idiopathic thrombocytopenic purpura. Eur J Haematol 1989;42:431-5.
38. Suarez CR, Rademaker D, Hasson A, Mongogna L. High-dose steroids in childhood acute idiopathic thrombocytopenia purpura. Am J Pediatr Hematol Oncol 1986;8:111-15.
39. Carcao MD, Zipursky A, Butchart S, et al. Short-course oral prednisone therapy in children presenting with acute immune thrombocytopenic purpura (ITP). Acta Paediatr 1998;424(Suppl):71-4.
40. Blanchette VS, Luke B, Andrew M, et al. A prospective, randomized trial of high-dose intravenous immune globulin G therapy, oral prednisone therapy, and no therapy in childhood acute immune thrombocytopenic purpura. J Pediatr 1993;123:989-95.
41. Blanchette V, Imbach P, Andrew M, et al. Randomized trial of intravenous immunoglobulin G, intravenous anti-D, and oral prednisone in childhood acute immune thrombocytopenic purpura. Lancet 1994;344:703-7.
42. Imbach P, Berchtold W, Hirt A, et al. Intravenous immunoglobulin versus oral corticosteroids in acute immune thrombocytopenic purpura in childhood. Lancet 1985;464-8.
43. Sartorius JA. Steroid treatment of idiopathic thrombocytopenic purpura in children. Am J Pediatr Hematol Oncol 1984;6:165-9.
44. Albayrak D, Islek I, Kalayci AG, Gurses N. Acute immune thrombocytopenic purpura: A comparative study of very high oral doses of methylprednisolone and intravenously administered immune globulin. J Pediatr 1994;125:1004-7.

45. Rosthoj S, Nielson S, Pederson FK. Randomized trial comparing intravenous immunoglobulin with methylprednisolone pulse therapy in acute idiopathic thrombocytopenic purpura. Acta Paediatr 1996;85:910-15.
46. van Hoff J, Ritchey K. Pulse methylprednisolone therapy for acute childhood idiopathic thrombocytopenic purpura. J Pediatr 1998;113:563-6.
47. Imbach P, d'Apuzzo V, Hirt A, et al. High-dose intravenous gammaglobulin for idiopathic thrombocytopenic purpura in childhood. Lancet 1981:1228-31.
48. Fehr J, Hofmann V, Kappeler CM. Transient reversal of thrombocytopenia in idiopathic thrombocytopenic purpura by high-dose intravenous gamma globulin. N Engl J Med 1982;306:1254-8.
49. Kurlander RJ. Reversible and irreversible loss of Fc receptor function of human monocytes as a consequence of interaction with immunoglobulin G. J Clin Invest 1980;66:773-81.
50. Kimberly RP, Salmon JE, Bussel JB, et al. Modulation of mononuclear phagocyte function by intravenous γ-globulin. J Immunol 1984;132:745-50.
51. Zimmerman SA, Malinoski FJ, Ware RE. Immunologic effects of anti-D (WinRho-SD) in children with immune thrombocytopenic purpura. Am J Hematol 1998;131-8.
52. Salama A, Mueller-Eckhardt, Kiefel V. Effect of intravenous immunoglobulin in immune thrombocytopenia. Competitive inhibition of reticuloendothelial system function by sequestration of autologous red blood cells? Lancet 1983;193-5.
53. Tsubakio T, Kurata Y, Katagiri S, et al. Alteration of T cell subsets and immunoglobulin synthesis in vitro during high dose γ-globulin therapy in patients with idiopathic thrombocytopenic purpura. Clin Exp Immunol 1983;53:697-702.
54. Dammacco F, Iodice G, Campobasso N. Treatment of patients with idiopathic thrombocytopenic purpura with intravenous immunoglobulin: Effects on circulating T cell subsets and PWM-induced antibody synthesis in vitro. Br J Haematol 1986;62:125-35.
55. Delfraissy JF, Tchernia G, Laurian Y, et al. Suppressor cell function after intravenous gammaglobulin treatment in adult chronic idiopathic thrombocytopenic purpura. Br J Haematol 1985;60:315-22.
56. Stohl W. Cellular mechanisms in the in vitro inhibition of pokeweed mitogen-induced B cell differentiation by immunoglobulin for intravenous use. J Immunol 1986;136:4407-13.
57. Imbach P, Barandun S, Hirt A, Wagner HP. Intravenous immunoglobulin for idiopathic thrombocytopenic purpura (ITP) in childhood. Am J Pediatr Hematol Oncol 1984;6:171-4.
58. Rosthoj S, Steffensen GK, Glud TK. Simplified immunoglobulin treatment of idiopathic thrombocytopenic purpura. Acta Paediatr Scand 1987;76:631-5.

59. Tarantino MD, Madden RM, Fennewald DL, et al. Treatment of childhood acute immune thrombocytopenic purpura with anti-D immune globulin or pooled immune globulin. J Pediatr 1999;134:21-6.
60. Warrier I, Bussel JB, Valdez L, et al. Safety and efficacy of low-dose intravenous immune globulin (IVIG) treatment for infants and children with immune thrombocytopenic purpura. J Pediatr Hematol Oncol 1997;19: 197-201.
61. Kattamis AC, Shankar S, Cohen AR. Neurologic complications of treatment of childhood acute immune thrombocytopenic purpura with intravenously administered immunoglobulin G. J Pediatr 1997;130:281-3.
62. Tsiouris J, Tsiouris N. Hemiplegia as a complication of treatment of childhood immune thrombocytopenic purpura with intravenously administered immunoglobulin (letter). J Pediatr 1998;133:717.
63. Sekul EA, Culper EJ, Dalakas MC. Aseptic meningitis with high-dose intravenous immunoglobulin therapy: Frequency and risk factors. Ann Intern Med 1994;121:259-62.
64. Jayabose S, Mahmoud M, Levendoglu-Tugal O, et al. Corticosteroid prophylaxis for neurologic complications of intravenous immunoglobulin G therapy in childhood immune thrombocytopenic purpura. J Pediatr Hematol Oncol 1999;21:514-17.
65. Bresee JS, Mast EE, Coleman PJ, et al. Hepatitis C virus infection associated with administration of intravenous immune globulin: A cohort study. JAMA 1996;276:1563-7.
66. Bussel JB, Graziano JN, Kimberly RP, et al. Intravenous anti-D treatment of immune thrombocytopenic purpura: Analysis of efficacy, toxicity, and mechanism of effect. Blood 1991;77:1884-93.
67. Freiburg A, Mauger D. Efficacy, safety, and dose response of intravenous anti-D immune globulin (WinRho SDF) for the treatment of idiopathic thrombocytopenic purpura in children. Semin Hematol 1998;35(Suppl 1):23-7.
68. Gaines AR. Acute onset hemoglobinemia and/or hemoglobinuria and sequelae following Rh_0(D) immune globulin intravenous administration in immune thrombocytopenic purpura patients. Blood 2000;95:2523-9.
69. Imbach P, Kuhne T. Sequelae of treatment of ITP with anti-D (Rh_0) immunoglobulin (commentary). Lancet 2000;356:447-8.
70. Mantadakis E, Buchanan GR. Elective splenectomy in children with idiopathic thrombocytopenic purpura. J Pediatr Hematol Oncol 2000;22: 148-53.
71. Lammi AT, Lovric VA. Idiopathic thrombocytopenic purpura: An epidemiologic study. J Pediatr 1973;83:31-6.
72. Schiavotto C, Ruggeri M, Rodeghiero F. Failure of repeated courses of high-dose intravenous immunoglobulin to induce stable remission in patients with chronic idiopathic thrombocytopenic purpura. Ann Hematol 1995;70:89-90.

73. Anderson JC. Response of resistant idiopathic thrombocytopenic purpura to pulsed high-dose dexamethasone therapy. N Engl J Med 1994;330:1560-4.
74. Kuhne T, Freedman J, Semple JW, et al. Platelet and immune responses to oral cyclic dexamethasone therapy in childhood chronic immune thrombocytopenic purpura. J Pediatr 1997;130:17-24.
75. Borgna-Pignatti C, Rugolotto S, Nobili B, et al. A trial of high-dose dexamethasone therapy for chronic idiopathic thrombocytopenic purpura in childhood. J Pediatr 1997;130:13-16.
76. Adams DM, Kinney TR, O'Branski-Rupp E, Ware RE. High dose oral dexamethasone therapy for chronic childhood idiopathic thrombocytopenic purpura. J Pediatr 1996;128:281-3.
77. Chen JS, Wu JM, Chen YJ, Yeh TF. Pulsed high dose dexamethasone therapy in children with chronic idiopathic thrombocytopenic purpura. J Pediatr Hematol Oncol 1997;19:526-9.
78. Reid MM. Chronic idiopathic thrombocytopenic purpura: Incidence, treatment and outcome. Arch Dis Child 1995;72:125-8.
79. Weinblatt ME, Ortega JA. Steroid responsiveness. A predictor of the outcome of splenectomy in children with chronic immune thrombocytopenic purpura. Am J Dis Child 1982;136:1064-6.
80. Law C, Marcaccio M, Tam P, et al. High-dose intravenous immune globulin and the response to splenectomy in patients with idiopathic thrombocytopenic purpura. N Engl J Med 1997;336:1494-8.
81. Benham ES, Taft LI. Idiopathic thrombocytopenic purpura in children: Results of steroid therapy and splenectomy. Aust Paediatr J 1972;8: 311-17.
82. Walker RW, Walker W. Idiopathic thrombocytopenia, initial illness and long term follow-up. Arch Dis Child 1984;59:316-22.
83. Akatsuka JI, Fujisawa K, Ishidoya N, et al. Long-term follow-up study of children with chronic ITP. Blut 1989;59:105-8.
84. Cohn J. Thrombocytopenia in childhood: An evaluation of 433 patients. Scand J Haematol 1976;16:226-40.
85. Weinblatt ME, Kochen J, Ortega J. Danazol for children with immune thrombocytopenic purpura. Am J Dis Child 1988;142:1317-19.
86. Tarantino MD. Treatment options for chronic immune (idiopathic) thrombocytopenia purpura in children. Semin Hematol 2000;37(Suppl 1):35-41.
87. Moskowitz IPG, Gaynon PS, Nasrollah TS, Cripe TP. Low-dose cyclosporin A therapy in children with refractory immune thrombocytopenic purpura. J Pediatr Hematol Oncol 1999;21:77-9.
88. Schultz KR, Warrier I. Cyclosporin A therapy of immune-mediated thrombocytopenia in children (letter). Blood 1995;85:1406-8.
89. Stasi R, Pagano A, Stipa E, Amadori S. Rituximab chimeric anti-CD20 monoclonal antibody treatment for adults with chronic idiopathic thrombocytopenic purpura. Blood 2001;98:952-7.

In: Herman JH, Manno CS, eds.
Pediatric Transfusion Therapy
Bethesda, MD: AABB Press, 2002

17

Apheresis vs Whole-Blood-Derived Platelets for Pediatric Transfusion

DAVID F. FRIEDMAN, MD

PLATELET PRODUCTS FOR TRANSFUSION may be derived from whole blood, or they may be collected by apheresis technique. Both processes yield blood components consisting of platelets suspended in citrated plasma, at concentrations approximately 5 to 10 times the concentration of platelets in normal whole blood. Both components may therefore be considered "concentrates" of normal platelets that are suitable for transfusion to patients with appropriate indications for platelets. In the United States, the demand for platelets is rising faster than demand for red cells, and there has been a trend toward increased use of platelets col-

David F. Friedman, MD, Associate Director, Transfusion Service, The Children's Hospital of Philadelphia, Philadelphia, Pennsylvania

lected by apheresis.[1] However, both whole-blood-derived and apheresis platelets are likely to remain part of the blood inventory for the foreseeable future.

This chapter compares these two types of platelet products,[2] and discusses how their similarities and differences may influence the selection of platelet products for transfusion in infants and children.

Definitions

There are several commonly used terms and abbreviations for the available components,[3(p89)] and the terminology may be confusing. The clearest terms are those that describe how each component is produced. "Apheresis platelets" are produced when an individual donor undergoes a standard donor plateletpheresis procedure, and "whole-blood-derived platelets" are produced when platelets are isolated from the red cell and plasma elements of a unit of donated whole blood. Table 17-1 gives explanations of terminology that may be encountered in the literature and in practice.

Comparison of Platelet Products

Whole-blood-derived platelets and apheresis platelets are roughly equivalent with respect to their principal characteristic, the concentration of platelets. Both methods of preparing platelet concentrates result in average platelet concentrations of about 1.5×10^9 platelets per mL.[2] However, there is significant variability in the platelet concentration among platelet products of both types, and an understanding of the reasons for this variability is important for their optimal use.

Sources of Variation

The peripheral blood platelet count in normal adult blood donors may vary from 150,000 to 450,000/μL, more than a threefold range of platelet concentrations. This wide variation in donor platelet count gives rise to broad variation in the platelet content of both whole-blood-derived and apheresis platelets. Blood

Table 17-1. Terminology Used to Describe Platelet Products

Term	Explanation or Usual Meaning
Apheresis platelets (also called single-donor platelets)	Because apheresis platelets are not usually pooled, each unit represents only one donor exposure.
HLA-matched platelets	Apheresis platelets from a donor whose HLA type is known and was selected to be as close as feasible to the HLA type of the intended recipient.
Whole-blood-derived platelets (also called random-donor platelets)	The term random-donor platelets is often used in contrast to the term "single-donor platelets." This usage may be misleading because it implies that the donor of a "single" apheresis platelet product was selected by criteria more specific to the recipient than the donor of the "random" whole-blood-derived platelets, which is usually not the case.
Platelet concentrates	This term usually refers to whole-blood-derived platelets, but is an equally appropriate description of apheresis platelets, because both contain platelets in concentrations higher than in peripheral blood.
Buffy-coat-derived platelets	Whole-blood-derived platelets produced using the high speed centrifugation first, sedimenting the platelets into the buffy coat. This is the method for manufacturing platelet products from whole blood in Europe.
Platelet-rich-plasma-derived platelets	Whole-blood-derived platelets produced using the low speed centrifugation first, leaving the platelets suspended in platelet-rich plasma. This is the method for manufacturing platelet products from whole blood in the United States and Canada.

(continued)

Table 17-1. Terminology Used to Describe Platelet Products (continued)

Term	Explanation or Usual Meaning
Platelets	Labeling required by the US Food and Drug Administration for one unit of whole-blood-derived platelets issued individually, not in a pool.
Platelets Pooled	Labeling required by the US Food and Drug Administration for two or more units of whole-blood-derived platelets issued as a pooled product.
Platelets Pheresis	Labeling required by the US Food and Drug Administration for a portion of or the entire apheresis platelet product drawn from one donor.
Leukocyte-reduced platelets	Platelet product from which the leukocytes have been removed, either by passage through an adhesion filter or by a collection method that includes a centrifugal chamber that separates white cells from platelets during collection.
Concentrated platelets, or plasma-removed platelets	A platelet product subjected to centrifugation and removal of some of the plasma, rendering the concentration of platelets higher, and the volume of the product lower, than in the original product. This modification of the platelet product is used for patients requiring meticulous fluid restriction.
Saline-suspended platelets	Same as plasma removed, with a volume of normal saline added to restore the original volume of the product, diluting the residual plasma.

centers may attempt to limit this variability by choosing not to accept platelet donations from donors with counts on the lower end of the normal range, below 200,000/μL for example. The techniques used to isolate the platelets from the other components of blood may also affect the final content of platelets in the product. For example, if the parent unit of whole blood is destined to be stored in the preservatives CPD or CPDA, more plasma must be left with the red cells than if it is destined to be stored in the additive solutions AS-1, -3, or -5. For the platelet-rich-plasma method of harvesting whole blood derived, this means that more platelets are left behind with the CPDA red cells than with the AS-1 red cells, and fewer find their way to the platelet product. For apheresis platelets, several aspects of collection technique may have significant effects on platelet yield, including the collection chamber (bowl vs channel), the number of collection cycles or duration of continuous collection, and the donor's tolerance of the procedure. The choice of leukocyte reduction technique may also affect platelet yield. There may be as much as a 20% loss of platelet content depending on the deadspace volume of the filter, storage age of the component at the time of leukocyte reduction, and other factors.[4] Inventory management decisions may also affect the content of platelet units—in some collection centers, a mandate to increase production may influence the collection staff to strive for "double components" that can be divided to yield two separate platelet products. The platelet content of the divided products would still be within the acceptable range for platelet yield, but at the lower end of that range, compared with a product that was not split.

Variation in Platelet Content

The platelet content of a product is the number of platelets in the bag, regardless of the volume. One unit of whole-blood-derived platelets should contain at least 5.5×10^{10} platelets,[3(p35)] but may contain twice that number or more. The platelet content of a unit of apheresis platelets should contain at least 3.0×10^{11} platelets, but depending on several donor and technical factors discussed above, may contain two or more times that number. Furthermore, these lower limits of platelet content are often quality control standards measured on a small sample of the platelet products collected each month, so that a few products may have platelet contents below the "minimum."[3(p35)] This potential for variation in the number of platelets given in a single dose may have an important effect on the expected increase in the recipient's platelet count.

Variation in Volume

The volume of a platelet product is determined by the amount of plasma in which the platelets are suspended. For whole-blood-derived platelets, the volume of one unit is 40 to 60 mL, with variation due to factors including the eventual anticoagulant-preservative solution for the red cells in that whole blood donation, and the technique of the individual who prepares the component. For apheresis platelets, the volume of one platelet collection may vary from 200 to over 500 mL, depending on the donor's count, the type of separator, the number of draw cycles, the rate at which citrate anticoagulant is added to the apheresis circuit, and other factors. The potential for variation in the volume of a platelet product is especially important for younger children weighing less than 30 kg, for whom an apheresis platelet product near the high end of the range of variation might result in the rapid administration of 15 to 20 mL/kg or more. Variations in the platelet product volume, platelet content, and concentration are compared in Table 17-2.

Table 17-2. Comparison of Average Values for Characteristics of Platelet Products

	Whole Blood-Derived	Apheresis
Platelet content	7×10^{10} platelets	4×10^{11} platelets
Volume	50 mL	300 mL
Concentration	1.5×10^{9}/mL	1.5×10^{9}/mL

Modified from Chambers and Herman[2]

Leukocyte Content

Platelet concentrates derived from whole blood or apheresis collections contain a significant number of donor leukocytes. Whole-blood-derived platelets typically contain a larger number of leukocytes (around 10×10^7 white cells per 40 to 60 mL) than apheresis platelets, which contain 2 to 10×10^7 white cells per 225 to 500 mL. Both can be effectively leukocyte reduced using current third-generation leukocyte reduction filters to levels below 5.5×10^6 white cells per product.[4,5] The benefits of leukocyte reduction of blood components include prevention of HLA alloimmunization, reduction of cytomegalovirus risk, and reduction of the rate of febrile transfusion reactions.

There are some differences between whole-blood-derived platelets and apheresis platelets with respect to the practical aspects of implementing leukocyte reduction. Some plateletpheresis methods incorporate a second centrifugal chamber that separates leukocytes from platelets during the collection procedure, while others incorporate a leukocyte filtration step immediately after collection. In either case, the component is modified before storage and requires no subsequent manipulation to reduce white cell content.[5] In contrast, whole-blood-derived platelets are typically passed through leukocyte reduction filters after they are pooled, which means that the leukocyte reduction step is performed either in the blood bank or at the bedside. The consistency and quality control of leukocyte reduction may therefore be superior for apheresis platelets compared with whole-blood-derived platelets.[6]

This difference in the time of leukocyte reduction has a broader impact for platelet transfusion in children for whom small volumes are required. Consider, for example, a platelet transfusion for an infant who requires leukocyte-reduced blood and in whom 50 mL is the appropriate dose. This dose can be provided easily by removing an aliquot of 50 mL from an apheresis platelet product that has been leukocyte reduced before storage. Filling the same order using 1 unit of whole-blood-derived platelets might require leukocyte filtration of a small volume. Even if a pediatric size leukocyte reduction filter were used, the loss of platelets within the dead space of the filter may be a large fraction of the starting volume of the component. In practice, two whole-blood-derived platelet units may have to be pooled to compensate for this loss, doubling the number of donor exposures and increasing the preparation time further. In summary, although both apheresis and whole-blood-derived platelets can be effectively leukocyte reduced, apheresis platelets have some practical advantages within the blood bank, especially in the context of providing small volumes for pediatric patients.

Red Cell Content

The red cell content of whole-blood-derived and apheresis platelets is very low, such that crossmatching is not required. However, the level of residual red cells can be sufficient to cause red cell alloimmunization, especially to the highly antigenic D antigen in D-negative recipients. Although the risk of immunization to the D antigen is low, especially in immunosuppressed oncology and hematology patients,[7] some pediatric transfusion services provide D-negative platelets for D-negative recipients. In practice, this policy often limits the availability of platelets for D-negative patients.

Posttransfusion Increments

The ultimate clinical outcome measure for the efficacy of platelet transfusion is reduction of thrombocytopenic bleeding. However, because occult bleeding is difficult to quantify and overt bleeding is relatively uncommon, and most platelet transfusions are given prophylactically to prevent bleeding, most studies focus on the posttransfusion platelet count increment as the endpoint measurement. When measured within 60 minutes after a transfusion and corrected for the number of platelets transfused and the size of the patient, the corrected count increment is a measure of immediate platelet recovery. Some studies also focus on platelet survival by measuring the interval between transfusions or the total platelet requirement over time.[8-10]

Several factors—some intrinsic to the product, some intrinsic to the recipient—have an impact on the rise in the recipient's platelet count after transfusion. Among the product variables that affect posttransfusion increments are the platelet content, the storage age, activation during storage, and ABO blood group compatibility with the recipient. Among the recipient variables that affect posttransfusion increments are the presence of fever, infection, bleeding, consumptive coagulopathy, splenomegaly, and degree of HLA alloimmunization.[2,11,12] Studies that have attempted to control for these variables have concluded that apheresis platelets and whole-blood-derived platelets have roughly equivalent clinical efficacy as measured by platelet count increment.[13,14]

In the clinical practice of platelet transfusions, neither the product-related variables, the patient-related variables described above, or the timing of posttransfusion platelet counts are easily controlled. The availability of platelets at the time of need is often the main determinant of which component is transfused. The most fundamental variable, the number of platelets transfused, is not usually controlled precisely because of the wide variability among components in platelet content and volume. The underlying disease processes that affect platelet recovery and survival—infection, consumptive coagulopathy, and bleeding—are also subject to change. For these reasons, posttransfusion platelet increments are often highly variable from one transfusion to the next and from one patient to the next.

Risks

Bacterial Contamination

Bacterial contamination of platelet products is the most common cause of septic reactions related to blood transfusion. The risk is in the range of 1:4,000 to 1:12,000 platelet units.[15] The likelihood of bacterial contamination of a platelet unit increases with storage age, suggesting that bacterial contaminants, usually skin organisms, are most often introduced at the time of collection, and then grow during storage at 22 C.[16] There are, however, studies that suggest that whole-blood-derived platelets are associated with higher rates of contamination than apheresis platelets.[17] The possible explanations for this difference include bacterial contamination during open pooling procedures, and the increased chance of a contaminant related to the number of components used in the pool. However, it is also possible that whole-blood-derived platelets are transfused, on average, at a more advanced storage age than apheresis platelets, and are therefore more likely to be contaminated at a level that is clinically apparent. Because the organisms most commonly associated with contaminated platelets are typical skin organisms such as *Staphylococcus* species, it is difficult to determine whether the origin of contamination was the donation, the pooling, or a contaminant introduced at the time of culturing. In conclusion, bacterial contamination is a low but real risk associated with platelet transfusion. It is not a clear reason to prefer apheresis over whole-blood-derived components.

Volume Overload

There is significant variation in the volume of individual platelet products—as much as two- to three-fold. Whole-blood-derived platelets may range from 40 to 60 mL per unit, with the range of variation reduced somewhat by averaging (because of pooling); apheresis platelets range from 200 to 450 mL per unit.[18] For whole-blood-derived platelets, the source of this variation is related to donor's platelet count and to the technique of component preparation. For apheresis platelets, additional variables related to the cell separator used, the number of draw cycles, and subsequent splitting of the collection all affect the final volume of a single unit.

While these variables also affect the platelet concentration and content of the products, for pediatric transfusions, the variation in volume probably represents the most immediate risk. Specifically, if orders for platelets are specified as numbers of, or fractions of, units and the volume that the patient will receive is not specified or limited, then the patient will be exposed to the volume variations inherent in platelet products. Because platelets are typically infused rapidly, a patient who receives an unusually large unit may receive 15 to 20 mL/kg of colloid fluid or more, and may suffer an episode of volume overload. If, on the other hand, the more prudent practice of specifying the volume is used for ordering platelets, then the patient is exposed to the inherent variation in platelet content. In this case, the posttransfusion platelet count increment will be less predictable because of the variation in number of platelets given.

Allergic Transfusion Reactions

Allergic transfusion reactions occur in association with 1% to 3% of platelet transfusions, and are usually mild, with itching and hives as the most frequent clinical manifestations. Less commonly, wheezing, airway edema, and anaphylaxis may occur. Allergic reactions are thought to be mediated by antigens in the plasma portion of a platelet concentrate, rather than the platelets themselves, and occur when the recipient has a preformed antibody of the IgE class against an allergen in the donor plasma. In the special case of a truly IgA-deficient recipient, the allergen responsible for the reaction is known to be the IgA in the donor's plasma. Complete IgA deficiency is rare, but these patients can produce IgE antibodies with anti-IgA specificity, and can experience life-threatening anaphylactic reactions when exposed to blood components that contain IgA. For the more common, milder allergic reactions, however, the allergen is not identified, and may be a polymorphic difference in a serum protein between donor and recipient, or a drug the donor has taken, or an allergen derived from food the donor has recently ingested. Therefore, mild allergic type reactions to platelet transfusions are usually idiosyncratic and unpredictable.

On a theoretic basis, pools of whole-blood-derived platelets might be predicted to have a greater risk of allergic reactions because more than one potential source of allergens is involved. On the other hand, apheresis platelets would contain a large amount of a given allergen because all the plasma in the product is derived from one donor. In clinical studies, the risk of allergic transfusion reactions is the same for whole-blood-derived and apheresis platelets.[19]

Febrile Reactions and Hypotensive Reactions

Febrile transfusion reactions, usually defined as a rise in the recipient's temperature by more than 1 C, occur following almost 30% of platelet transfusions.[20] These reactions are thought to be mediated by donor leukocytes in the component, but the risk of reactions is not directly correlated with the number of leukocytes. Febrile reactions are probably caused by cytokines, including interleukins and gamma interferon, released from leukocytes in the blood component. These pro-inflammatory cytokines are released from leukocytes into the plasma portion of the component during storage[21] so that the storage age is a primary determinant of the risk of febrile reactions.[22] Leukocyte reduction, especially when performed close to the time of collection, removes the source of the cytokines and reduces this risk. Whole-blood-derived platelets have been associated with higher rates of febrile transfusion reactions than apheresis platelets, possibly because they are transfused, on average, at a later time in their storage life, and because some are leukocyte reduced at or near the time of transfusion rather than at the time of collection.

Hypotensive reactions not associated with anaphylaxis or sepsis have also been described following platelet transfusions.[23] As with febrile reactions, these hypotensive reactions are thought to be caused by soluble mediators that accumulate in the plasma during storage. However, the mediators of hypotensive reactions may be complement fragments or vasoactive byproducts of activation of the coagulation cascade, rather than cytokines released from leukocytes.

Hemolysis from Out-of-Group Plasma

Although it is preferable to transfuse ABO type-specific platelets, the limitations of platelet availability often make this impossible. Many institutions select platelet products without regard for minor incompatibility, between the plasma in the unit and the recipient's red cells.[24] Posttransfusion platelet increments following out-of-group platelet transfusions are reduced to only a minor degree relative to transfusion within group.

However, life-threatening hemolytic episodes, including deaths in pediatric patients, have been reported following out-of-group platelet transfusions.[25-27] This risk is primarily related to group O donors whose plasma contains anti-A or anti-B hemagglutinins in unusually high titers, or with unusually high avidity, or with an unusually high capacity to fix complement. Hemolysis from such platelet donors is estimated to occur in 1 in 10,000 transfusions,[26] and there is no reliable screening method to identify donors at risk. For this risk, whole-blood-derived platelets may be slightly safer than apheresis platelets because the plasma from the group O donor of whole blood may be diluted or neutralized by pooling with other platelet units. If a group O donor donates an apheresis platelet unit, the group A or B recipient of that unit will receive a larger dose of the hemolytic antibody.

Risks Related to Donor Exposures

Several other risks of transfusion, including transfusion-transmitted infectious diseases, HLA alloimmunization and platelet refractoriness, and transfusion-associated acute lung injury are discussed in other chapters. Each of these risks is related primarily to the number of different donors to whom a patient is exposed. In the context of the choice between whole-blood-derived and apheresis platelets, there is at least a theoretical reason to prefer apheresis platelets because they are drawn from one donor, while whole-blood-derived platelets are transfused as pooled products. For neonates whose dose of platelets could be filled by one unit of whole-blood-derived platelets, this advantage of reduced numbers of donor exposures is lost when a single transfusion is considered. However, for a child who will receive several platelet transfusions within the time frame of the shelf life of a platelet concentrate, the number of donor exposures can be reduced by the use of apheresis platelets if an effort is made to reserve one unit for the patient and take several aliquots from that unit.

The real benefit to the patient of efforts to minimize the number of donor exposures is relatively small, especially for patients who must receive multiple transfusions because of their underlying illness. For instance, because the residual risk of human immunodeficiency disease per donor exposure is 1 in half a million or less, the absolute difference in risk between 30 donor exposures and 50 donor exposures is very small compared with the increased cost of apheresis platelets, as much as double the cost of whole-blood-derived platelets.[28]

Transfusion-Associated Graft-vs-Host Disease

Transfusion-associated graft-vs-host disease is a rare, but fatal, complication of transfusion in which viable T cells from the blood component proliferate in an immunocompromised recipient, giving rise to immunologic attack on host tissues. The syndrome has been described in association with platelets as well as red cells, granulocytes, and unfrozen plasma. The patient populations at risk include oncology patients and marrow transplant recipients, and in pediatric practice, patients with congenital immunodeficiencies such as severe combined immunodeficiency syndromes, Wiskott-Aldrich syndrome, and DiGeorge syndrome. Gamma irradiation of blood components before transfusion effectively eliminates this risk by inducing DNA damage in the T cells, rendering them unable to proliferate. Because platelet recovery and function are not affected by the doses of gamma irradiation, 1500 to 2500 cGy necessary to eliminate this risk, platelets can be irradiated for specific patients or universally for all patients with little concern except for the time and expense required to perform the irradiation. There is no difference between whole-blood-derived platelets and apheresis platelets with regard to this risk or the effect of gamma irradiation.

Summary

The comparison between whole-blood-derived platelets and apheresis platelets suggests that they have similar efficacy as sources of platelets with hemostatic activity, and can in general be substituted for each other when necessary. Apheresis platelets have the general advantages of fewer donor exposures, fewer febrile transfusion reactions, and lower risk of bacterial contamination. Whole-blood-derived platelets are generally less expensive and more available, although these advantages are dependent on the practices and logistics of the local blood supplier(s). Whole-blood-derived platelets may also be safer from the standpoint of adjusting dose to patient size and avoiding volume overload, but this advantage depends upon the blood ordering and issuing protocols of the transfusion service. An understanding of the differences between these two components is important in optimizing the safety of platelet transfusions for pediatric patients.

References

1. Wallace E, Churchill WH, Surgenor DM, et al. Collection and transfusion of blood and blood components in the United States, 1994. Transfusion 1998;38:625-36.
2. Chambers LA, Herman JH. Considerations in the selection of a platelet component: Apheresis versus whole blood-derived. Transfus Med Rev 1999;13:311-22.
3. Gorlin JB, ed. Standards for blood banks and transfusion services, 21st ed. Bethesda, MD: American Association of Blood Banks, 2002.
4. Kao KJ, Mickel M, Braine HG, et al. White cell reduction in platelet concentrates and packed red cells by filtration: A multicenter clinical trial. Transfusion 1995;35:13-19.
5. Sweeney JD, Holme S, Stromberg RR, Heaton WAL. In vitro and in vivo effects of prestorage filtration of apheresis platelets. Transfusion 1995; 35:125-30.
6. Williamson LM, Wimperis JZ, Williamson P, et al. Bedside filtration in the prevention of HLA alloimmunization—a prospective randomized study. Blood 1994;83:3028-35.
7. Molnar R, Johnson R, Sweat L, et al. Absence of D alloimmunization in D– pediatric oncology patients receiving D-incompatible single-donor platelets. Transfusion 2002;42:177-82.
8. Herman JH, Klumpp TR, Christman RA, et al. The effect of platelet dose on the outcome of prophylactic platelet transfusion (abstract). Transfusion 1995;35(Suppl):46S.
9. Klumpp TR, Herman JH, Gaughan JP, et al. Clinical consequences of alternations in platelet transfusion dose: A prospective, randomized double-blind trial. Transfusion 1999;39:674-81.
10. Klumpp TR, Herman JH, Innis S, et al. Factors associated with response to platelet transfusions following hematopoietic stem cell transplantation. Bone Marrow Transplant 1996;17:1035-41.

11. Herman JH, Kamel HT. Platelet transfusion: Current techniques, remaining problems, and future prospects. Am J Pediatr Hematol/Oncol 1987; 9:272-86.
12. Slichter SJ. Platelet transfusion therapy. Hematol/Oncol Clin North Am 1990;4:291-311.
13. Anderson NA, Gray S, Copplestone JA, et al. A prospective randomized study of three types of platelet concentrates in patients with haematological malignancy: Corrected platelet count increments and frequency of nonhaemolytic febrile transfusion reactions. Transfus Med 1997; 7:33-9.
14. Slichter SJ, Grabowski M, Townsent-McCall D, et al. Prospective randomized transfusion trial to directly compare fresh and stored apheresis platelets (AP) and pooled random donor platelet concentrates (PC) in thrombocytopenic patients (abstract). Blood 1998;92(Suppl 1):672a.
15. Dodd RY. Adverse consequences of blood transfusion: Quantitative risk estimates. In: Nance ST, ed. Blood supply: Risks, perceptions and prospects for the future. Bethesda, MD: American Association of Blood Banks, 1994:1-24.
16. Braine HG, Kickler RS, Charache P, et al. Bacterial sepsis secondary to platelet transfusions: An adverse effect of extended storage at room temperature. Transfusion 1986;26:391-3.
17. Yomtovian R, Lazarus HM, Goodnough LT, et al. A prospective microbiologic surveillance program to detect and prevent the transfusion of bacterially contaminated platelets. Transfusion 1993;33:902-9.
18. Rebulla P. In vitro and in vivo properties of various types of platelets. Vox Sang 1998;74(Suppl 2):217-22.
19. Federowicz I, Barrett BB, Andersen JW, et al. Characteristics of reactions after transfusions of cellular blood components that are white cell reduced before storage. Transfusion 1996;36:21-8.
20. Miller JP, AuBuchon JP. Leukocyte-reduced and cytomegalovirus-reduced-risk blood components. In: Mintz PD, ed. Transfusion therapy: Clinical principles and practice. Bethesda, MD: AABB Press, 1999:313-39.
21. Heddle NM, Klama L, Singer J, et al. The role of the plasma from platelet concentrates in transfusion reactions. N Engl J Med 1994;331:625-8.
22. Heddle NM, Klama LN, Griffith L, et al. A prospective study to identify the risk factors associated with acute reactions to platelet and red cell transfusions. Transfusion 1993;33:794-7.
23. Hume HA, Popovsky MA, Benson K, et al. Hypotensive reactions: A previously uncharacterized complication of platelet transfusion? Transfusion 1996;36:904-9.
24. Lin Y, Callum JL, Coovadia AS, Murphy PM. Transfusion of ABO-nonidentical platelets is not associated with adverse clinical outcomes in cardiovascular surgery patients. Transfusion 2002;42:166-72.
25. Larsson LG, Welsh VJ, Ladd DJ. Acute intravascular hemolysis secondary to out-of-group platelet transfusion. Transfusion 2000;40:902-6.

26. Mair B, Benson K. Evaluation of changes in hemoglobin levels associated with ABO-incompatible plasma in apheresis platelets. Transfusion 1998; 38:51-5.
27. Pierce RN, Reich LM, Mayer K. Hemolysis following platelet transfusions from ABO-incompatible donors. Transfusion 1985;25:60-2.
28. Sweeney JD, Petrucci J, Yankee R. Pooled platelet concentrates: Maybe not fancy, but fiscally sound and effective. Transfus Sci 1997;18:575-83.

In: Herman JH, Manno CS, eds.
Pediatric Transfusion Therapy
Bethesda, MD: AABB Press, 2002

18

Transfusion Support in Pediatric Oncology and Hematopoietic Transplantation

JED GORLIN, MD, AND STEPHAN GRUPP, MD, PhD

MOST TRANSFUSION REQUIREMENTS FOR THE PEDIATRIC oncology patient or recipient of a marrow or peripheral blood progenitor cell (PBPC) transplant are not unique. However, frequency of transfusion, the array of different components required, and the immunocompromised state of many of the recipients provide special challenges.

Jed Gorlin, MD, Medical Director, Memorial Blood Centers, Minneapolis, and Assistant Professor, Department of Laboratory Medicine, University of Minnesota, Minneapolis, Minnesota, and Stephan Grupp, MD, PhD, Director, Stem Cell Biology, Division of Oncology, Children's Hospital of Philadelphia, and Assistant Professor of Pediatrics, University of Pennsylvania, Philadelphia, Pennsylvania

Sequelae of Frequent Transfusion

Platelet Alloimmunization

Although the rate of platelet alloimmunization observed in pediatric oncology patients is lower than that observed in adults, it still may represent a substantial problem for patient care. One report observed a higher rate of alloimmunization in pediatric acute myelogenous leukemia (AML) than in acute lymphocytic leukemia (ALL) patients, reflecting either the greater immunosuppression associated with ALL regimens or the greater transfusion requirements of the former group.[1] That disease- and therapy-specific observation aside, the more the patient is transfused, the more opportunities exist for development of HLA antibodies. Presumably, the observations of the Trial to Reduce Alloimmunization to Platelets (TRAP) study also apply to pediatric patients.[2] Specifically, provision of prestorage leukocyte-reduced blood is likely to slow the rate of alloimmunization by diminishing allogeneic HLA exposure. Because the subset of participants in the TRAP study of multiparous women began with a baseline rate of sensitization, the pediatric population would be most analogous to the never previously transfused males—for whom a clear benefit of leukocyte-reduced components was easiest to demonstrate. Thus, most pediatric oncology programs try to provide prestorage leukocyte-reduced components when possible. Because pediatric oncology patients often represent a large percentage of the pediatric patients who receive platelet transfusions, many facilities have adopted universal leukocyte reduction, ie, providing leukocyte-reduced cellular components to all patients, if only to avoid the logistical difficulties of trying to manage two inventories.

Red cell alloimmunization is also less common among pediatric as opposed to adult transfusion recipients.[3] Whether it has to do with less mature immune systems (children are more tolerant of adults than vice versa) or the greater degree of immunosuppression of many pediatric transfusion recipients, it simply is an empirical observation that red cell immunization among pediatric patients is less common than in adults. A notable exception may be highly transfused sickle cell patients, whose optimal management is discussed in Chapter 11.

Immune Compromise: Cytomegalovirus

Immunosuppressed patients are at risk from overwhelming infection with cytomegalovirus (CMV), a herpes family virus. Because CMV is a transfusion-transmitted virus that is usually carried in leukocytes, transfusion transmission is associated only with transfusion of cellular components. Alternative strategies to provide CMV-reduced-risk components include either providing cellular components from donors found to be negative for evidence of exposure to CMV on antibody screening or to provide leukocyte-reduced components. While the entire issue of providing CMV reduced-risk components is the subject of Chapter 8, suffice it to say that neither strategy can entirely preclude the transmission of CMV.[4] In addition, depending upon the prevalence of CMV in the donor population (which may vary geographically between 50% and 80%), the rate of false-negative results using conventional enzyme immunoassays currently available approaches 3%.[5] Most transfusion services have policies equating prestorage leukocyte-reduced components with antibody-screened components as equivalent in risk of transmitting CMV.

Immune Compromise: Transfusion-Associated Graft-vs-Host Disease

While Chapter 7 addresses the issues of transfusion-associated graft-vs-host disease (TA-GVHD) in general, it is worthwhile to add that in addition to neonates, the pediatric patients at most risk from TA-GVHD are those receiving directed donor transfusions and immunosuppressed patients such as pediatric oncology or transplant patients. In fact, one of the largest groups for which case reports exist are advanced stage pediatric neuroblastoma patients who typically receive very aggressive and immunosuppressive chemotherapy.[6] With the advent of many new highly immunosuppressive chemotherapy agents including fludarabine and 2-CDA, many B-cell lymphoma patients (largely adults) who were not formerly considered candidates for receiving irradiated blood, have been documented to have acquired TA-GVHD.[7,8] Many pediatric oncology programs have simply defaulted to the practice of irradiating all cellular components for all patients receiving chemotherapy, as opposed to trying to pick and choose which protocols require provision of irradiated components. Whether or not the advent of pathogen inactivation strategies that also prevent lymphocyte division will abrogate the need to use irradiation has yet to be established. Multiple studies confirm the efficacy of T-cell inactivation in the prevention of TA-GVHD both in animal and in-vitro models.[9]

A situation that is unique to allogeneic hematopoietic transplantation is the potential for TA-GVHD to occur when the marrow or PBPC donor receives unirradiated cellular component transfusions prior to or during the collection of hematopoietic cells. This either may occur intraoperatively during marrow harvest or as a part of priming the apheresis collection device for a pediatric PBPC collection.[10] When transfused cells may be collected with the marrow or peripheral blood, it is advisable to delay operative red cell transfusion during marrow harvest or PBPC collection until the procedure is complete. Most transplant collection centers require that only irradiated components be given to donors, despite the fact that the allogeneic hematopoietic cell donor, per se, is not immunocompromised.

Transfusion Support

There are no scientifically based transfusion triggers for red cell and platelet transfusion that are unique to pediatrics. The most definitive recommendations come from consensus statements as opposed to being derived from objective randomized trials. An editorial challenging the 20,000/µL trigger for prophylactic platelet transfusions in pediatric patients resulted in some lively debate.[11,12] Subsequent studies in adults documented the relative safety of withholding platelet transfusions from nonbleeding adult oncology patients until platelet counts fall below 10,000/μL, resulting in decreased transfusion requirements, but no increased incidence of problematic bleeding episodes.[13] In a 1992 AABB survey, 69% of pediatric platelet transfusions were labeled as prophylactic as opposed to therapeutic in contrast to only 58% of adult transfusions. However, even then, over 17% of institutions treating pediatric patients were using platelet transfusion triggers of less than 20,000/μL.[14] Perhaps the greatest effect of lowering the transfusion trigger is that now more children actually have counts around 20,000/μL when receiving prophylactic transfusion than the historically higher counts that may have resulted in transfusion "just in case." Guidelines for "difficult patients" have been proposed, allowing accommodation for some of the special needs of pediatric and other special patients.[15] Two examples of this include the practice of higher platelet transfusion trigger for brain tumor patients with bulk disease and marrow transplant patients with severe hypertension.

ABO Matching of Components Containing Platelets and Plasma

Although the importance of not giving group A red cells to a group O recipient is straightforward, transfusion services are often faced with the dilemma of not having ABO-identical platelets available for transfusion, especially in frequently transfused patients, such as pediatric oncology patients. The exact importance of providing ABO-identical platelets is less well founded, and often as a pragmatic matter, incompatible platelets and plasma are administered.

The problems potentially associated with administration of out-of-group platelet transfusions include: decreased platelet count increment,[16] acute hemolysis from incompatible plasma,[17] and transfusion reaction symptoms associated with acute hemolysis of residual incompatible red cells in pooled platelets from whole blood. Less well-defined issues such as rate of development of alloimmunization and immunomodulatory effects of receiving or creating circulating immune complexes are also potential problems.

With respect to posttransfusion platelet count increment, various studies, largely in adults, observed varying outcomes of out-of-group platelet transfusions. Some studies observed no difference in increment, whereas other studies observed a significantly lower increment if either the plasma or the platelets were not compatible with the recipient.[18] For example, one study observed a 64% higher corrected count increment in patients receiving only ABO-identical platelets in comparison to patients receiving out-of-group transfusions.[16]

Clearly there are both recipient- and donor-specific characteristics related to the ABO system that may affect platelet count increment. Specifically, if either the donor or recipient is group O and has an especially high anti-A titer and there is a group O vs group A incompatibility, then these transfusions are associated with lower increments or greater risk of acute reactions.[19] This is especially relevant for pediatric recipients of multiple transfusions. For example, a 1999 report detailed adverse outcomes in three infants receiving incompatible plasma in platelet transfusions.[20] Infants and small, frequently-transfused pediatric recipients may be at greatest risk because the amount transfused relative to their size is often greater than an adult would receive. (Very few adults receive 15 to 20 mL/kg of incompatible plasma during a platelet transfusion, a common transfusion volume of platelet-rich plasma for neonates.)

In addition, group A or B infants normally have lower levels of circulating A or B substance and frequently-transfused pediatric patients may have had their circulating A,B group substances depleted, thereby diminishing the buffering capacity of the substance to adsorb A,B antibody. Finally, analogous to the greater risk from a plateletpheresis donor with high titer anti-A, such infants are more likely to receive an unpooled transfusion, ie, apheresis platelets from a single donor with high-titer anti-A in contrast to plasma diluted in a pool of 5-6 platelets if transfused to an adult.

Other effects of receiving out-of-group transfusions should be noted. Transfusion services should be aware that a frequent complication of administration of incompatible plasma is the likelihood of a positive direct antiglobulin test (DAT).[21] More controversial was a report by Benjamin and Antin of decreased survival of allogeneic marrow transplant recipients receiving marrow from out-of-group ABO donors who also received platelet transfusions incompatible with the recipient's original ABO group.[22] This information was not confirmed by other studies.[23] Finally, another report describes a higher rate of venoocclusive disease in children undergoing autologous hematopoietic transplantation who received ABO-mismatched platelets. The study does not control for the fact that those most likely to receive the out-of-group transfusions may have been the sickest, ie, those requiring the most transfusions may simply also be those at greatest risk for veno-occlusive disease.[24]

Rh Matching of Platelet Components

Because oncology and transplant patients are frequently transfused, having ready access to sufficient supplies of D-negative RBC units for patients requiring them is important. Conversely, the necessity to always have D-negative platelets on hand is far more controversial. Simply put, platelets do not express the Rh antigens. Thus, for a component such as apheresis platelets whose red cell content is extremely small, it may not even be necessary to consider Rh. Indeed, one study of adult transplant patients documented failure to observe any development of new D antibodies in 67 consecutive D-negative patients who received both D-positive and D-negative platelets during their entire treatment course.[25]

Because pooled platelets derived from whole blood may visibly contain red cells, there is greater risk of sensitization. However, especially in the course of the immuno-suppression associated with transplant therapy, the rates of sensitization may be lower than otherwise expected. One study observed a 19% rate (3 of 16) of anti-D sensitization in D-negative patients receiving large numbers of D-positive (whole-blood-derived) platelets during the course of autologous transplant. They had received 50 to 100 D-positive components during the course of transplantation and developed antibodies 13 to 83 days after the procedure. Two of the three also developed anti-C.[26] Hence, the development of an antibody, even when it does occur, may appear sufficiently far into the transplantation that it occurs after receipt of most of the red cell units anyway. Because the worst outcome of sensitization is that further red cell transfusions would require a full (as opposed to an abbreviated) crossmatch, the risks engendered by not always providing D-negative platelets are small. In addition, with the advent of the availability of an intravenous form of anti-D immunoglobulin, one can simply provide the smallest available dose, 120 μg (which covers infusion of up to approximately 7 mL of red cells—far more than would occur in even the bloodiest pool of random-donor platelets) to female patients of current or future childbearing potential. (Note: One can no longer presume that the chemotherapy and radiation administered during the course of transplantation will preclude future childbearing potential, as more than one such patient has stored oocytes or used other donor oocytes with the plan for subsequent childbearing should the transplant be successful. There are also case reports of women conceiving after high-dose chemotherapy and stem cell rescue even after total body irradiation.) In short, recognizing that D-negative platelets—especially apheresis platelets—may not always be available, policies and procedures should be in place to allow the use of platelets from D-positive donors, and provision of Rh immune globulin for the patients that warrant it.

Allogeneic Transplantation—Unique Issues

ABO Nonidentity Between Donor and Recipient

When the hematopoietic cell donor and recipient are not identical with respect to ABO group, the transfusion service faces special challenges that are best addressed before transplantation.[27] First, there is a risk of acute hemolytic transfusion reactions either during the hematopoietic cell infusion itself (due to clinically significant volumes of either incompatible red cells or plasma), or due to ongoing blood component support. More insidious are issues of delayed hemolysis or delay in red cell engraftment that may occur as a result of the changing ABO groups.[28] Indeed, while few blood bankers generally regard delayed hemolytic transfusions with the same concern as acute reactions, there are published cases where engraftment of donor lymphocytes resulted in hemolysis so severe that exchange transfusion by apheresis was required.[29] In fact, some physicians have advocated red cell exchange prophylactically to avoid this occurrence.[30] Allogeneic PBPC transplants across ABO types can also cause hemolysis following engraftment of a minor incompatible (eg, group O donor and group A patient) transplant.[31] Indeed, patients who receive PBPCs are more likely than marrow recipients to have high-titer donor-derived anti-A and/or anti-B and other red cell alloantibodies detectable in their serum during the first 30 days after transplantation.[32] Major incompatible allogeneic donations (eg, a group A donor and a group O recipient) may also be associated with considerable, but selective delay in red cell engraftment.[33] One should anticipate larger red cell transfusion requirements in recipients of such mismatches if they have already developed a significant titer before the transplant.

In short, the general rule is to provide blood components immediately before and after admission for a hematopoietic transplant that are ideally compatible with both the donor and recipient types (see Tables 18-1 and 18-2). In practice, this may be difficult in that it may functionally require a disproportionately large use of components containing group O red cells and group AB plasma. Because group AB platelets are typically in limited supply, this often simply requires judicious use of volume reduction when a plasma-containing component that is mutually compatible with donor and recipient alike is not available. Finally, with regard to platelet selection, there are far fewer and less severe complications associated with group A plasma being given to a patient with group B or AB red cells than with group O plasma being given to a patient with group A red cells. In most settings (including pediatric transfusion), group B recipients tolerate larger volumes of incompatible group A plasma and group A recipients tolerate more incompatible group B plasma than a group A recipient would tolerate group O plasma.

Table 18-1. Suggested RBC Components When PBPC Donor and Recipient Are of Different ABO Groups

	Donor			
Patient	**O**	**A**	**B**	**AB**
O	O	O	O	O
A	O	A/O	O	A/O
B	O	O	B/O	B/O
AB	O	A/O	B/O	ANY*

*While any ABO group red cells may be administered, one must consider platelet transfusions (see Table 18-2). In the event that apheresis platelets are to be transfused, the availability of group AB apheresis units, or the need to volume-reduce the plasma if no group AB apheresis units should be considered. A practical alternative is to consider using group A red cells, which in turn allows the use of group A platelet donations that will be much more available and preclude the need to volume-reduce.)

Nonidentical Rh Components in Hematopoietic Transplantation

With a D-positive donor and a D-negative recipient, there is no need to provide D-negative components, because the new im-

Table 18-2. Suggested Plasma-Containing Components When Donor and Recipient Are of Different ABO Groups

	Donor			
Patient	**O**	**A**	**B**	**AB**
O	ANY	A	B/AB	AB*
A	A	A	AB	AB*
B	B	AB/A*	B/AB	AB*
AB	AB/A*/B*	AB/A*	AB	AB*

*Recognizing that there may be limited availability of group AB platelet components, the option to volume-reduce to minimize the volume of incompatible plasma may be considered (see text).

mune system will become tolerized to D-positive red cells. While it is possible to begin administering D-positive cells at the time of admission, most transfusion services prefer to ensure consistency for their staff by not providing positive components until the recipient's type is officially designated as D-positive. In practice, some centers will transfuse at least some D-positive components, such as platelets, from the time of admission, whereas others may wait until there is evidence of engraftment before providing D-positive red cells.

Conversely, with a D-negative donor and a (formerly) D-positive recipient, there is a possibility that when the new immune system engrafts, there could be a vigorous delayed hemolytic transfusion reaction. Depending upon the residual content of D-positive cells, up to the entire red cell mass of the patient could be subject to hemolysis.[34,35] Many facilities provide D-negative red cell components from the time of admission, or even shortly beforehand.

With respect to platelet transfusion, see the discussion earlier in this chapter.

Alternatives to Transfusion

With the relative vanquishing of transfusion-transmitted viral disease risks, the urgency to find alternatives to transfusion has decreased. Indeed, recently published data following implementation of nucleic acid amplification testing put the current residual risk of human immunodeficiency virus and hepatitis C virus at less than one chance in a million.[36] Hence, the use of growth factors to diminish transfusion support requirements has seen little application in pediatric protocols outside of those that use granulocyte colony-stimulating factor to mobilize PBPCs or to diminish the length of time a patient is profoundly neutropenic and at greater risk of infection.

Anecdotally, many clinicians have treated children whose parents have religious objections to transfusion, eg, Jehovah's witnesses, where the judicious use of erythropoietin has successfully prevented transfusions altogether in pediatric patients being treated on relatively non-transfusion-intensive protocols, such as those for brain tumors. In adults and in children, the use of erythropoietin to decrease red cell transfusion needs is limited,[37] because most of these patients will already have high-to-normal erythropoietin levels and will therefore have modest responses to the drug. Similarly, platelet-specific growth factors are in limited use. Interleukin (IL)-11 is active in thrombopoiesis[38] and has been shown to decrease platelet transfusion requirements during dose-intensive chemotherapy.[39] The platelet effects of IL-11 have not justified the cost, inconvenience, or side effects such as dilutional anemia in most clinician's minds. Thrombopoietin, an extremely active stimulator of platelet production in normal individuals,[40] has had disappointing efficacy in the setting of intensive chemotherapy. One form of thrombopoietin has induced thrombopoietin antibodies[41] (resulting in aplastic anemia or chronic idiopathic thrombocytopenic purpura) in a small number of patients receiving this agent. Many protocols for autologous transplantation in adult patients do not include transfusion.[42]

Directed Donations

While the pros and cons of directed donations have been debated, their use for oncology and transplantation patients may be particularly problematic, because of the many logistic issues encountered as well as more theoretical concerns about immunologic sensitization. The logistic issues relate to the frequent transfusions required by this patient population, the practical impossibility of linking all donations to a patient from just one or a few donors, and the urgency with which many of the transfusions are given. Because a directed donation often requires at least 24 hours for processing and testing prior to being available (even longer if it doesn't pass all required tests on the first round of testing), there is the danger that a well-intentioned parent may, in fact, inhibit prompt care by insisting on a directed donation that may be quite delayed in its administration. Most programs have found these logistic prohibitions so great that they simply preclude the ordering of directed donor apheresis platelet components for all the reasons stated above.

More important, one of the complications of frequent platelet transfusion is platelet alloimmunization due usually to HLA antibodies. Because development of HLA antibodies could both theoretically increase the risk of graft rejection, and diminish the effectiveness of family-related platelet donations, most programs try to avoid using family members as blood donors prior to transplants.[43] This is especially important since the advent of platelet crossmatching, in that if the patient is demonstrating signs of alloimmunization (poor platelet count increments and demonstration of HLA antibodies) many programs may turn to family members as potential apheresis platelet donors as they are the most likely to share HLA antigens that the recipient is not yet sensitized to. The early use of family members as donors may preclude the ability to use them later when they could, in fact, be most useful.

Autologous Donations

With a single exception, there is little relevance of autologous donation of red cells in transfusion support of pediatric oncology patients. The exception occurs in the setting of allogeneic marrow transplantation where a donor of sufficient size and maturity (typically greater than 80 pounds and 10 years of age) may agree to autologous blood collection before a marrow harvest. As an alternative, in the setting of major mismatched (ie, group A donor and group O recipient), red cell depletion of the allogeneic marrow collection is typically performed before infusion. Depending upon the separation method used, a deviation from standard practice may be considered to allow rescue of the red cells removed from the marrow to be reinfused into the donor. Reports of successful application of this practice have been published, albeit prior to the currently highly regulated transfusion environment.[44]

Cord Blood

Umbilical cord blood as a source for hematopoietic cells for transplantation has greatly increased over the last decade. While both related and unrelated donors have been used, the largest growth has followed the establishment of many unrelated cord blood banks as an alternative for patients for whom another matched donor is not available. Perhaps their greatest utility is the observation that perhaps due to the relative immunologic immaturity of the lymphocytes included in the graft, the degree of TA-GVHD does not appear to be any higher despite relatively less well-matched transplants. Specifically, several studies have not observed any greater frequency or severity of Grade II, III, or IV GVHD in cord blood transplants with one to three mismatched loci than case-controlled unrelated allogeneic marrow transplants with full matches.[45]

If immunologic tolerance is the boon of cord blood transplantation, delayed engraftment is its bane. While patients appear to be supportable throughout the transplant procedure, the delay in WBC engraftment puts the recipients at higher risk for infection due to granulocytopenia, as well as delayed immunologic reconstitution from apparent delays in CD8 activity. Median day to neutrophil engraftment is around 4 weeks in several series.[46] The marked delays in platelet and red cell engraftment put the recipient at risk for far greater transfusion requirements than with transplants using other hematopoietic sources. Specifically, the median day to platelet recovery (>20,000/µL for at least 7 days without transfusion) was 58 (range 35 to 142) and for red cells the median day was 60, (range 21 to 273). These delays result in marked increases in the amount of transfusion support required for cord blood transplant recipients, especially as these transplants have been extended to larger and older recipients.[47]

PBPCs vs Marrow: Implications for Transfusion

At least one pediatric study documented a significant economic advantage for PBPCs as the hematopoietic progenitor source in comparison with marrow. Specifically, the more rapid engraftment with the former led to fewer neutropenic days, shorter length of stay, fewer days of treatment with antibiotics, and considerably fewer transfusions.[48]

Table 18-3. Complications of Transfusion in Hematopoietic Transplantation

Reaction/Complication Type	Etiology	Therapy
Coagulopathy	Excessive heparin in allogeneic marrow	Volume reduction of marrow
Hemolysis	Either incompatible red cells or plasma in hematopoietic cell product	Red cell depletion of marrow, or volume reduction or washing to remove incompatible plasma
Sepsis	Bacterial contamination	Process controls in marrow harvest treat with antibiotics
Volume overload	Excessive volume	Volume reduction of marrow
Line occlusion	Particulate clumping within infused product	Use of a 170-micron filter for reinfusion of marrow or PBPCs
Nausea, vomiting, cough, cardiac arrhythmias, neurologic symptoms, hypo- or hypertension	DMSO in cryopreserved hematopoietic cell reinfusion	Thaw-wash protocols to remove excessive DMSO or limiting the amount and rate of reinfusion

Acute Transfusion Reactions and Complications Associated with Hematopoietic Therapy

Many different types of adverse reactions or complications are associated with infusion of hematopoietic progenitors.[49] Many, if not most, of these are associated with previously cryopreserved components and can, in turn, be linked to the cryoprotectant dimethyl sulfoxide (DMSO). Table 18-3 delineates different types of reactions, their apparent etiologies, and strategies to either avoid or treat the reaction or complication.

Conclusion

In summary, pediatric oncology and hematopoietic transplantation patients form but a subset of all pediatric patients. Rules and guidelines within institutions for transfusing such patients should be set with all transfused pediatric patients in mind, yet reflect the flexibility and resources available to meet the special needs of these challenging yet rewarding patients. With the ongoing successes in treatment of various oncologic maladies, strategies need to include the possibility—even the probability—that these patients may live another 70 years after transfusion. Therefore, all reasonable measures to preclude viral transmission and alloimmunization are going to be most cost-effective within this special group. Indeed, cost-effectiveness studies with adults concluded that apheresis platelets are wasted on oncology patients and should instead better be used on adults undergoing cardiac bypass, because of the low likelihood of cure and relatively short posttreatment survivals.[50] In contrast, the high likelihood of cure and long survival following successful treatment for pediatric ALL, if plugged into these same formulae, would suggest that minimizing donor exposure still may have a role in the treatment of pediatric patients.

References

1. DeCoteau J, Haddad S, Blanchette V, Poon A. Refractoriness to platelet transfusions in children with acute leukemia. J Pediatr Hematol Oncol 2001;17(4):306-10.

2. TRAP. Leukocyte reduction and ultraviolet B irradiation of platelets to prevent alloimmunization and refractoriness to platelet transfusions. N Engl J Med 1997;337:1861-9.
3. Floss AM, Strauss RG, Goeken N, Knox L. Multiple transfusions fail to provoke antibodies against blood cell antigens in human infants. Transfusion 2001;26:419-22.
4. Bowden RA. Cytomegalovirus: Transmission by blood components and measures of prevention. In: Nance SJ, ed. Blood safety: Current challenges. Bethesda, MD: American Association of Blood Banks, 1992.
5. Dumont LJ, Luka J, Vanden Broeke T, et al. The effect of leukocyte-reduction method on the amount of human cytomegalovirus in blood products—a comparison of apheresis and filtration methods. Blood 2001;97:3640-7.
6. Hume H, Preiksaitis J. Transfusion associated graft-versus-host disease, cytomegalovirus infection and HLA alloimmunization in neonatal and pediatric patients. Transfus Sci 1999;21(1):73-95.
7. Zulian GB, Roux E, Tiercy JM, et al. Transfusion-associated graft-versus-host disease in a patient treated with Cladribine (2-chlorodeoxyadenosine): Demonstration of exogenous DNA in various tissue extracts by PCR analysis. Br J Haematol 1995;89(1):83-9.
8. Williamson LM, Lowe S, Love EM, et al. Serious hazards of transfusion (SHOT) initiative: Analysis of the first two annual reports. Br Med J 1999;319:16-19.
9. Luban N. Prevention of transfusion-associated graft-versus-host disease by inactivation of T cells in platelet components. Semin Hematol 2001; 38:34-45.
10. Wadsworth LD, Herd SL, Stanley CE. Unique aspects of marrow collection, processing and transplantation in pediatric patients. In: Sacher R, AuBuchon J, eds. Marrow transplantation: Practical and technical aspects of stem cell reconstitution. Bethesda, MD: American Association of Blood Banks, 1992:129-56.
11. Beutler E. Platelet transfusions: The 20,000/μL trigger. Blood 1993;81 (6):1411-13.
12. Kelleher JF. When to give platelet transfusions. Blood 1993;82(2):682, 683.
13. Sagmeister M, Oec L, Gmur J. A restrictive platelet transfusion policy allowing long-term support of outpatients with severe aplastic anemia. Blood 1999;93(9):3124-6.
14. Pisciotto P, Benson K, Hume H, et al. Prophylactic versus therapeutic platelet transfusion practices in hematology and/or oncology patients. Transfusion 1995;35:498-502.
15. Rebulla P. Platelet transfusion trigger in difficult patients. Transfus Clin Biol 2001;8(3):249-54.
16. Heal JM, Rowe JM, Blumberg N. ABO and platelet transfusion revisited. Ann Hematol 1993;66:309-14.

17. Larsson LG, Welsh VJ, Ladd DJ. Acute intravascular hemolysis secondary to out-of-group platelet transfusion. Transfusion 2001;40:902-6.
18. Lee EJ, Schiffer CA. ABO Compatibility can influence the results of platelet transfusion: Results of a randomized trial. Transfusion 1989;29: 384-9.
19. Friedberg R, Donnelly SF, Boyd JC, et al. Clinical and blood bank factors in the management of platelet refractoriness and alloimmunization. Blood 2001;81:3428-34.
20. Duguid JKM, Minards J, Bolton-Maggs HB. Lesson of the week: Incompatible plasma transfusions and haemolysis in children. Br Med J 1999;318:176-7.
21. Shanwell A, Ringden O, Wiechel B, et al. A study of the effect of ABO incompatible plasma in platelet concentrates transfused to bone marrow transplant recipients. Vox Sang 1991;60:23-7.
22. Benjamin RJ, Antin JH. ABO-incompatible bone marrow transplantation: The transfusion of incompatible plasma may exacerbate regimen-related toxicity. Transfusion 1999;39:1273-4.
23. Butch S, Hoffman SK, Krijanovski OI, Davenport RD. Does transfusion of ABO incompatible plasma with platelet transfusions decrease platelet survival? (abstract). Transfusion 2000;40(Suppl):133S.
24. Lapierre V, Mahe C, Stambouli F, et al. Transfusion of ABO-incompatible plasma with platelet concentrates is a risk factor for hepatic veno-occlusive disease after autologous haematopoietic stem cell transplantation in young children (abstract). Blood 2000;96(11):818a.
25. Klumpp TR, Herman J, Innis S, et al. Factors associated with response to platelet transfusion following hematopoietic stem cell transplantation. Bone Marrow Transplant 1996;17(6):1035-41.
26. McLeod BC, Piehl MR, Sassetti RJ. Alloimmunization to RhD by platelet transfusions in autologous bone marrow transplant recipients. Vox Sang 1990;59(3):185-9.
27. Bensinger WI, Buckner CD, Thomas ED, Clift RA. ABO-incompatible marrow transplants. Transplantation 1982;33(4):427-9.
28. Hows J, Beddow K, Gordon-Smith E, et al. Donor-derived red blood cell antibodies and immune hemolysis after allogeneic bone marrow transplantation. Blood 1986;67(1):177-81.
29. Greeno E, Ilstrup S, Perry E, Weisdorf D. Total erythrocyte hemolysis following ABO donor incompatible bone marrow transplantation: Rapid appearance of donor-derived red cell antibodies (abstract). Blood 1992;80 (Suppl):484a.
30. Sniecinski I, Delaney G, Aldridge L, Nowicki B. Successful approach to prevention of the delayed immune hemolysis following minor ABO-mismatched marrow transplantation (abstract). J Clin Apheresis 1994; 9:85.

31. Bolan C, Childs R, Proctor J, et al. Massive immune haemolysis after allogeneic peripheral blood stem cell transplantation with minor ABO incompatibility. Br J Haematol 2001;112(3):787-95.
32. Lapierre V, Oubouzar N, Auperin A, et al. Influence of the hematopoietic stem cell source on early immunohematologic reconstitution after allogeneic transplantation. Blood 2001;97(9):2580-6.
33. Bolan CD, Leitman SF, Griffith LM, et al. Delayed donor red cell chimerism and pure red cell aplasia following major ABO-incompatible nonmyeloablative hematopoietic stem cell transplantation. Blood 2001; 98(6):1687-94.
34. Klumpp T. Immunohematologic complications of bone marrow transplantation. Bone Marrow Transplant 1991;8:159-70.
35. Franchini M, deGironcoli M, Gandini G, et al. Transmission of an anti-RhD alloantibody from donor to recipient after ABO-incompatible BMT. Bone Marrow Transplant 1998;21:1071-3.
36. Busch MP. Closing the windows on viral transmission by blood transfusion. In: Stramer S, ed. Blood safety in the new millennium. Bethesda, MD: American Association of Blood Banks, 2001:33-54.
37. Bottomley A, Thomas R, van SK, et al. Human recombinant erythropoietin and quality of life: A wonder drug or something to wonder about? Lancet Oncol 2002;3:145-53.
38. Braithwaite K, Abu-Ghosh A, Anderson L, Cairo MS. Treatment of severe thrombocytopenia with IL-11 in children with Wiskott-Aldrich syndrome. J Pediatr Hematol Oncol 2002;24:323-6.
39. Tepler I, Elias L, Smith JW, et al. A randomized placebo-controlled trial of recombinant human interleukin-11 in cancer patients with severe thrombocytopenia due to chemotherapy. Blood 1996;87:3607-14.
40. Kaushansky K, Drachman JG. The molecular and cellular biology of thrombopoietin: The primary regulator of platelet production. Oncogene 2002;21:3359-67.
41. Basser RL, O'Flaherty E, Green M, et al. Development of pancytopenia with neutralizing antibodies to thrombopoietin after multicycle chemotherapy supported by megakaryocyte growth and development factor. Blood 2002;99:2599-602.
42. Ballen K, Ford P, Waitkus H. Successful autologous bone marrow transplant without the use of blood product support. Bone Marrow Transplant 2000;26:227-9.
43. Kaminski ER, Hows JM, Goldman JM, Batchelor JR. Pretransfused patients with severe aplastic anemia exhibit high numbers of cytotoxic T lymphocyte precursors probably directed at non-HLA-antigens. Br J Haematol 1990;76:401-5.
44. Pleschourt S, Harbaugh C, Pineda A. Transfusion of residual red blood cells derived from a bone marrow harvest reduces allogeneic exposures (abstract). Transfusion 1994;34(Suppl):51S.

45. Barker JN, Davies SM, DeFor T, et al. Survival after transplantation of unrelated donor umbilical cord blood is comparable to that of human leukocyte antigen-matched unrelated donor bone marrow: Results of a matched-pair analysis. Blood 2001;97:2957-61.
46. Weinberg K, Blazar B, Wagner J, et al. Factors affecting thymic function after allogeneic hematopoietic stem cell transplantation. Blood 2001; 97(5):1458-66.
47. Laughlin M, Barker J, Bambach B, et al. Hematopoietic engraftment and survival in adult recipients of umbilical-cord blood from unrelated donors. N Engl J Med 2001;344(24):1860-1.
48. Vicent M, Madero L, Chamorro L, et al. Comparative cost analysis of autologous peripheral blood progenitor cell and bone marrow transplantation in pediatric patients with malignancies. Haematologica 2001; 86(10):1087-94.
49. Gorlin JB. Transfusion reactions associated with hematopoietic progenitor cell reinfusion. In: Popovsky MA, ed. Transfusion reactions, 2nd ed. Bethesda, MD: American Association of Blood Banks, 2001:235-54.
50. Lopez-Plaza I, Weissfeld J, Triulzi DJ. The cost-effectiveness of reducing donor exposures with single donor versus pooled random-donor platelets. Transfusion 1999;39(9):925-32.

In: Herman JH, Manno CS, eds.
Pediatric Transfusion Therapy
Bethesda, MD: AABB Press, 2002

19

Pediatric Peripheral Blood Progenitor Cell Transplantation

STEPHAN A. GRUPP, MD, PhD, AND JED GORLIN, MD

UNTIL RECENTLY, THE PRIMARY source of hematopoietic progenitor cells (HPCs) for use in autologous and allogeneic transplantation has been marrow. Over the past decade, there has been an increasing use of peripheral blood containing mobilized stem and progenitor cells for transplantation (Table 19-1).[1,2] This product is variously referred to as peripheral blood stem cells (PBSCs), peripheral blood progenitor cells (PBPCs), or given the shorthand designation "stem cells."

Stephan A. Grupp, MD, PhD, Director, Stem Cell Biology, Division of Oncology, Children's Hospital of Philadelphia, and Assistant Professor of Pediatrics, University of Pennsylvania, Philadelphia, Pennsylvania, and Jed Gorlin, MD, Medical Director, Memorial Blood Centers, Minneapolis, and Assistant Professor, Department of Laboratory Medicine, University of Minnesota, Minneapolis, Minnesota

Table 19-1. Cellular Characteristics of Various Hematopoietic Cell Sources

	Cell Source			
Characteristic	**Marrow**	**Peripheral Blood**	**G-CSF Primed Marrow**	**Umbilical Cord Blood**
Stem cell content	++	++	++	+
Progenitor cell content	++	++++	+++	+
T-cell content	+	++++	+	+/Functionally immature
Risk of tumor cell contamination in autologous transplant	++++	+	Not applicable	Not applicable

Plus marks connote relative degree of the stated effect or number.

The use of PBPCs has advantages and disadvantages, and the relative balance between these differs depending on the type of transplantation being performed, the disease state being treated, and the age and physiologic status of both donor and recipient. This chapter explores the indications for the use of PBPCs, drawing distinctions between well-established and more experimental use of these cells. Practical approaches to the collection and processing of PBPCs are discussed, with particular reference to special issues in pediatric transplantation.

Techniques for PBPC Mobilization

Although early attempts to collect PBPCs used steady-state peripheral blood as the source, it soon became apparent that large increases in the number of circulating stem and progenitor cells occur at the point of recovery from myelosuppressive chemotherapy, at which time large numbers of these cells are mobilized from the marrow. This typically occurs at a point when the absolute neutrophil count (ANC) has reached 1000 after the chemotherapy-induced nadir and is increasing rapidly. The exact point of maximal cell mobilization is difficult to predict and highly patient-dependent.

Chemotherapy-induced mobilization is possible using a large variety of myelosuppressive regimens. The most commonly used approach is to give cyclophosphamide (often at a total dose of 4 g/m^2 over 2 days). Multiple-drug regimens that are used in the treatment of the primary disease can also be used to induce a nadir after which PBPC collection is possible. PBPCs can be collected successfully after most chemotherapy regimens, including topoisomerase inhibitors such as etoposide. However, there is a concern that the DNA damage that occurs after treatment with etoposide may occur in hematopoietic cells, and this damage may increase the risk of secondary (treatment-related) leukemia in a patient who is reconstituted with these cells. In one study, use of PBPCs collected after etoposide resulted in a 7- to 12-fold relative risk of secondary leukemia,[3] with other studies also demonstrating an increased risk attributable more to the prior chemotherapy than to the preparative regimen used for the

HPC transplant.[4,5] This effect, together with the observation that multiple cycles of chemotherapy reduce the yields of PBPC collection,[6] argue that PBPCs should be collected as early in treatment as possible, but after sufficient therapy (usually two or three cycles of chemotherapy) to clear circulating tumor cells.[7]

The use of chemotherapy to mobilize PBPCs may not be possible or desirable in every patient, has a risk of toxicity during the nadir, and is clearly not appropriate for normal allogeneic donors in whom the chemotherapy has no potential benefit. An alternative approach—the use of hematopoietic growth factors (HGFs)—is in widespread use.[8] Donors are placed on a daily regimen of HGF injections, followed by initiation of PBPC collection on day 4 or 5 of treatment. HGF treatment continues until the apheresis is complete. There are several choices of HGF doses and regimens (Table 19-2). Filgrastim (rHuG-CSF) is the most common HGF used for this purpose. Doses given vary widely. There is a modest dose-response effect between 2 and 16 μg/kg of G-CSF. Although doses as high as 24 μg/kg/day have been used for mobilization, there is little evidence that these very high doses are more efficacious and they have the disadvantage of greater cost and higher incidence of side effects,[9] especially bone pain.

Table 19-2. Regimens for PBPC Mobilization

- Cyclophosphamide 2000 mg/m^2/day over 2 days, followed by G-CSF 5 μg/kg/day subcutaneously from day 3 to the end of apheresis
- G-CSF 5 μg/kg/day subcutaneously for 3 to 4 days, followed by apheresis on days 4 and 5 and following.
- GM-CSF 250 μg/m^2/day subcutaneously for 3 to 4 days, followed by apheresis on days 4 and 5 and following.
- Combination of G-CSF 5-10 μg/kg/day (subcutaneously in morning) and GM-CSF 250 μg/m^2/day (subcutaneously in afternoon) for 4 days, apheresis starting on day 5.
- Other chemotherapy/hematopoietic growth factor combinations.

Sargramostim (rHuGM-CSF) is an alternative. Comparisons of G-CSF and GM-CSF as single agents reveal either no significant advantage of one HGF over the other in terms of PBPC collection efficiency or extent of progenitor cell mobilization,[10] or a modest advantage for G-CSF.[11,12] Laboratory studies have suggested that PBPCs collected after G-CSF mobilization may have a polarization in T-cell response toward the more suppressive T-helper lymphocyte type 2 (Th2) response.[13,14] This may in turn have an impact on 1) the recovery of cellular immunity after HPC transplantation and 2) the risk of graft-vs-host disease (GVHD) after allogeneic HPC transplantation,[15] but this has not been proven in a clinical trial. The extent to which GM-CSF may not cause this Th2 polarization has not been well studied. The combination of G-CSF and GM-CSF may be superior to either alone, although one pediatric study failed to show an advantage for the combination.[16] In any case, most donors will mobilize well with a single HGF and will not require this combination.

The one setting in which the combination of G-CSF plus GM-CSF may be superior is when a patient has had inadequate numbers of HPCs collected over several apheresis procedures. In these so-called "poor mobilizers," combination HGF regimens may improve the likelihood that adequate PBPCs can be collected.[17,18] Other HGFs have been tested as PBPC mobilizers and work as well,[19] including stem cell factor[17,20,21] and thrombopoietin,[22] but there is no evidence to suggest superiority in terms of clinical outcome during transplantation over the standard use of G-CSF, even when higher numbers of CD34+ cells are collected. On the other hand, collection of higher numbers of CD34+ cells has the potential to reduce the number of large-volume leukapheresis (LVL) procedures a donor must undergo, which is a benefit in terms of cost, convenience, and potential donor exposure, especially in pediatric practice. Balanced against this is the high cost of HGFs, and the fact that adding a second HGF doubles this cost.[16] In patients who are receiving myelosuppressive chemotherapy, HGFs such as filgrastim are often used to improve recovery. The concurrent use of chemotherapy and an HGF improves PBPC mobilization as well,[23,24] although a randomized trial did not show this improved mobilization to have an impact on survival or engraftment.[25] Thus, any patient receiving chemotherapy after which PBPC collection is planned should be treated with an HGF, even if similar courses during the treatment are not supported by an HGF.

PBPC Collection

After mobilization, the PBPCs are collected through the use of apheresis technology, which can separate specific components from whole blood continuously and in real time by centrifugation. Any component can be targeted for relatively specific removal—plasma, red cells, platelets, or white cells. After venous blood is collected and processed through the apheresis machine, the nontargeted components are returned to the patient. Significant advances in the techniques employed in pediatric apheresis have allowed collection from donors as small as 6 to 10 kg.[26]

In order to allow continuous blood processing for PBPC collection, two ports of vascular access are necessary. In most adults, this can be accomplished using two antecubital lines. In 5% to 10% of adults and most children, percutaneous antecubital large-bore access is not possible and an apheresis catheter is used instead. A veno-arterial approach, utilizing an arterial line to draw blood and a conventional venous catheter to return it to the patient, has also been described.[27,28] Although there are many configurations, the apheresis catheter is generally a two-lumen catheter with offset proximal and distal ports and side holes along the tip of the catheter. This offset configuration minimizes mixing of processed and unprocessed blood and maximizes the efficiency of the collection. Conventional Broviac-type catheters are difficult to use for apheresis, especially in pediatric sizes, because the lumen collapses under the negative pressure used to draw blood at a useful rate for apheresis (generally 2 mL/kg/minute). Thus, an apheresis catheter is designed to allow faster draw rates using a combination of larger lumen size, shorter catheter length, and stiffer walls. This general design is similar to that of dialysis catheters and these catheters can be, and are, used for apheresis purposes. However, as the flow rates required for apheresis are lower than those required for dialysis, a dialysis-type catheter is generally larger and stiffer than a catheter specifically designed for apheresis.

Apheresis catheters are available both for temporary and tunneled insertion. For smaller patients (as small as 10 kg, depending on the operator's assessment of the patient), an 8 Fr cuffed tunneled apheresis catheter (MedComp, Harleysville, PA) can be used. Smaller patients generally require femoral line placement. The concern in smaller patients is threefold: 1) the risk of partial or complete vessel occlusion with the catheter, 2) the risk of vessel erosion and perforation, which may be greater with stiffer catheters in small vessels,[29] and 3) the difficulty in placing an offset catheter in a short vessel where, if the proximal port is in an adequate position, the distal port may be too far advanced. Femoral catheters are short, allowing faster collection rates for a given diameter. However, a patient with a percutaneous nontunneled femoral catheter cannot walk, necessitating admission to the hospital for what is otherwise an outpatient procedure. Also, the perceived risk of complication (especially infection) with a femoral catheter is higher.[30] For both of these reasons, femoral catheters are generally placed only temporarily, except in unusual circumstances.[31] Another approach used at some institutions is to place a single-lumen 7 Fr Broviac-type central venous catheter on the opposite side of the patient's existing double-lumen catheter. The single-lumen line is then used as the draw line and the smaller double-lumen catheter is used as the return line.

Even in a mobilized patient, the number of HPCs circulating in the entire blood volume may be inadequate to provide engraftment. Thus, processing of multiple blood volumes, often over more than 1 day, is required for many patients to collect adequate numbers of cells.[32] The minimum required for most patients is 1 LVL procedure, which represents approximately 20 L in an adult or between three and four blood volumes in a child. This volume is the typical goal for a single apheresis session, although some physicians continue the procedure until six or more blood volumes are collected.[33] Depending on the collection goal and effectiveness of mobilization, patients will often undergo 2 or more days of apheresis. This is most often true in patients serving as autologous donors who have been extensively pretreated with chemotherapy. On the other hand, an untreated and healthy allogeneic donor, equal to or larger than the size of the recipient, will often require only one session.

There are two issues in PBPC collection that require special consideration in children. First is the issue of priming. Even with devices that minimize extracorporeal volume, apheresis for smaller children will require priming of the machine with red cells to prevent unacceptable dilutional anemia. Second is the issue of anticoagulation. In older patients, anticoagulation required for the apheresis procedure is accomplished using ACD. Although the effects of ACD are rapidly reversible, ACD creates a higher risk of symptomatic hypocalcemia in young patients. These patients are managed with a combination of ACD and heparin to achieve anticoagulation, or they receive a calcium infusion in the apheresis return line.

Target Dose for PBPC Infusion

When marrow is collected, most operators target a final volume, or more commonly, a volume and a nucleated cell dose. Because of the high variability in stem and progenitor cell content in PBPCs, a more direct assay is needed to ensure that adequate numbers for reliable engraftment have been collected. There is no well-established assay for human stem cells, although stem cell activity is likely to be found in a portion of cells that are detected by the long-term culture-initiating cell assay[34] or the SCID mouse repopulating cell assay.[35] Progenitor cell content can be assessed by the colony-forming unit–granulocyte/monocyte (CFU-GM) assay. The presence of 2 to 10 × 10^4 CFU-GM/kg of recipient weight is predictive of engraftment,[36] but the assay is laborious, expensive, and difficult to standardize. It also takes 14 days to complete, making it useless to assess PBPC collections in real time. For all these reasons, most centers have discontinued the use of CFU-GM assays.[37]

A major advance in the use of PBPCs was the recognition that most (although perhaps not all[38,39]) of the cells in the hematopoietic stem and progenitor cell compartment bear the antigen CD34, regardless of lineage.[40] Enumeration of CD34+ cells allows for more accurate assessment of engraftment potential provided by a given number of mononuclear cells. There is a threshold for reliable engraftment and a rough correlation between number of CD34+ cells collected above the threshold and the speed of engraftment (Table 19-3). The threshold for reliable engraftment is generally thought to be 1×10^6 CD34+ cells/kg.[41] Below this threshold, the likelihood of delayed engraftment of neutrophils and especially platelets increases.[42,43] Increasing the minimum acceptable number to 2 to 2.5×10^6 CD34+ cells/kg decreases this likelihood somewhat further,[44] and this is the threshold that most transplant centers attempt to achieve. Some authors have advocated a goal (rather than a minimum) of between 5 and 15×10^6 CD34+ cells/kg.[17] This higher goal is unrealistic in many patients, especially patients who have been treated with multiple cycles of chemotherapy prior to collection, and has the potential to significantly increase the cost and length of apheresis.

Table 19-3. Choosing Doses of PBPCs for Transplantation

Dose Level	CD34+ Cells/kg of Recipient Weight	Notes
Minimum	1×10^6	At this dose, there is some risk of prolonged neutropenia and extended platelet transfusion requirements
Optimum	2 to 2.5×10^6	Threshold dose for many centers
Ideal	5×10^6	There is a limited dose-response effect at doses $>2.5 \times 10^6$ cells, and this target may increase number of apheresis procedures needed and cost

CD34+ cells in the marrow can range from 1% to 4% of the total cells, while CD34+ cells in mobilized apheresis products can range from 0.1% (in a poor mobilizer) to >1%. The assay for CD34+ cells is a flow cytometric assay,[45,46] and this technique is inherently inaccurate at low percentages. This means that the number of CD34+ cells based on a measured frequency of 0.1% could easily be off by twofold in either the direction of more or fewer cells. This variation must be borne in mind when clinicians are assessing when to stop apheresis procedures in patients with poor collections. In collections that have undergone CD34 selection (see Processing), the CD34 purity is generally >60% and these determinations are extremely accurate. Another consideration is that PBPC collections with low CD34 cell counts often may have a higher granulocyte content, which can complicate freezing/thawing and therefore have an impact on yield of cells actually infused after storage.

There are many different approaches to determining optimal timing of apheresis for the highest number of PBPCs. The goals are to obtain adequate numbers of PBPCs as defined above, preferably in a single collection procedure. When HGF regimens alone are used, timing is simple: the donor undergoes apheresis on either the fourth or fifth day of HGF administration. After chemotherapy, the point at which the best collection can be obtained is more difficult to predict. Peripheral WBC count is a poor predictor of stem cell mobilization.[47] There is some theoretical concern for donor safety and possible hyperleukocytosis at WBC counts of more than 70×10^9/L, and some advocate G-CSF dose reductions for donors whose WBC count reaches this level.[48] Many centers use some variation on the following algorithm: 1 to 3 days after the ANC reaches 1000 after the nadir, at a point where there is some evidence of platelet recovery, PBPC collection begins. Rather than using a rising neutrophil count to trigger apheresis, some centers with access to rapid-turnaround, quantitative (or "absolute") CD34+ cell counts use the increase in peripheral CD34+ cells to schedule the initiation of collection. Detection of <5 CD34+ cells/μL of blood is highly predictive of poor PBPC collection, whereas >10 to 20 CD34+ cells/μL correlates well with the likelihood of collecting $>2.5 \times 10^6$ CD34 cells/kg in a single LVL procedure.[47,49]

Processing and Storage of PBPCs

Most PBPC preparations collected to support transplant procedures are autologous, and must be cryopreserved for later use. In the allogeneic setting, products can be collected before the start of pretransplant conditioning in the recipient or they can be collected on the day of intended infusion. In addition to cryopreservation, other processing options exist, depending on the purpose for which the PBPCs will be used. Specific engineering of the graft is possible to remove or expand desired cell populations. For patients undergoing allogeneic PBPC transplantation, cells are collected from normal donors (see below). Because the donor does not undergo the conditioning for the transplant, these cells can be collected at the time of use and do not need to be cryopreserved. The advantage of this "just in time" strategy is that there is no cell loss due to freezing and thawing. The disadvantage is that, if there is trouble collecting PBPCs, either because of access issues or because the donor is a poor mobilizer, the recipient has already been conditioned and there is considerable time pressure to accomplish any back-up measures (line placement, alternative mobilization strategies, or marrow harvest).

After collection, the PBPC product is taken to the processing laboratory. This is where procedures to ensure quality of the product take place, including determination of CD34+ cell content (see Target Dose), viability determinations, mononuclear cell counts, and confirmation of sterility. The various procedures involved in HPC processing have attracted more scrutiny from the Food and Drug Administration (FDA). Voluntary standards for HPC collection and processing have been promoted by both the Foundation for the Accreditation of Cellular Therapy (FACT)[50] and the AABB.[51] FACT has also established voluntary standards for the clinical care of donors and recipients.[50]

Options for stem cell processing[52] include 1) depletion of granulocytes by density gradient centrifugation,[53] 2) depletion of potential tumor cells by a direct purging technique or

CD34 selection,[54] and 3) depletion of T cells in an allogeneic product to decrease the risk of GVHD.[55] Many of the processing steps described here and below, with the notable exception of CD34 selection, were developed using marrow products and all are made somewhat more complicated by the considerably higher number of cells found in peripheral blood compared with marrow.

Cell Selection Techniques

All of these processing procedures either depend on negative selection (removal of the cell type that is unwanted) or positive selection (selection of stem/progenitor cells, leaving all other cells behind). CD34 selection is the primary positive selection technique available. CD34 is a cellular antigen that is expressed on stem cells, as well as progenitor cells of all hematopoietic lineages. Automated processes that select the CD34+ cell population[56] away from the 99% of PBPCs that are irrelevant for engraftment are available, and one of these technologies, the Isolex 300i device (Nexell Therapeutics, Irvine, CA),[57] is FDA-approved. An alternative device, the CliniMACS device (Miltenyi Biotec, Hamburg, Germany),[58,59] is approved in Europe and may become available in the United States. In general, CD34 cell selection will result in a product that is 60% to 95% CD34+ cells, removing more than 99% of T cells[60,61] and tumor cells,[62-64] providing that the tumor cells do not express the CD34 antigen. Hematopoietic tumors such as acute leukemias often express CD34[65,66] and are therefore not depleted by CD34 cell selection.

Negative selection procedures, by contrast, are tumor- or cell-type specific. Many techniques have been developed to negatively select T cells or T-cell subsets away from stem and progenitor cells in marrow and peripheral blood.[67] One technique uses a variety of monoclonal antibodies directed against T cells[68,69] such as OKT3 (anti-CD3),[70] Campath-1 (anti-CDw52),[71] and T10B9 (anti-TCR)[72,73] with or without complement. This type of procedure is technically difficult in PBPCs given the large number of T cells collected in the graft. Other techniques include counterflow centrifugal elutriation,[74] which separates lymphocytes based on physical characteristics, sheep red cell rosetting,[75,76] and immunomagnetic removal of T cells. Some of these procedures allow for more specific graft engineering by removing specific T-cell subsets such as CD8+ T cells[77] or T cells expressing activation markers such as CD25 or CD69.[78,79]

Depletion of Tumor Cells

It is also possible to deplete tumor cells using tumor-specific monoclonal antibodies, often followed by a magnetic depletion step. This approach has been proven to purge tumor cells from HPC products collected from patients with B cell lymphomas[80] and neuroblastoma,[81,82] among others. Gene marking studies have shown that tumor-contaminating products may contribute to relapse. In these studies, a marrow aliquot was transfected with a marker gene and infused after transplantation. Tumor cells at sites of relapse were found to contain the marker gene, suggesting that clonogenic tumor had been infused with the graft.[83] In follicular lymphoma, inability to detect tumor cells in the HPC product after purging is associated with improved outcome after autologous transplant,[80,84] but no study has shown that purging itself improves outcome. Compared with marrow, peripheral blood from a patient receiving high-dose chemotherapy and stem cell rescue (HDC/SCR) for a malignancy is less likely to contain tumor cells[85,86] and have a lower content of tumor cells if any are present. Therefore, tumor cells are more likely to be purged successfully from PBPC collections.[87]

Cryopreservation

After processing, PBPCs are cryopreserved for later infusion. Controlled-rate freezing with temperature curve monitoring is required. Products are stored in the vapor phase of liquid nitrogen until they are required for infusion.[88] Usually the storage period is weeks to months, but HPC products have provided adequate engraftment when infused 8 to 10 years after cryopreservation.[89] After thawing, PBPCs again are checked for viability.

Granulocytes do not survive cryopreservation, so loss of this cell fraction from the collection is expected. In order to allow cells to survive freezing and thawing, they are placed in a medium containing 7.5% to 10% dimethyl sulfoxide. Hematopoietic cells lose viability over time in this medium,[90] so it is important to infuse the cells immediately after thawing.

Indications for Autologous PBPC Transplantation

Commonly referred to as autologous transplantation, the use of the patient's own HPCs to support recovery from high-dose chemotherapy is more properly referred to as high-dose chemotherapy with stem cell rescue. The HDC regimen used to prepare the patient is usually myeloablative, meaning that no marrow recovery is possible without SCR. There are also submyeloablative HDC regimens, in which the SCR is used to speed recovery, decrease toxicity, and decrease treatment interval without being absolutely required for engraftment.[91,92]

Compared with autologous marrow, peripheral blood provides faster hematopoietic recovery from HDC; this in turn results in lower infection risk, more rapid resolution of mucositis, earlier discharge from the hospital, and less risk of prolonged need for transfusion, especially platelet transfusion. The use of PBPCs, along with other advances in prophylaxis and supportive care, have decreased the treatment-related mortality rate in autologous transplant to <5% in many studies. As a result, the use of autologous marrow to support HDC/SCR has very limited indications and has all but disappeared.[93] This improvement in treatment-related mortality has properly returned the focus of clinical studies in autologous transplantation to the issue of disease control. In the area of disease control, results have been more mixed. The general paradigm for HDC/SCR is that in chemosensitive disease, many or most patients can be put into complete remission (CR). However, in high-risk malignancies, the CR rate, which can be high, does not translate into a high 3- or 5-year event-free survival (EFS) rate. A good example of this is high-risk neuroblastoma, in which 80% of patients have responsive disease but <20% are long-term survivors with conventional chemotherapy.

There are several well-established indications for autologous HDC/SCR. One is relapsed Hodgkin's disease. Patients who relapse after modern combined modality therapy (multiagent chemotherapy plus involved field radiotherapy), are at very high risk for further progression. This is not true of patients who are treated with a single modality, in whom salvage rates are good. However, especially in the pediatric population where there is an increasing emphasis on decreasing the morbidity and risks of radiation therapy, many more patients are now treated with combined modality therapy. The high risk of subsequent relapse is seen even in the 70% of patients who successfully achieve a second CR. Use of HDC/SCR in relapsed Hodgkin's increases EFS to approximately 40% to 60%.[94] Achievement of CR before HDC/SCR confers improved prognosis,[95] although patients who are not in a complete remission prior to transplant but who achieve remission after transplant also benefit from the procedure.[94] The most commonly used conditioning regimen for Hodgkin's disease is BCNU, cyclophosphamide, and etoposide. There is a high risk of pulmonary fibrosis with this regimen, which can be largely but not completely avoided by ensuring that mantle (or any pulmonary) irradiation occurs after the HDC/SCR procedure, or that at least 3 months pass between radiotherapy involving the lung and the administration of high-dose BCNU.[96]

Another indication for HDC/SCR is high-risk neuroblastoma. Several studies have indicated that autologous marrow transplantation may improve the EFS in children with this disease.[97-99] More recently, the Children's Cancer Group 3891 study[100] showed improved EFS in children who underwent marrow transplantation compared with those treated with conventional chemotherapy. This study also showed a survival advantage for patients receiving the drug 13-cis-retinoic acid after the chemotherapy or transplantation was complete, and patients receiving both a transplant and cis-retinoic acid had an EFS at 3 years of approximately 40%.[100] This concept has been extended using the more rapid recovery and lower tumor burden afforded by PBPCs in a study that used two sequential cycles of HDC/SCR. The approach is called tandem transplant and allows for greater dose intensification in the consolidation phase. Three-year EFS in this multi-institution phase II study was 56% in patients with high-risk neuroblastoma.[101,102]

The role of HDC/SCR in the treatment of patients with metastatic sarcoma is less clear. Attempts to improve outcome for children with metastatic rhabdomyosarcoma have been an unequivocal failure. Some pilot studies of HDC/SCR in high-risk Ewing sarcoma patients have indicated improved EFS compared with historical controls but other studies have not and HDC/SCR has not been tested in a randomized study.[103] Similarly, pilot studies have suggested a survival advantage for patients with relapsed germ cell tumors,[104] but the approach has not been proven. HDC/SCR in single or multiple cycles is being tested in children with high-risk, chemosensitive brain tumors such as medulloblastoma,[105,106] but this remains entirely investigational. Finally, a number of limited clinical trials have been published using HDC/SCR (or, less frequently, allogeneic transplant) for high-risk autoimmune and rheumatologic diseases.[107] Although responses have been observed in patients with intractable disease, this is an indication best explored in the context of a controlled clinical trial.

Allogeneic Transplantation Using PBPCs

Although the use of PBPCs to support HDC/SCR is well established, using PBPCs instead of marrow-derived cells for allogeneic transplant is more investigational,[108-111] especially in pediatric practice,[112] although it is fast becoming a standard in adult transplantation.[93] PBPCs have higher numbers of progenitor cells, which result in faster engraftment in the autologous setting. PBPCs also have 10-fold higher T-cell content than marrow (Table 19-1), which carries with it the potential to increase the risk of acute and chronic GVHD.[113] PBPCs also have advantages and disadvantages in terms of collection as compared with marrow-derived cells.

From the point of view of engraftment, the higher CD34 content of PBPCs provides a modest improvement over marrow. This improvement in engraftment speed is somewhat less pronounced than that seen with HDC/SCR. Various studies of allogeneic PBPC transplants have shown that the time to achieve an ANC >500 improves from 1 to 6 days. Platelet engraftment also occurs between 4 and 7 days earlier with use of PBPCs. The degree of response is further improved by targeting higher CD34+ cell doses in PBPC collections, although this goal requires more collection time. Faster engraftment can result in shorter hospital stays, and studies have shown that patients supported with PBPCs are discharged up to 5 days earlier than patients receiving marrow. Graft failure, an uncommon complication of marrow transplantation using an unmanipulated product for grafting, may or may not be less likely with PBPCs.

Infusion of more T cells with a PBPC graft may increase the risk of GVHD. Most studies have not shown a significant increase in the risk of acute (prior to posttransplant day 100) GVHD with the use of PBPCs. The use of G-CSF to mobilize the PBPCs may decrease the risk of acute GVHD. On the other hand, there is a clear increase in chronic GVHD,[113,114] as well as an increase in the proportion of extensive, as opposed to limited, chronic GVHD. Extensive chronic GVHD is a devastating and often life-threatening complication of allogeneic transplantation. This complication has provided the principal barrier to wider adoption of PBPCs over marrow for allogeneic transplant. Because GVHD may decrease the risk of relapse in some patients with leukemia, the effect of PBPC support on relapse risk is being studied. However, there is not yet strong evidence that PBPC transplantation decreases leukemic relapse. An interesting intermediate option between mobilized PBPCs and marrow collected at steady state has recently emerged. This option is G-CSF-primed marrow collection,[115] with the justification being that this approach might increase progenitor cell dose without significantly increasing T-cell dose compared with steady-state marrow.[116] Early studies in this area show promise, with a recent randomized comparison of G-CSF-primed marrow and PBPCs in adults showing similar engraftment kinetics with significantly decreased rates of both acute and chronic GVHD in the patients receiving G-CSF-primed marrow.[117] Even with lower rates of GVHD, however, this 57-patient study did not detect a survival difference between the two study arms.

Marrow is usually collected under general anesthesia in the operating room from multiple punctures of the posterior iliac crest. Donors often stay overnight, and there is some residual discomfort for 5 to 14 days after the procedure. Strenuous exertion is not recommended for a week or so after harvesting. PBPC collection does not require general anesthesia or an inpatient stay for most patients. The actual collection procedure lasts 4 to 6 hours daily over 1 to 4 days, with the majority of donors only requiring 1 or 2 days of collection. The HGFs used for mobilization can cause moderate to severe bone pain in up to 50% to 70% of adults,[118-121] although this may be less frequent (or reported less frequently) in children receiving a growth factor.[122] Life-threatening events are very rare for either procedure, although general anesthesia carries a small risk. Splenic rupture, an unusual complication of G-CSF administration, has been described in patients with myeloid malignancies undergoing treatment including G-CSF,[123] as well as normal donors receiving G-CSF.[124-126] A retrospective study of 1488 allogeneic PBPC collections from normal donors found no fatalities.[127] There is also a small risk of bleeding in patients undergoing PBPC collection who start with a lower platelet count, as PBPC collection often causes temporary thrombocytopenia. Donors for pediatric patients are often children themselves, and this changes the risk/benefit consideration for choice of peripheral blood vs marrow from the donor's point of view.[112] Most pediatric PBPC donors will require apheresis catheter placement, usually under general anesthesia, with the attendant risks of pneumothorax and, remotely, infection. It may be that these risks are higher, lower, or similar to those experienced in the collection of marrow under general anesthesia. Many investigators feel that it is premature to routinely utilize PBPC collection in pediatric donors outside of the context of a controlled clinical trial until the risk/benefit relationship for these younger donors has been better defined.[128]

Cord Blood

In addition to marrow and peripheral blood, an alternative source of hematopoietic cells is umbilical cord blood.[34,129] As with peripheral blood, cord blood has certain advantages or disadvantages as a hematopoietic cell source. Cord blood is used almost exclusively for allogeneic transplantation.[130] The primary advantage of cord blood is that its use results in a somewhat lower risk of GVHD compared with marrow or peripheral blood. Thus, for a given degree of HLA matching, cord blood may have a lower risk of GVHD than marrow, although this risk is not abrogated.[129,131] This fact allows for a larger degree of HLA disparity to be tolerated in a cord blood transplant than a marrow transplant. A single HLA mismatch (out of six to eight relevant HLA loci) between donor and recipient would be tolerated at many centers performing marrow transplantation. The lower risk of GVHD seen with cord blood allows the use of a two-antigen mismatched product. Controversy exists concerning the use of a haplotype-mismatched cord blood unit (ie, 3/6 or 4/8 HLA matches). Some investigators believe that the risk of GVHD in such a haplotype-mismatched cord blood transplant is acceptable, while others feel that this use of such a product confers an unacceptably high risk of GVHD.

In addition to the possibility of GVHD, there are other issues to be considered in the choice of cord blood over marrow or peripheral blood. The first is that the volume of cord blood is limited to that which can be collected from the placenta after birth. Although the relative number of hematopoietic cells in cord blood is far higher than that seen in unmobilized peripheral blood in a child or adult,[132,133] the total number of cells is also very limited. Practically speaking, this limits the use of cord blood as a stem cell source to recipients who weigh less than 40 kg. The lower number of progenitor cells results in slower engraftment of neutrophils and especially platelets after transplantation, especially in a larger recipient receiving a relatively lower number of cells per unit body weight.[132,133] This in turn results in longer hospitalizations, a greater need for transfusions, and potentially higher risks for infection. For this reason, many transplant centers routinely administer G-CSF after cord blood transplantation.[134] A second issue concerns cord blood as a source of unrelated donor stem cells for transplant. Patients who do not have an HLA-matched sibling are considered for unrelated donor transplantation. The National Marrow Donor Program, which contains HLA information on more than 4 million potential marrow donors, has experienced a relatively lower success rate in finding unrelated marrow donors for African-American patients than for Caucasian patients. Design of a program to collect cord blood units for unrelated donation has therefore focused on attracting as many minority donors as possible in the hope of further improving the success rates for finding unrelated-donor stem cells for minority patients.

References

1. Korbling M, Dorken B, Ho AD, et al. Autologous transplantation of blood-derived hemopoietic stem cells after myeloablative therapy in a patient with Burkitt's lymphoma. Blood 1986;67:529-32.
2. Kessinger A, Armitage JO, Landmark JD, Weisenburger DD. Reconstitution of human hematopoietic function with autologous cryopreserved circulating stem cells. Exp Hematol 1986;14:192-6.
3. Krishnan A, Bhatia S, Slovak ML, et al. Predictors of therapy-related leukemia and myelodysplasia following autologous transplantation for lymphoma: An assessment of risk factors. Blood 2000;95:1588-93.
4. Kollmannsberger C, Beyer J, Droz JP, et al. Secondary leukemia following high cumulative doses of etoposide in patients treated for advanced germ cell tumors. J Clin Oncol 1998;16:3386-91.
5. Pedersen-Bjergaard J, Pedersen M, Myhre J, Geisler C. High risk of therapy-related leukemia after BEAM chemotherapy and autologous stem cell transplantation for previously treated lymphomas is mainly related to primary chemotherapy and not to the BEAM-transplantation procedure. Leukemia 1997;11:1654-60.
6. Jerjis S, Croockewit S, Preijers F, et al. Impact of chemotherapy on the mobilisation, harvest and economic costs of autologous peripheral stem cell transplantation in patients with multiple myeloma. Leuk Lymphoma 2000;37:551-60.
7. Moss TJ, Sanders DG, Lasky LC, Bostrom B. Contamination of peripheral blood stem cell harvests by circulating neuroblastoma cells. Blood 1990;76:1879-83.

8. Law P, Lane TA. Mobilization of allogeneic peripheral blood progenitor cells. Cancer Treat Res 2002;110:51-77.
9. Kroger N, Renges H, Sonnenberg S, et al. Stem cell mobilisation with 16 μg/kg vs 10 μg/kg of G-CSF for allogeneic transplantation in healthy donors. Bone Marrow Transplant 2002;29:727-30.
10. Gazitt Y. Comparison between granulocyte colony-stimulating factor and granulocyte-macrophage colony-stimulating factor in the mobilization of peripheral blood stem cells. Curr Opin Hematol 2002;9:190-8.
11. Bolwell BJ, Goormastic M, Yanssens T, et al. Comparison of G-CSF with GM-CSF for mobilizing peripheral blood progenitor cells and for enhancing marrow recovery after autologous bone marrow transplant. Bone Marrow Transplant 1994;14:913-18.
12. Weaver CH, Schulman KA, Buckner CD. Mobilization of peripheral blood stem cells following myelosuppressive chemotherapy: A randomized comparison of filgrastim, sargramostim, or sequential sargramostim and filgrastim. Bone Marrow Transplant 2001;27(Suppl 2):S23-29.
13. Sloand EM, Kim S, Maciejewski JP, et al. Pharmacologic doses of granulocyte colony-stimulating factor affect cytokine production by lymphocytes in vitro and in vivo. Blood 2000;95:2269-74.
14. Volpi I, Perruccio K, Tosti A, et al. Postgrafting administration of granulocyte colony-stimulating factor impairs functional immune recovery in recipients of human leukocyte antigen haplotype-mismatched hematopoietic transplants. Blood 2001;97:2514-21.
15. Gyger M, Stuart RK, Perreault C. Immunobiology of allogeneic peripheral blood mononuclear cells mobilized with granulocyte-colony stimulating factor. Bone Marrow Transplant 2000;26:1-16.
16. Madero L, Gonzalez-Vicent M, Molina J, et al. Use of concurrent G-CSF + GM-CSF vs G-CSF alone for mobilization of peripheral blood stem cells in children with malignant disease. Bone Marrow Transplant 2000;26:365-9.
17. Stiff PJ. Management strategies for the hard-to-mobilize patient. Bone Marrow Transplant 1999;23(Suppl 2):S29-33.
18. Bashey A, Corringham S, Gilpin E, et al. Simultaneous administration of G-CSF and GM-CSF for re-mobilization in patients with inadequate initial progenitor cell collections for autologous transplantation. Cytotherapy 2000;2:195-200.
19. Gazitt Y. Recent developments in the regulation of peripheral blood stem cell mobilization and engraftment by cytokines, chemokines, and adhesion molecules. J Hematother Stem Cell Res 2001;10:229-36.
20. Glaspy JA, Shpall EJ, LeMaistre CF, et al. Peripheral blood progenitor cell mobilization using stem cell factor in combination with filgrastim in breast cancer patients. Blood 1997;90:2939-51.
21. Facon T, Harousseau JL, Maloisel F, et al. Stem cell factor in combination with filgrastim after chemotherapy improves peripheral blood pro-

genitor cell yield and reduces apheresis requirements in multiple myeloma patients: A randomized, controlled trial. Blood 1999;94: 1218-25.
22. Somlo G, Sniecinski I, ter Veer A, et al. Recombinant human thrombopoietin in combination with granulocyte colony-stimulating factor enhances mobilization of peripheral blood progenitor cells, increases peripheral blood platelet concentration, and accelerates hematopoietic recovery following high-dose chemotherapy. Blood 1999;93:2798-806.
23. Knudsen LM, Gaarsdal E, Jensen L, et al. Improved priming for mobilization of and optimal timing for harvest of peripheral blood stem cells. J Hematother 1996;5:399-406.
24. Levine JE, Boxer LA. Clinical applications of hematopoietic growth factors in pediatric oncology. Curr Opin Hematol 2002;9:222-7.
25. Narayanasami U, Kanteti R, Morelli J, et al. Randomized trial of filgrastim versus chemotherapy and filgrastim mobilization of hematopoietic progenitor cells for rescue in autologous transplantation. Blood 2001;98:2059-64.
26. Gorlin JB, Humphreys D, Kent P, et al. Pediatric large-volume peripheral blood progenitor cell collections from patients under 25 kg: A primer. J Clin Apheresis 1996;11:195-203.
27. Takaue Y, Watanabe T, Abe T. Experience with peripheral blood stem cell collection for autografts in children with active cancer. Bone Marrow Transplant 1992;10:241-8.
28. Takaue Y, Kawano Y, Abe T, et al. Collection and transplant of peripheral blood stem cells in very small children weighing 20 kg or less. Blood 1995;85:372-80.
29. Welch RH, Gravenstein N, Blackshear RH. Multilumen central venous catheters in children: Relative potential to perforate vessels. An in vitro study. J Clin Monit 1997;13:75-9.
30. Merrer J, De Jonghe B, Golliot F, et al. Complications of femoral and subclavian venous catheterization in critically ill patients: A randomized controlled trial. JAMA 2001;286:700-7.
31. Chow KM, Szeto CC, Leung CB, et al. Cuffed-tunneled femoral catheter for long-term hemodialysis. Int J Artif Organs 2001;24:443-6.
32. Rowley SD, Yu J, Gooley T, et al. Trafficking of CD34+ cells into the peripheral circulation during collection of peripheral blood stem cells by apheresis. Bone Marrow Transplant 2001;28:649-56.
33. Gorlin JB, Vamvakas EC, Cooke E, et al. Large-volume leukapheresis from pediatric patients: Processing more blood volumes diminishes the apparent magnitude of intra-apheresis recruitment. Transfusion 1996; 36:879-85.
34. Broxmeyer HE, Douglas GW, Hangoc G, et al. Human umbilical cord blood as a potential source of transplantable hematopoietic stem/ progenitor cells. Proc Natl Acad Sci U S A 1989;86:3828-32.

35. Wang JC, Doedens M, Dick JE. Primitive human hematopoietic cells are enriched in cord blood compared with adult bone marrow or mobilized peripheral blood as measured by the quantitative in vivo SCID-repopulating cell assay. Blood 1997;89:3919-24.
36. Rowley SD, Zuehlsdorf M, Braine HG, et al. CFU-GM content of bone marrow graft correlates with time to hematologic reconstitution following autologous bone marrow transplantation with 4-hydroperoxycyclophosphamide-purged bone marrow. Blood 1987;70:271-5.
37. Papadopoulos KP, Ayello J, Tugulea S, et al. Harvest quality and factors affecting collection and engraftment of CD34+ cells in patients with breast cancer scheduled for high-dose chemotherapy and peripheral blood progenitor cell support. J Hematother 1997;6:61-8.
38. Goodell MA, Rosenzweig M, Kim H, et al. Dye efflux studies suggest that hematopoietic stem cells expressing low or undetectable levels of CD34 antigen exist in multiple species. Nat Med 1997;3:1337-45.
39. Dick JE. Absence of CD34 on some human SCID-repopulating cells. Ann N Y Acad Sci 1999;872:211-17; discussion 217-19.
40. Krause DS, Fackler MJ, Civin CI, May WS. CD34: Structure, biology, and clinical utility. Blood 1996;87:1-13.
41. Shpall EJ, Champlin R, Glaspy JA. Effect of CD34+ peripheral blood progenitor cell dose on hematopoietic recovery. Biol Blood Marrow Transplant 1998;4:84-92.
42. Weaver CH, Potz J, Redmond J, et al. Engraftment and outcomes of patients receiving myeloablative therapy followed by autologous peripheral blood stem cells with a low CD34+ cell content. Bone Marrow Transplant 1997;19:1103-10.
43. Diaz MA, Villa M, Madero L, et al. Analysis of engraftment kinetics in pediatric patients undergoing autologous PBPC transplantation. J Hematother 1998;7:367-73.
44. Weaver CH, Hazelton B, Birch R, et al. An analysis of engraftment kinetics as a function of the CD34 content of peripheral blood progenitor cell collections in 692 patients after the administration of myeloablative chemotherapy. Blood 1995;86:3961-9.
45. Trischmann TM, Schepers KG, Civin CI. Measurement of CD34+ cells in bone marrow by flow cytometry. J Hematother 1993;2:305-13.
46. Sutherland DR, Anderson L, Keeney M, et al. The ISHAGE guidelines for CD34+ cell determination by flow cytometry. International Society of Hematotherapy and Graft Engineering. J Hematother 1996;5:213-26.
47. Yu J, Leisenring W, Bensinger WI, et al. The predictive value of white cell or CD34+ cell count in the peripheral blood for timing apheresis and maximizing yield. Transfusion 1999;39:442-50.
48. Anderlini P, Przepiorka D, Korbling M, Champlin R. Blood stem cell procurement: Donor safety issues. Bone Marrow Transplant 1998;21(Suppl 3):S35-9.

49. Linn YC, Heng KK, Rohimah S, Goh YT. Peripheral blood progenitor cell mobilization in three groups of subjects: A comparison of leukapheresis yield and timing. J Clin Apheresis 2000;15:217-23.
50. Rowley SD. Regulation of hematopoietic stem cell processing and transplantation. Int J Hematol 2002;75:237-45.
51. Haley NR, ed. Standards for hematopoietic progenitor cell and cellular product services, 3rd ed. Bethesda, MD: American Association of Blood Banks, 2002.
52. Rowley SD. Processing of hematopoietic stem cell components for transplantation: Variations in current practice. Transfusion 1998; 38:1-4.
53. Rowley SD, Davis JM, Piantadosi S, et al. Density-gradient separation of autologous bone marrow grafts before ex vivo purging with 4-hydroperoxycyclophosphamide. Bone Marrow Transplant 1990;6:321-7.
54. Civin CI, Strauss LC, Fackler MJ, et al. Positive stem cell selection—basic science. Prog Clin Biol Res 1990;333:387-401.
55. Martin PJ, Rowley SD, Anasetti C, et al. A phase I-II clinical trial to evaluate removal of CD4 cells and partial depletion of CD8 cells from donor marrow for HLA-mismatched unrelated recipients. Blood 1999; 94:2192-9.
56. Strauss LC, Trischmann TM, Rowley SD, et al. Selection of normal human hematopoietic stem cells for bone marrow transplantation using immunomagnetic microspheres and CD34 antibody. Am J Pediatr Hematol Oncol 1991;13:217-21.
57. Stainer CJ, Miflin G, Anderson S, et al. A comparison of two different systems for CD34+ selection of autologous or allogeneic PBSC collections. J Hematother 1998;7:375-83.
58. Despres D, Flohr T, Uppenkamp M, et al. CD34+ cell enrichment for autologous peripheral blood stem cell transplantation by use of the CliniMACs device. J Hematother Stem Cell Res 2000;9:557-64.
59. Schumm M, Lang P, Taylor G, et al. Isolation of highly purified autologous and allogeneic peripheral CD34+ cells using the CliniMACS device. J Hematother 1999;8:209-18.
60. O'Donnell PV, Myers B, Edwards J, et al. CD34 selection using three immunoselection devices: Comparison of T-cell depleted allografts. Cytotherapy 2001;3:483-8.
61. Beelen DW, Peceny R, Elmaagacli A, et al. Transplantation of highly purified HLA-identical sibling donor peripheral blood CD34+ cells without prophylactic post-transplant immunosuppression in adult patients with first chronic phase chronic myeloid leukemia: Results of a phase II study. Bone Marrow Transplant 2000;26:823-9.
62. Donovan J, Temel J, Zuckerman A, et al. CD34 selection as a stem cell purging strategy for neuroblastoma: Preclinical and clinical studies. Med Pediatr Oncol 2000;35:677-82.

63. Klein JL, Hamm C, Dansey RD, et al. High-dose chemotherapy and CD34-selected peripheral blood progenitor cell transplantation for patients with breast cancer metastatic to bone and/or bone marrow. Bone Marrow Transplant 2001;28:1023-9.
64. Mohr M, Dalmis F, Hilgenfeld E, et al. Simultaneous immunomagnetic CD34+ cell selection and B-cell depletion in peripheral blood progenitor cell samples of patients suffering from B-cell non-Hodgkin's lymphoma. Clin Cancer Res 2001;7:51-7.
65. Borowitz MJ, Shuster JJ, Civin CI, et al. Prognostic significance of CD34 expression in childhood B-precursor acute lymphocytic leukemia: A Pediatric Oncology Group study. J Clin Oncol 1990;8:1389-98.
66. Borowitz MJ, Gockerman JP, Moore JO, et al. Clinicopathologic and cytogenic features of CD34 (My 10)-positive acute nonlymphocytic leukemia. Am J Clin Pathol 1989;91:265-70.
67. Ho VT, Soiffer RJ. The history and future of T-cell depletion as a graft-versus-host disease prophylaxis for allogeneic hematopoietic stem cell transplantation. Blood 2002;98:3192-204.
68. Keever-Taylor CA, Craig A, Molter M, et al. Complement-mediated T-cell depletion of bone marrow: Comparison of T10B9.1A-31 and Muromonab-Orthoclone OKT3. Cytotherapy 2001;3:467-81.
69. Champlin RE, Passweg JR, Zhang MJ, et al. T-cell depletion of bone marrow transplants for leukemia from donors other than HLA-identical siblings: Advantage of T-cell antibodies with narrow specificities. Blood 2000;95:3996-4003.
70. Gilmore MJ, Prentice HG, Jones EP, et al. Allogeneic bone marrow transplantation: The monitoring of granulocyte macrophage colonies following the collection of bone marrow mononuclear cells and after the subsequent in-vitro cytolysis of OKT3 positive lymphocytes. Br J Haematol 1983;55:587-93.
71. Waldmann H, Polliak A, Hale G, et al. Elimination of graft-versus-host disease by in-vitro depletion of alloreactive lymphocytes with a monoclonal rat anti-human lymphocyte antibody (CAMPATH-1). Lancet 1984;2:483-6.
72. Godder KT, Hazlett LJ, Abhyankar SH, et al. Partially mismatched related-donor bone marrow transplantation for pediatric patients with acute leukemia: Younger donors and absence of peripheral blasts improve outcome. J Clin Oncol 2000;18:1856-66.
73. Drobyski WR, Ash RC, Casper JT, et al. Effect of T-cell depletion as graft-versus-host disease prophylaxis on engraftment, relapse, and disease-free survival in unrelated marrow transplantation for chronic myelogenous leukemia. Blood 1994;83:1980-7.
74. Wagner JE, Santos GW, Noga SJ, et al. Bone marrow graft engineering by counterflow centrifugal elutriation: Results of a phase I-II clinical trial. Blood 1990;75:1370-7.

75. Reisner Y, Kapoor N, Kirkpatrick D, et al. Transplantation for acute leukaemia with HLA-A and B nonidentical parental marrow cells fractionated with soybean agglutinin and sheep red blood cells. Lancet 1981;2:327-31.
76. Reisner Y, Kapoor N, Kirkpatrick D, et al. Transplantation for severe combined immunodeficiency with HLA-A,B,D,DR incompatible parental marrow cells fractionated by soybean agglutinin and sheep red blood cells. Blood 1983;61:341-8.
77. Champlin R, Ho W, Gajewski J, et al. Selective depletion of CD8+ T lymphocytes for prevention of graft-versus-host disease after allogeneic bone marrow transplantation. Blood 1990;76:418-23.
78. Koh MB, Prentice HG, Lowdell MW. Selective removal of alloreactive cells from haematopoietic stem cell grafts: Graft engineering for GVHD prophylaxis. Bone Marrow Transplant 1999;23:1071-9.
79. Fehse B, Goldmann M, Frerk O, et al. Depletion of alloreactive donor T cells using immunomagnetic cell selection. Bone Marrow Transplant 2000;25(Suppl)2:S39-42.
80. Freedman AS, Neuberg D, Mauch P, et al. Long-term follow-up of autologous bone marrow transplantation in patients with relapsed follicular lymphoma. Blood 1999;94:3325-33.
81. Reynolds CP, Seeger RC, Vo DD, et al. Model system for removing neuroblastoma cells from bone marrow using monoclonal antibodies and magnetic immunobeads. Cancer Res 1986;46:5882-6.
82. Seeger RC, Vo DD, Ugelstad J, Reynolds CP. Removal of neuroblastoma cells from bone marrow with monoclonal antibodies and magnetic immunobeads. Prog Clin Biol Res 1986;211:285-93.
83. Rill DR, Santana VM, Roberts WM, et al. Direct demonstration that autologous bone marrow transplantation for solid tumors can return a multiplicity of tumorigenic cells. Blood 1994;84:380-3.
84. Zwicky CS, Maddocks AB, Andersen N, Gribben JG. Eradication of polymerase chain reaction detectable immunoglobulin gene rearrangement in non-Hodgkin's lymphoma is associated with decreased relapse after autologous bone marrow transplantation. Blood 1996;88:3314-22.
85. Dominici C, Deb G, Angioni A, et al. Peripheral blood stem cells in children with solid tumors. Part II. Immunocytologic detection of tumor cells in bone marrow and peripheral blood stem cell harvests. Anticancer Res 1993;13:2573-5.
86. Ladetto M, Omede P, Sametti S, et al. Real-time polymerase chain reaction in multiple myeloma. Quantitative analysis of tumor contamination of stem cell harvests. Exp Hematol 2002;30:529-36.
87. Ladetto M, Sametti S, Donovan JW, et al. A validated real-time quantitative PCR approach shows a correlation between tumor burden and successful ex vivo purging in follicular lymphoma patients. Exp Hematol 2001;29:183-93.

88. Rowley SD. Hematopoietic stem cell cryopreservation: A review of current techniques. J Hematother 1992;1:233-50.
89. Attarian H, Feng Z, Buckner CD, et al. Long-term cryopreservation of bone marrow for autologous transplantation. Bone Marrow Transplant 1996;17:425-30.
90. Rowley SD, Anderson GL. Effect of DMSO exposure without cryopreservation on hematopoietic progenitor cells. Bone Marrow Transplant 1993;11:389-93.
91. Kletzel M, Katzenstein HM, Haut PR, et al. Treatment of high-risk neuroblastoma with triple-tandem high-dose therapy and stem-cell rescue: Results of the Chicago Pilot II Study. J Clin Oncol 2002;20: 2284-92.
92. Kreissman SG, Rackoff W, Lee M, Breitfeld PP. High dose cyclophosphamide with carboplatin: A tolerable regimen suitable for dose intensification in children with solid tumors. J Pediatr Hematol Oncol 1997;19:309-12.
93. Horowitz MM. Uses and growth of hematopoietic cell transplantation. In: Thomas ED, Blume KG, Forman SJ, eds. Hematopoietic cell transplantation, 2nd ed. Malden, MA: Blackwell 1999:12-32.
94. Lazarus HM, Loberiza FR, Jr, Zhang MJ, et al. Autotransplants for Hodgkin's disease in first relapse or second remission: A report from the autologous blood and marrow transplant registry (ABMTR). Bone Marrow Transplant 2001;27:387-96.
95. Lazarus HM, Rowlings PA, Zhang MJ, et al. Autotransplants for Hodgkin's disease in patients never achieving remission: A report from the Autologous Blood and Marrow Transplant Registry. J Clin Oncol 1999; 17:534-45.
96. Tsang RW, Gospodarowicz MK, Sutcliffe SB, et al. Thoracic radiation therapy before autologous bone marrow transplantation in relapsed or refractory Hodgkin's disease. PMH Lymphoma Group, and the Toronto Autologous BMT Group. Eur J Cancer 1999;35:73-8.
97. Matthay KK, Harris R, Reynolds CP, et al. Improved event-free survival for autologous bone marrow transplantation vs chemotherapy in neuroblastoma: A Children's Cancer Group study. Med Pediatr Oncol 1998;31:191-207.
98. Matthay KK. Impact of myeloablative therapy with bone marrow transplantation in advanced neuroblastoma. Bone Marrow Transplant 1996; 18:S21-4.
99. Matthay KK, O'Leary MC, Ramsay NK, et al. Role of myeloablative therapy in improved outcome for high risk neuroblastoma: Review of recent Children's Cancer Group results. Eur J Cancer 1995;31A:572-5.
100. Matthay KK, Villablanca JG, Seeger RC, et al. Treatment of high-risk neuroblastoma with intensive chemotherapy, radiotherapy, autologous

bone marrow transplantation, and 13-cis-retinoic acid. N Engl J Med 1999;341:1165-73.

101. Grupp SA, Stern JW, Bunin N, et al. Tandem high-dose therapy in rapid sequence for children with high-risk neuroblastoma. J Clin Oncol 2000;18:2567-75.
102. Grupp SA, Stern JW, Bunin N, et al. Rapid sequence tandem transplant for children with high-risk neuroblastoma. Med Ped Oncol 2000; 35:696-700.
103. Burdach S, van Kaick B, Laws HJ, et al. Allogeneic and autologous stem-cell transplantation in advanced Ewing tumors. An update after long-term follow-up from two centers of the European Intergroup study EICESS. Stem-Cell Transplant Programs at Dusseldorf University Medical Center, Germany and St. Anna Kinderspital, Vienna, Austria. Ann Oncol 2000;11:1451-62.
104. Ayash LJ, Clarke M, Silver SM, et al. Double dose-intensive chemotherapy with autologous stem cell support for relapsed and refractory testicular cancer: The University of Michigan experience and literature review. Bone Marrow Transplant 2001;27:939-47.
105. Dunkel IJ, Finlay JL. High-dose chemotherapy with autologous stem cell rescue for brain tumors. Crit Rev Oncol Hematol 2002;41:197-204.
106. Papadakis V, Dunkel IJ, Cramer LD, et al. High-dose carmustine, thiotepa and etoposide followed by autologous bone marrow rescue for the treatment of high risk central nervous system tumors. Bone Marrow Transplant 2000;26:153-60.
107. Barron KS, Wallace C, Woolfrey CEA, et al. Autologous stem cell transplantation for pediatric rheumatic diseases. J Rheumatol 2001;28: 2337-58.
108. Anderlini P, Korbling M. The use of mobilized peripheral blood stem cells from normal donors for allografting. Stem Cells 1997;15:9-17.
109. Korbling M, Anderlini P. Peripheral blood stem cell versus bone marrow allotransplantation: Does the source of hematopoietic stem cells matter? Blood 2001;98:2900-8.
110. Bensinger WI, Martin PJ, Storer B, et al. Transplantation of bone marrow as compared with peripheral-blood cells from HLA-identical relatives in patients with hematologic cancers. N Engl J Med 2001;344: 175-81.
111. Bensinger WI, Storb R. Allogeneic peripheral blood stem cell transplantation. Rev Clin Exp Hematol 2001;5:67-86.
112. Levine JE, Wiley J, Kletzel M, et al. Cytokine-mobilized allogeneic peripheral blood stem cell transplants in children result in rapid engraftment and a high incidence of chronic GVHD. Bone Marrow Transplant 2000;25:13-18.

113. Storek J, Gooley T, Siadak M, et al. Allogeneic peripheral blood stem cell transplantation may be associated with a high risk of chronic graft-versus-host disease. Blood 1997;90:4705-9.
114. Champlin RE, Schmitz N, Horowitz MM, et al. Blood stem cells compared with bone marrow as a source of hematopoietic cells for allogeneic transplantation. IBMTR Histocompatibility and Stem Cell Sources Working Committee and the European Group for Blood and Marrow Transplantation (EBMT). Blood 2000;95:3702-9.
115. Slowman S, Danielson C, Graves V, et al. Administration of GM-/G-CSF prior to bone marrow harvest increases collection of CD34+ cells. Prog Clin Biol Res 1994;389:363-9.
116. Serody JS, Sparks SD, Lin Y, et al. Comparison of granulocyte colony-stimulating factor (G-CSF)-mobilized peripheral blood progenitor cells and G-CSF-stimulated bone marrow as a source of stem cells in HLA-matched sibling transplantation. Biol Blood Marrow Transplant 2000;6:434-40.
117. Morton J, Hutchins C, Durrant S. Granulocyte-colony-stimulating factor (G-CSF) primed allogeneic bone marrow: Significantly less graft-versus-host disease and comparable engraftment to G-CSF-mobilized peripheral blood stem cells. Blood 2002;98:3186-91.
118. Martinez C, Urbano-Ispizua A, Marin P, et al. Efficacy and toxicity of a high-dose G-CSF schedule for peripheral blood progenitor cell mobilization in healthy donors. Bone Marrow Transplant 1999;24:1273-8.
119. Fortanier C, Kuentz M, Sutton L, et al. Healthy sibling donor anxiety and pain during bone marrow or peripheral blood stem cell harvesting for allogeneic transplantation: Results of a randomised study. Bone Marrow Transplant 2002;29:145-9.
120. Rowley SD, Donaldson G, Lilleby K, et al. Experiences of donors enrolled in a randomized study of allogeneic bone marrow or peripheral blood stem cell transplantation. Blood 2001;97:2541-8.
121. Murata M, Harada M, Kato S, et al. Peripheral blood stem cell mobilization and apheresis: Analysis of adverse events in 94 normal donors. Bone Marrow Transplant 1999;24:1065-71.
122. Ayan I, Kebudi R, Dogan S, et al. Granulocyte colony-stimulating factor in neutropenic, pediatric solid tumor patients following chemotherapy. Pediatr Hematol Oncol 1996;13:417-24.
123. Zimmer BM, Berdel WE, Ludwig WD, et al. Fatal spleen rupture during induction chemotherapy with rh GM-CSF priming for acute monocytic leukemia. Clinical case report and in vitro studies. Leuk Res 1993;17: 277-83.
124. Falzetti F, Aversa F, Minelli O, Tabilio A. Spontaneous rupture of spleen during peripheral blood stem-cell mobilisation in a healthy donor (letter). Lancet 1999;353:555.

125. Brown SL, Dale DC. Spontaneous splenic rupture following administration of granulocyte colony-stimulating factor (G-CSF): Occurrence in an allogeneic donor of peripheral blood stem cells. Biol Blood Marrow Transplant 1997;3:341-3.
126. Becker PS, Wagle M, Matous S, et al. Spontaneous splenic rupture following administration of granulocyte colony-stimulating factor (G-CSF): Occurrence in an allogeneic donor of peripheral blood stem cells. Biol Blood Marrow Transplant 1997;3:45-9.
127. Anderlini P, Rizzo JD, Nugent ML, et al. Peripheral blood stem cell donation: An analysis from the International Bone Marrow Transplant Registry (IBMTR) and European Group for Blood and Marrow Transplant (EBMT) databases. Bone Marrow Transplant 2001;27:689-92.
128. Gross TG, Egeler RM, Smith FO. Pediatric hematopoietic stem cell transplantation. Hematol Oncol Clin North Am 2001;15:795-808.
129. Gluckman E, Rocha V, Boyer-Chammard A, et al. Outcome of cord-blood transplantation from related and unrelated donors. Eurocord Transplant Group and the European Blood and Marrow Transplantation Group. N Engl J Med 1997;337:373-81.
130. Ebbeson P, Gratwohl A, Hows J, ten Have H. Autologous cord blood transplantation. A procedure with potential beyond bone marrow replacement? Bone Marrow Transplant 2000;26:1129-30.
131. Wagner JE, Kernan NA, Steinbuch M, et al. Allogeneic sibling umbilical-cord-blood transplantation in children with malignant and nonmalignant disease. Lancet 1995;346:214-19.
132. Kurtzberg J, Laughlin M, Graham ML, et al. Placental blood as a source of hematopoietic stem cells for transplantation into unrelated recipients. N Engl J Med 1996;335:157-66.
133. Wagner JE, Rosenthal J, Sweetman R, et al. Successful transplantation of HLA-matched and HLA-mismatched umbilical cord blood from unrelated donors: Analysis of engraftment and acute graft-versus-host disease. Blood 1996;88:795-802.
134. Cairo MS, Wagner JE. Placental and/or umbilical cord blood: An alternative source of hematopoietic stem cells for transplantation. Blood 1997;90:4665-78.

In: Herman JH, Manno CS, eds.
Pediatric Transfusion Therapy
Bethesda, MD: AABB Press, 2002

20

Pediatric Therapeutic Apheresis

ANNE F. EDER, MD, PhD, AND HAEWON C. KIM, MD

THERAPEUTIC APHERESIS IS first-line treatment or valuable adjunctive therapy for a variety of diseases and conditions occurring in children.[1-5] Although the basic principles of apheresis are the same regardless of the age of the patient, techniques designed to treat adults must be modified for infants and small children to minimize untoward effects of the procedure.[1] Key technical factors in performing a safe and effective apheresis procedure in pediatric populations include establishment of adequate vascular access,

Anne F. Eder, MD, PhD, Director, Hematology Laboratory and Assistant Director, Blood Bank and Apheresis Service, Department of Pathology and Clinical Laboratories, The Children's Hospital of Philadelphia; and Haewon C. Kim, MD, Director, Apheresis Service, Division of Hematology, The Children's Hospital of Philadelphia, and Associate Professor of Pediatrics, University of Pennsylvania School of Medicine, Philadelphia, Pennsylvania

maintenance of intravascular fluid and red cell volume, and prompt recognition of adverse reactions. An understanding of age-appropriate behavior, pediatric psychology, and social dynamics among children and their parents or caretakers is also essential to a successful procedure.

Therapeutic apheresis involves separating whole blood into its components and selectively removing undesired cells or plasma from patients with disease (Fig 20-1). The cellular components that can be specifically removed from circulating blood include red cells by erythrocytapheresis; white cells, including blasts, by leukapheresis; and platelets by plateletpheresis. Plasmapheresis is the bulk removal of plasma; various modifications of the procedure allow more specific removal of plasma constituents, such as immune complexes or low-density lipoprotein. In contrast to therapeutic apheresis procedures intended to remove abnormal blood components causing or contributing to a disease state, preparative or donor apheresis procedures are performed to col-

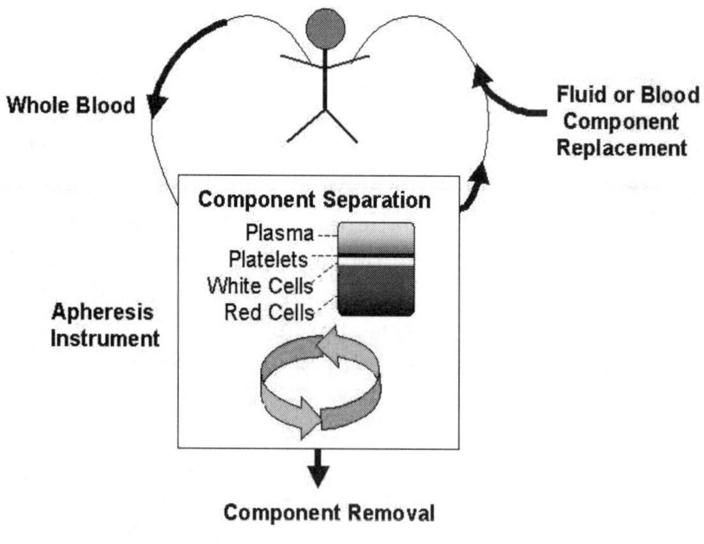

Figure 20-1. Schematic diagram of therapeutic apheresis.

lect normal blood components, such as hematopoietic progenitor cells, for subsequent infusion to patients. This chapter addresses therapeutic rather than preparative procedures utilized in pediatric clinical settings.

Therapeutic apheresis has been used to treat many of the same diseases in children that also affect adults. The application of therapeutic apheresis in both adults and children, however, is often based on theoretical rationale, experience and empiric data rather than prospective, randomized controlled trials. In general, research to evaluate the efficacy of therapeutic apheresis is sparse, largely due to the fact that clinical circumstances often impede controlled study. The procedures are used to treat rare diseases, life-threatening conditions unresponsive to conventional therapy, or diseases for which therapeutic response is difficult to assess due to variable diagnostic criteria, unpredictable clinical course, concomitant therapies, and subjective evaluation of response.[6] Despite these limitations, several randomized controlled studies have been performed to evaluate the efficacy of therapeutic apheresis. These data are derived primarily from adults; less information is available on children. Although some conclusions drawn from adult studies may be extrapolated to the pediatric population, caution is urged because the natural course of a disease and the response to treatment may differ in children compared with adults.[7] Consequently, there is often a lack of universally accepted indications, treatment schedules, and clinical endpoints for therapeutic apheresis procedures, especially for pediatric applications.

To provide guidance on the use of therapeutic apheresis, two professional organizations, the American Association of Blood Banks (AABB) and the American Society for Apheresis (ASFA) independently reviewed the available current literature to classify clinical indications into four categories.[8-13] Category I includes disorders for which therapeutic apheresis is standard and acceptable, either as primary or adjunctive therapy based on well-designed, randomized controlled trials or a broad and noncontroversial base of published experience. Category II includes disorders for which there is sufficient evidence to suggest efficacy, usually as adjunctive therapy, based mostly on small case series or informative case studies. Category III includes disorders for which there is inconclusive evidence of efficacy or uncertain risk/benefit ratio. Category IV includes disorders for which controlled trials have demonstrated a lack of efficacy. Those diseases encountered in pediatrics are shown in Table 20-1.

This chapter discusses technical considerations unique to pediatric patients and focuses on the role of therapeutic apheresis in the treatment of pediatric diseases, with emphasis on those most commonly encountered in a tertiary children's hospital and new applications of apheresis in pediatrics.

Technical and Physiologic Considerations

Careful consideration of several practical aspects of therapeutic apheresis procedures is essential to ensure safe and effective treatment of pediatric patients.[1] The most important factors are establishment of adequate vascular access, maintenance of intravascular fluid volume and circulating red cell mass, and prompt recognition of adverse reactions related to volume shifts, anticoagulants, transfused blood components, or anxiety. Continuous-flow apheresis systems such as the COBE Spectra (Gambro BCT Inc, Lakewood, CO) are preferred for pediatric use because of their smaller extracorporeal volume compared with that of intermittent-flow devices. Continuous-flow entails withdrawing whole blood and returning the processed blood components and replacement fluids or cells simultaneously. Intermittent-flow involves first withdrawing whole blood, processing it into components, then returning appropriate fractions with replacement fluids or cells. Both devices use centrifugation to separate blood into its components based on cellular density and require the use of anticoagulants to prevent occlusion of the extracorporeal circuit. Citrate, heparin,[4] or both may be used in pediatric apheresis procedures, with citrate being the primary anticoagulant used at most institutions.[1,3]

In planning therapeutic apheresis procedures, the patient's total blood volume (TBV), plasma volume, and/or red cell volume should be calculated to predict the net fluid and red cell volume shift (Table 20-2). The total blood volume of a child greater than

Table 20-1. Pediatric Diseases Treated with Apheresis: ASFA and AABB Indication Categories*

Plasmapheresis	Cytapheresis
Category I: Standard and acceptable primary or adjunctive therapy	
Chronic inflammatory demyelinating polyradiculonephropathy	**Leukocytosis** **Sickle cell disease**
Acute inflammatory demyelinating polyradiculonephropathy (Guillain-Barré syndrome)	**Thrombocytosis**
Familial hypercholesterolemia (plasmapheresis with selective adsorption; AABB-NR)	
Myesthenia gravis	
Phytanic acid storage disease (Refsum's disease)	
Thrombotic thrombocytopenic purpura	
Rheumatoid arthritis (plasmapheresis with protein A immunoadsorption; AABB-NR)	
Category II: Sufficient evidence to suggest efficacy usually as adjunctive therapy	
Coagulation factor inhibitors (AABB-III)	Erythrocytosis/polycythemia vera (AABB-NR)
Familial hypercholesterolemia (AABB-I)	Rheumatoid arthritis (AABB-III)
Lambert-Eaton myasthenic syndrome	
Rapidly progressive glomerulonephritis	
Idiopathic thrombocytopenia purpura (ITP) (plasmapheresis with protein A immunoadsorption; AABB-III)	
Category III: Inconclusive evidence of efficacy or uncertain risk benefit ratio	
Overdose poisoning (AABB-II)	**Malaria/babesiosis (AABB-II)**
Hemolytic-uremic syndrome (AABB-II)	
Hepatic failure (acute) (AABB-IV)	
Renal transplantation, recurrent focal segmental glomerulosclerosis (AABB-NR)	

(continued)

Table 20-1. Pediatric Diseases Treated with Apheresis: ASFA and AABB Indication Categories* (continued)

Plasmapheresis	Cytapheresis
Renal transplantation, presensitization (AABB-NR)	
Systemic lupus erythematosus (AABB-NR)	
Rasmussen's encephalitis	
Autoimmune hemolytic anemia	
Category IV: Lack of efficacy in controlled trials	
Renal transplantation, rejection	
Rheumatoid arthritis	

*Only diseases encountered in pediatrics are included; refer to the AABB and ASFA comprehensive guidelines for diseases that primarily affect adults.[8,13] Diseases in bold are discussed in greater detail in the text. If the category ratings differ between the organizations, then the indication is included in the ASFA category and the AABB rating is given in parentheses.
NR = not rated.

3 months old may be estimated as 65 to 75 mL/kg; younger infants have greater blood volumes of approximately 80 to 100 mL/kg.[14] Total blood volume varies with body composition; consequently, weight-based calculations overestimate the blood volume of obese individuals and underestimate the blood volume of lean or muscular individuals. Automated apheresis devices use more complex algorithms to calculate total blood volume on the basis of gender, height, and weight; however, the calculation performed by the COBE Spectra has been shown to be inaccurate in male children.[15] For example, prepubescent boys under 10 to 12 years old or weighing less than 30 kg have smaller blood volumes than predicted by the algorithm.[15] Consequently, the TBV calculated automatically must be verified against a manual weight-based estimate.

Table 20-2. Sample Calculations and Predictions

Formula	Calculation	Net Volume
Calculations		
Total blood volume (TBV) 70 mL/kg × wt	(70 mL/kg) × (10 kg)	700 mL
Red cell volume (RV) Hct ×TBV	(0.3) × (700 mL)	210 mL
Plasma volume (PV) (1 – Hct) × TBV	(1 – 0.3) × (700 mL)	490 mL
Predictions with Standard Procedure*		
A. Extracorporeal blood volume (EBV)		
Intraprocedure volume loss Device- and procedure-specific	Table 20-4	–150 mL
Percent EBV (EBV ÷ TBV) × 100	$\frac{150\text{ mL}}{700\text{ mL}} \times 100$	21%
B. Extracorporeal red cell volume (ERV)		
Extracorporeal red cell volume (ERV) loss Device- and procedure-specific COBE Spectra = 68 mL COBE SpectraTherm blood warmer ECV = 36 mL	68 mL + (36 mL × 0.3)	–79 mL
Percent ERV (ERV ÷ RV) × 100 = %ERV	$\frac{79\text{ mL}}{210\text{ mL}} \times 100$	38%
Intraprocedure Hct $\frac{(\text{RV} - \text{ERV})}{\text{TBV}} \times 100 = \text{IH}$	$\frac{(210 - 79)\text{ mL}}{700\text{ mL}} \times 100$	19%

*Plasmapheresis, COBE Spectra, dual-needle operation, diverting prime saline ERV equals COBE Spectra red cell requirement to establish the plasma-red cell interface within the channel (68 mL) in addition to the red cells in the blood warmer [ECV x Hct of blood in warmer]. This standard procedure is not acceptable for this child because the extracorporeal blood volume (EBV) exceeds 10% to 15% of total blood volume (TBV) and the extracorporeal red cell volume (ERV) exceeds 30% of circulating red cell volume (RV). Consequently, the procedure should be modified to include blood prime and ensure fluid and red cell balance throughout the procedure.

In addition to the calculated blood volume, the kinetics and vascular distribution of the constituent being removed has important implications for planning procedures with respect to the exchange volume and the scheduled frequency. Red cell exchange targets whole or partial red cell volumes, depending on the desired extent of depletion of native red cells, expressed as the fraction of cells remaining in circulation. The life span of transfused red cells is 2 to 4 months in the absence of immune hemolysis; consequently, the procedure would not be repeated in an acute setting. For chronic transfusion regimens, the procedure would be repeated on a specific schedule depending primarily on the desired clinical goals for an individual patient and the survival kinetics of the transfused red cells. Like red cells, some plasma components remain entirely in the intravascular space with no equilibration with the extravascular space (ie, IgM, fibrinogen), and a one-volume exchange will remove approximately 65% of the solute, and a two-volume exchange will remove approximately 85% of the solute. These "ideal solutes" are removed efficiently with only one procedure; consideration of the half-life of the plasma protein will govern when, or if, the procedure will need to be repeated. Plasma constituents that equilibrate between the intravascular and extravascular space, such as IgG, are not removed as efficiently as ideal solutes, necessitating daily or alternate day treatment regimens to allow for equilibrium between vascular compartments. Because the efficiency of cellular or solute depletion with therapeutic apheresis is logarithmic, not linear, the incremental benefit derived from the procedure diminishes when performing greater volume exchanges, with 65%, 85%, and 95% removed after 1.0, 2.0, and 3.0 volume exchanges, respectively. Consequently, in this context, 1 to 1.5 plasma volumes are usually exchanged with each procedure on the desired schedule.

Vascular Access

Adequate vascular access, a prerequisite for all therapeutic apheresis procedures, is more difficult to obtain in children than in adults. Continuous-flow apheresis devices require dual vascular access with 18-gauge or larger caliber needles for the draw line and at least 22-gauge intravenous catheters for the return line. The antecubital veins of large children and adolescents may accommodate the necessary needles or catheters. Peripheral access is often not an option, however, for young children and infants whose veins cannot support the use of such lines. In these cases, central venous access is required. Depending on the urgency of the clinical situation and the expected frequency and duration of the treatment, a femoral line may be placed for either a single use or until a central venous catheter is available. For a child requiring chronic apheresis therapy, a surgically implanted central venous catheter with a double lumen is appropriate for long-term use.

Blood is withdrawn at a high flow rate during therapeutic apheresis procedures; consequently, catheters must be rigid enough to withstand this negative pressure. Hemodialysis catheters with a large bore and double lumen, such as those from MedComp (MedComp, Inc., Harleysville, PA), VasCath (VasCath, Inc., Mississauga, Ontario, Canada), and Quinton (Mahurkar catheter or PermCath catheter, Quinton Instrument Co., Seattle, WA) are suitable for apheresis procedures. Although Hickman catheters, Infuse-a-Port, or peripherally inserted central venous catheters (PICC lines) can be used for returning replacement fluids during apheresis procedures, these types of catheters cannot be used to draw blood from a patient. Guidelines for catheter size according to the patient's weight are given in Table 20-3. Intravascular devices may be associated with complications including infection or thrombosis. The risks associated with line placement and maintenance should be weighed against the potential benefits of therapeutic apheresis.

Intravascular Volume Balance

A key to safe therapeutic apheresis in a child is maintenance of a constant intravascular volume. At the beginning of a standard plasma exchange procedure with the COBE Spectra, whole blood is drawn into the apheresis circuit and the saline contained in the tubing and centrifuge channel is diverted to a waste bag, re-

Table 20-3. Guidelines for Catheter Size*

Patient's Weight (kg)	Double-Lumen, Central Venous Catheter	Manufacturer
<10	7 Fr Med Comp	Med Comp, Inc., Harleysville, PA
10-20	8 Fr Med Comp or 8 Fr Quinton	Quinton Instrument Co., Seattle, WA
20-50	9 Fr Med Comp or 10 Fr Quinton	Vas-Cath, Inc., Mississauga, Ontario, Canada
>50	9 Fr or 11.5 Fr Med Comp; 10 Fr, 11.5 Fr, or 13.5 Fr Quinton; adult Vas-Cath or adult Vas-Cath	

*Adapted with permission from Kim.[1]

sulting in a temporary loss of 150 mL. This deficit persists until the cells and plasma in the extracorporeal circuit are returned to the patient during the rinseback phase at the completion of the procedure. The intravascular volume loss at the beginning of a procedure and rinseback volume will vary depending on the type of procedure, even with the same equipment (Table 20-4).

This volume shift must be carefully considered against the maximum blood loss that an individual patient can tolerate. Hemodynamically stable subjects can usually tolerate losing 10% to 15% of their total blood volume. Patients with cardiac, renal, or hepatic impairment; anemia; or dehydration may not tolerate this degree of hypovolemia. All patients will experience circulatory collapse with acute intravascular loss greater than 30% of the TBV. Conversely, volume overload should be avoided, especially in patients with impaired cardiac function or renal insufficiency.

For a 70-kg adult, with a total blood volume of about 5000 mL, losing 150 mL to the extracorporeal circuit at the beginning of an apheresis procedure is well tolerated, as it represents only 3%

Table 20-4. Intravascular Volume Shifts*

	Net Intravascular Volume Shift (mL)	
	Intraprocedure	Postprocedure
Plasma exchange	−150	+195
RBC exchange	−100	+245
Leukapheresis, version 4.7	−150 + AC − WBC	+263 + AC − WBC
Leukapheresis, version 6.0	−150 + AC − WBC	+185 + AC − WBC

*COBE Spectra, dual-needle operation, standard procedure (divert saline prime, perform rinseback)
AC = volume anticoagulant; WBC = volume of collected white blood cells.

of the TBV. In contrast, a 10-kg child has a total blood volume of about 700 mL, and acute loss of 150 mL of whole blood into the apheresis circuit would correspond to 21% of the TBV (Table 20-2). The default rinseback phase would result in a net positive volume shift of 195 mL, an increase of 30% of the TBV. These shifts would not be acceptable, and the standard procedure should be modified to ensure isovolemia during and after the procedure. This is accomplished by returning the prime saline, red cells, or other appropriate replacement fluid to the patient at the beginning of the procedure and omitting the rinseback phase.

Red Cell Volume Balance

Another consequence of drawing whole blood from the patient at the beginning of an apheresis procedure is the temporary loss of red cell mass with potential impairment of oxygen-carrying capacity. This red cell deficit remains throughout the procedure until the blood in the apheresis circuit is rinsed back to the patient. With the COBE Spectra, the initial red cell mass deficit is 68 mL for plasmapheresis and erythrocytapheresis procedures. Similar consideration must be given to red cell mass balance as intravascular volume balance for safe therapeutic apheresis (Table 20-5). The loss of red cells during the procedure may reduce

Table 20-5. Red Cell Volume Shifts

	Net Red Cell Volume Shift (mL)*	
	Intraprocedure	**Postprocedure**
Plasma exchange	–68	–15
RBC exchange	–68	–16
Leukapheresis, version 4.7	–114 – WBC	–24 – WBC
Leukapheresis, version 6.0	–66 – WBC	–9 – WBC

*COBE Spectra, dual-needle operation, standard procedure (divert saline prime, perform rinseback); volume of blood warmer or other devices added to the extracorporeal circuit is not included.

Average red cell volume in WBC collected = volume of WBC collected × hematocrit of WBC product/100.

circulating red cell mass to unacceptable levels. For example, a hematocrit of 30% in a 10-kg child would drop precipitously to a hematocrit of 19% with this red cell deficit (Table 20-2). This situation necessitates priming the circuit or the return line with red cells. To maintain a hematocrit of 30%, 79 mL of red cells should be administered to the patient. Assuming red cell units have a volume of approximately 300 mL and hematocrit of 60%, 131 mL or approximately half of the unit will be needed. If the red cell unit is divided with sterile technique, the remainder can be dedicated to this patient for later transfusion, within the shelf life of the unit, to limit the number of donor exposures the patient receives.

Red cell priming is generally recommended when 1) red cell volume depletion is greater than 30% of the original circulating red cell volume or 2) when any degree of reduction in the circulating red cell volume is deemed undesirable in hemodynamically unstable or anemic patients or in patients at risk of organ ischemia.[1] Infants and children weighing less than 20 kg or under the age of 5 or 6 years usually require blood priming prior to apheresis procedures, as do older children with anemia or underlying cardiopulmonary disease, hemodynamic instability, or tissue ischemia.

Adverse Reactions

Therapeutic apheresis procedures, even though they are often performed in critically ill patients, are relatively safe. Apheresis personnel must be able to recognize the early signs of adverse reactions and effectively manage these complications. A prospective, multicenter study reported that significant adverse effects occur in approximately 5% of therapeutic apheresis procedures.[16] Adverse reactions were more common in first-time procedures than in repeat procedures, and more common with blood component exchanges than for peripheral blood progenitor cell collections. The authors reported only "clinically troublesome reactions" and did not consider common reactions to therapeutic apheresis, such as peripheral or perioral paresthesia related to citrate anticoagulation or mild light-headedness. In descending order of occurrence were transfusion reactions (1.6%); citrate-related nausea and/or vomiting (1.2%); vasovagal reactions such as hypotension (1%), nausea and/or vomiting (0.5%), pallor and/or diaphoresis (0.5%); tachycardia (0.4%); respiratory distress (0.3%); citrate-related tetany or seizure (0.2%); and chills or rigors (0.2%).[16] No deaths resulted from therapeutic apheresis; three deaths were attributed to the underlying primary disease. The incidence of adverse reactions was not reported with respect to the age of the patient; however, citrate-related toxicity, transfusion reactions, and vasovagal reactions are among the most frequently encountered adverse effects in pediatric patients at The Children's Hospital of Philadelphia.

Citrate prevents coagulation of whole blood by chelating calcium ions and blocking calcium-dependent hemostasis. Citrate is rapidly metabolized in the liver; consequently, symptoms related to citrate-induced hypocalcemia are usually transient. Citrate toxicity is a greater problem with leukapheresis than with exchange procedures because virtually all of the administered anticoagulant is returned to the patient. In addition, small infants or children with liver disease may demonstrate increased sensitivity to citrate. In adults, the first symptoms of citrate toxicity are perioral and peripheral paresthesias. Children may also report the sensation of mouth or finger tingling in response to citrate, but more often manifest acute episodes of abdominal pain, nausea and/or vomiting, agitation, pallor, and sweating followed by tachycardia and hypotension. These toxic effects are usually avoided or minimized by careful monitoring of symptoms, blood pressure, and serum ionized calcium concentration; by reducing the flow rate; and/or by providing calcium supplementation.

If blood components, such as red cells or fresh frozen plasma, are used as replacement fluids, transfusion reactions may be difficult to distinguish clinically from other procedure-related reactions. Immediate adverse reactions to transfused components range from rare incidents of life-threatening acute intravascular hemolysis caused by incompatible red cell units or mechanical hemolysis, to more commonly reported and usually mild allergic or febrile reactions resulting from plasma constituents or cytokines in stored units. The signs and symptoms of transfusion reactions may be suggestive of a certain type of response, such as hives and urticaria in allergic responses or back pain in hemolytic reactions. More often, signs and symptoms are nonspecific with fever, chills, tachycardia, or hypotension being seen in hemolytic, allergic, febrile, and septic transfusion reactions. Consequently, an adverse reaction to blood product administration should not be attributed to a benign, febrile transfusion reaction, unless acute hemolysis and other, more serious reactions are eliminated as possibilities. The therapeutic apheresis procedure may need to be slowed, stopped temporarily, or discontinued until serologic studies are completed by the blood bank and the patient's symptoms resolve. Pretreatment with acetaminophen and administration of leukocyte-reduced red cells and platelets may prevent recurrent febrile reactions. For patients with a history of allergic reactions, premedication with antihistamines or washing of red cell units to remove residual plasma may be sufficient to prevent recurrent episodes.

Vasovagal reactions manifest as bradycardia, hypotension, diaphoresis, pallor, nausea, and apprehension. These reactions are managed by pausing the procedure and elevating the patient's legs. The changes in blood pressure usually resolve within a few minutes, allowing resumption and completion of the procedure. Vasovagal reactions may mimic reactions due to anxiety or hypovolemia with the exception that the former is usually associated with bradycardia, while the latter usually cause tachycardia. Distraction techniques, such as conversation, videos, or games, are used to divert the child's attention from the procedure and minimize anxiety.

Erythrocytapheresis

Erythrocytapheresis is used to remove excess or abnormal red cells from patients with hematologic, infectious, or metabolic disorders. Red cell reduction has been employed to alleviate symptoms attributable to increased red cell mass in polycythemia vera or secondary polycythemia resulting from cyanotic congenital heart disease, and to reduce iron stores in hemochromatosis.[10] Erythrocytapheresis may be preferable to simple phlebotomy for hemodynamically unstable patients because red cells can be removed rapidly while simultaneously returning autologous plasma along with saline or colloid solution to maintain constant intravascular volume. An application of erythrocytapheresis more common than isovolemic phlebotomy, however, is red cell exchange transfusion to remove abnormal red cells from patients with intrinsic and extrinsic red cell disorders and replace them with normal red cells. Intrinsic defects of red cells result from disorders of hemoglobin, the erythrocyte membrane, or red cell enzymes. The most common indication for red cell exchange is treatment of acute and chronic complications in sickle cell disease. Preoperative red cell exchange has also been used in patients with hemoglobin of abnormally high oxygen affinity, such as hemoglobin Rainier[17] or Bryn Mawr[18] to prevent potential tissue hypoxia, thromboembolic complications, and increased hemolysis during anesthesia. Finally, erythrocytapheresis can be a life-saving measure in patients with glucose-6-phosphate dehydrogenase deficiency following exposure to significant oxidant stress that causes refractory methemoglobinemia.[19] Extrinsic or acquired disorders treated with red cell exchange include infectious diseases, such as malaria and babesiosis, and incompatible transfusions.[20-23]

Sickle Cell Disease

Sickle cell anemia is a chronic illness of variable severity characterized by anemia and vascular occlusion in patients with homozygous hemoglobin S, hemoglobin SC, or hemoglobin S-beta thalassemia. The presence of hemoglobin S results in irreversibly sickled cells, with shortened survival and altered rheologic properties, including increased blood viscosity. Occlusion of small vessels by microvascular thrombi or sludging of sickled cells results in clinical infarctive crises; the manifestations and severity of such episodes are related to the location and magnitude of damaged tissue. These acute complications of sickle cell disease include painful episodes, acute chest syndrome, stroke, priapism, and splenic infarction and sequestration. Physiologic and hypoxic stress enhance the tendency of the red cells containing hemoglobin S to sickle and pose additional risk to patients with sickle cell disease. Individuals with sickle cell disease are predisposed to complications resulting from surgery and general anesthesia, and pregnant women with sickle cell disease are at risk for obstetric complications.

Chronic red cell transfusion therapy has been proven to reduce the rate of first and recurrent stroke among children with sickle cell anemia.[24,25] Conventional transfusion therapy strives to maintain hemoglobin S levels below 30%. A modified transfusion program that adjusts the hemoglobin S threshold to less than 50% after 3 years of transfusion still affords protection against stroke while reducing blood donor exposures and lowering the rate of iron accumulation.[26,27] After several years, however, tissue accumulation of transfusional iron ultimately may lead to significant morbidity, including diabetes, cirrhosis, cardiac arrhythmias, and failure. Although chelation therapy with deferoxamine effectively reduces tissue iron stores and prevents long-term complications, many patients are not compliant with the life-saving regimen.

Role of Therapeutic Apheresis

Red cell exchange transfusion is often a component of the emergent management of acute complications of sickle cell disease, such as acute chest syndrome and stroke, as well as chronic, prophylactic treatment to prevent first or recurrent stroke (Table 20-6). In both treatment settings, red cell exchange transfusion offers several distinctive advantages over simple transfusion. Because exchange transfusion removes sickled erythrocytes as normal red cells are transfused, the hemoglobin S concentration can be rapidly reduced without raising hematocrit or causing volume overload. Exchange transfusion avoids the simultaneous existence of high hemoglobin S and high hematocrit, a condition that increases blood viscosity and the risk of further vascular occlusion. For patients receiving chronic transfusion therapy, iron accumulation is prevented or markedly reduced with red cell exchange transfusion. Disadvantages of red cell exchange may include the lack of availability of an apheresis team experienced in

Table 20-6. Indications for Erythrocytapheresis in Sickle Cell Disease

Acute Management (Single procedure during acute episode)	**Chronic Treatment (Procedures over the course of several months to years)**
Acute thrombotic complications • Acute chest syndrome • Acute stroke • Retinal infarction • Acute hepatic crisis	Reduction of transfusional iron load with chronic transfusion regimen • Prevention of first or recurrent stroke • Prevention of recurrent complications (ie, stuttering priapism, debilitating painful episodes) • Chronic lung disease with arterial hypoxemia
Prophylactic transfusion prior to surgery	Prophylactic treatment during pregnancy

pediatric applications, increased technical complexity, and greater expense compared with simple transfusion.

Red cell exchange has been used as adjunctive therapy for severe, acute complications, including stroke, acute chest syndrome, retinal infarction, and acute hepatic crisis (Table 20-6).[1,10] The benefit of transfusion therapy for these indications has not been proven in randomized controlled trials. Supportive evidence comes from anecdotal reports and small series. Regardless, transfusion support in an attempt to alleviate or prevent acute life- or organ-threatening complications, such as stroke and acute chest syndrome, is widely accepted practice, and is classified as a Category I indication by both ASFA and AABB.[8,13] The choice of red cell exchange or simple transfusion for acute complications of sickle cell disease varies from center to center. In a recent study of acute chest syndrome involving 538 patients at 30 centers, 72% of patients received transfusions, with the majority (65%) being simple transfusions averaging 3 units. Both simple and exchange transfusion resulted in statistically significant improvements in oxygenation.

Although acute painful crises are usually managed without transfusion, red cell exchange may be used to treat chronic, debilitating pain and multiorgan failure syndrome associated with severe painful crises.[29] Unfortunately, it is not possible to predict which patients with pain crises are at risk for life-threatening complications. Exchange transfusion for priapism is controversial, and has been associated with central nervous system events occurring 1 to 14 days after the exchange.[30] The use of prophylactic red cell transfusions to prevent complications due to sickling in pregnancy is also controversial. However, red cell exchange may be appropriate in urgent situations such as preeclampsia, septicemia, and possibly general anesthesia and surgery.[31]

Prophylactic red cell transfusions are frequently given as a part of perioperative management of sickle cell patients, to prevent complications following surgery and general anesthesia. A prospective, randomized multicenter study demonstrated a conservative transfusion regimen to increase hemoglobin to 10 g/dL was as effective as an aggressive regimen to decrease the percentage of hemoglobin S to less than 30% in preventing perioperative complications in patients with sickle cell anemia.[32] The aggressive regimen was associated with a higher rate of red cell alloimmunization, resulting from increased blood usage in this group. Consequently, a conservative approach with the use of simple transfusion is recommended for prophylactic preoperative red cell transfusion in patients with sickle cell disease. Patients with hemoglobin SC or hemoglobin S-beta thalassemia who present with hemoglobin concentrations greater than 10 g/dL prior to surgery, however, may benefit from exchange transfusion rather than simple transfusion, to decrease the amount of sickle hemoglobin without increasing hematocrit and blood viscosity.

For chronically transfused patients, red cell exchange transfusion reduces or prevents iron accumulation and allows discontinuation of iron chelation therapy in some patients.[33-36] Kim et al[33] evaluated long-term erythrocytapheresis in 14 subjects with sickle cell disease and stroke or other complications as an alternative to simple transfusion. The goal with exchange transfusion was to decrease pretransfusion hemoglobin S to less than 50%, and patients were compared with historical controls treated with simple transfusion protocols with either conventional (target hemoglobin S <30%) or modified (target hemoglobin S <50%) goals. The mean annual iron load with erythrocytapheresis was 87% lower than with conventional simple transfusion and 82% lower than with modified simple transfusion. The major disadvantage of red cell exchange transfusion was the use of more donor blood. Donor blood usage with exchange transfusion increased 23% per year compared with conventional simple transfusion and 73% per year compared with modified simple transfusion. This increased annual requirement translates into 10 more units of red cells for erythrocytapheresis compared with conventional simple transfusion (hemoglobin S <30%) and 25 more units compared with modified simple transfusion (hemoglobin S <50%) for an adult subject who undergoes erythrocytapheresis every 3 weeks.[33]

Increased donor exposure has attendant risks of viral transmission and alloimmunization. Implementation of nucleic acid testing to directly detect HIV and HCV genetic material rather than the humoral immune response to infection has decreased the risk of viral transmission by identifying recently infected donors in the "window period" when antibodies to viral proteins are not yet detectable. The risk for human immunodeficiency virus is currently estimated as 1 in 1,930,000 units; for hepatitis B virus, 1 in 138,700 units; and for hepatitis C virus, 1 in 543,000 units.[37,38] Alloimmunization complicates identification of compatible blood for chronically transfused patients and may lead to significant delayed hemolysis. The risk of alloimmunization is primarily related to the number of red cell transfusions received. Strategies to reduce this risk include the use of racially matched blood or antigen matching for Rhesus, Kell, Duffy, and other red cell antigens.[39,40] The benefit of delaying or preventing iron-induced organ damage may outweigh these risks associated with increased donor exposure and may offset the increased cost of red cell exchange compared with simple transfusion with iron chelation therapy. At The Children's Hospital of Philadelphia, 34 patients with sickle cell disease currently undergo chronic exchange transfusion for prevention of stroke. Among the 28 patients who have been treated on a 3- or 4-week schedule for more than 1 year, nine have maintained a normal serum ferritin concentration and 17 have demonstrated significant decreases in serum ferritin concentration, obviating the need for iron chelation therapy.

Technical Aspects

The goals of red cell transfusion in treating new onset of stroke, acute chest syndrome, and other acute complications of sickle cell disease are to reduce or prevent sickling by lowering hemoglobin S concentration and to increase oxygen delivery to tissues by increasing the hematocrit. As a general guideline, hemoglobin S should be reduced to less than 30% of the total hemoglobin, and the hematocrit at the end of the procedure should be raised to 30% or greater, but not more than 36%. High hematocrit levels in sickle cell patients have been linked to serious thrombotic complications, most likely due to altered rheologic properties of the blood.[41] If the patient has not been transfused within the previous 3 months, the hemoglobin S level should be assumed to be 100%. Exchange of one blood volume should result in a hemoglobin A level of about 65% and lower the hemoglobin S to about 35%; consequently, approximately 1.5 red cell volumes are exchanged. For example, a 9-year old, 29-kg child with a blood volume of 2030 mL and a 25% hematocrit will require approximately 4 units of red cells. Patients with a first stroke are often placed on chronic transfusion therapy following resolution of the acute event. For these patients, the fraction of sickle cells remaining following red cell exchange should be even lower, with a target of 10% to 15%, to keep the patient's hemoglobin S below 30% for 3 to 4 weeks.[1] Post-exchange hematocrit and hemoglobin electrophoresis should be performed to validate the efficiency of the exchange.

The goal in the first 3 years of chronic transfusion therapy is to maintain hemoglobin S below 30% of the total hemoglobin concentration. If the patient is stable on this regimen for 3 years, the hemoglobin S threshold may be increased to 50%. For most patients, partial red cell exchange translates to 40% to 60% of their red cell volume, usually 2 to 4 units. A comparison of the COBE Spectra and Haemonetics V50 (Haemonetics Corporation, Braintree, MA) devices revealed that stepwise isovolemic hemodilution with the Haemonetics V50 required less donor blood to achieve the same reduction in hemoglobin S.[42] Consequently, procedures performed with the COBE Spectra at The Children's Hospital of Philadelphia have been modified to incorporate a depletion phase during which time the patient undergoes isovolemic hemodilution. If the goal of transfusion is to maintain hemoglobin S below 30%, the patient's initial hematocrit level is diluted to approximately 24% before donor red cell replacement is begun, by infusing normal saline to maintain isovolemia. Partial red cell exchange transfusion is performed every 3 to 4 weeks. If the goal of transfusion is to maintain hemoglobin S below 50%, isovolemic hemodilution is performed at the beginning of the procedure to decrease a patient's hematocrit to as low as 21%, and partial exchange transfusion is performed every 4 to 5 weeks. Regardless of the target hemoglobin S level, the target hematocrit following red cell exchange is either 27% or the same as the patient's pre-hematocrit but less than 36%, to optimally prevent hyperviscosity and iron accumulation.

Thalassemia Major

Complications in sickle cell disease result primarily from the presence of hemoglobin S rather than from anemia per se; in contrast, complications in thalassemia major result from severe anemia due to ineffective production of red cells secondary to the absence or decreased synthesis of the beta globin chain of hemoglobin. Patients with thalassemia major benefit from chronic red cell transfusion therapy as do patients with sickle cell disease, and likewise suffer from complications of transfusional iron overload. Red cell exchange transfusion as an alternative to simple transfusion has been investigated as a means to reduce the rate of iron accumulation in thalassemia patients. While the goal of transfusion in sickle cell disease is to reduce hemoglobin S levels more or less irrespective of the total hemoglobin level, the goal in treating patients with thalassemia major is to maintain a hemoglobin concentration of at least 9.0 g/dL. Berdoukas et al[43] evaluated 15 patients with thalassemia major who received automated exchange transfusions over a period of 6 to 7 months. Serum ferritin levels decreased by 20% during the treatment period with exchange transfusions, whereas serum ferritin levels rose by 12% during conventional transfusion therapy. The net rate of iron loading fell by 29%, but donor exposures increased 40% to 60%. Preliminary results in three patients, 26 to 30 years old, with beta thalassemia major suggest that iron accumulation can be reduced by a mean of 44% with exchange transfusion compared with simple transfusion at the expense of increasing donor blood utilization two- to threefold.[44] A prospective study is currently under way to evaluate the role of chronic, partial red cell exchange transfusions in reducing the rate of transfusional iron accumulation in patients with thalassemia major at The Children's Hospital of Philadelphia.

Acquired (Extracorpuscular) Red Cell Disorders

Red cell exchange has been used to replace abnormal red cells resulting from extracorpuscular disorders, such as protozoal infection in malaria and babesiosis.[19-21] Cerebral malaria is a life-threatening complication of *Plasmodium falciparum* infection. Although controlled trials have not been performed, case studies suggest red cell exchange in conjunction with antimalarial regimens results in more rapid reduction in peripheral parasite load and clinical improvement than pharmacotherapy alone.[19] Because the degree of parasitemia correlates with mortality, red cell exchange transfusion has been recommended for hyperparasitemia at levels exceeding 10% or 20%.[10,19,20] Red cell exchange has also been recommended for those patients, regardless of parasite burden, with severe complications of *P. falciparum* malaria, such as encephalopathy, disseminated intravascular coagulation (DIC), renal failure, and adult respiratory distress syndrome. Due to the paucity of data, the minimum effective volume of red cell exchange has not been determined and ranges from half-volume to two volumes in published cases.[10,19] Rather than a specified red cell volume exchange, the goal of the procedure should be directed at attaining a low parasite load (eg, <5%) and achieving clinical improvement.[10,20]

Plasmapheresis

Plasmapheresis efficiently reduces the plasma concentration of pathologic antibodies, plasma proteins, cytokines, lipoproteins, protein-bound drugs, and metabolic toxins. The majority of plasma exchange procedures are performed for immunologic diseases, when autoantibodies, alloantibodies, or immune complexes are implicated in the pathogenesis.[9,11,12] Plasmapheresis removes offending antibody and exerts other immunomodulatory effects to mitigate symptoms of autoimmune diseases. For example, serum autoantibodies against ganglioside are found in approximately 30% of patients with acute inflammatory demyelinating polyradiculoneuropathy, which is also known as the Guillain-Barré syndrome.[9] The titer of these antibodies has been correlated with the severity of the disease in small clinical series, and plasmapheresis may hasten clinical improvement by decreasing their concentration. However, patients without detectable antibodies are also effectively treated with plasmapheresis, implicating other beneficial immunomodulatory effects. A randomized controlled trial has demonstrated that intravenous immunoglobulin (IVIG) was as effective as plasmapheresis alone or plasmapheresis in combination with IVIG in alleviating disability associated with Guillain-Barré syndrome.[45] In contrast, some autoimmune diseases, such as rheumatoid arthritis, do not respond to plasmapheresis, but may be effectively treated with other therapeutic apheresis modalities such as lymphocytapheresis or Protein A immunoadsorption.[9]

Diseases resulting from excessive accumulation of normal plasma constituents or production of pathogenic factors are amenable to plasmapheresis. For example, patients with familial hypercholesterolemia or severely dyslipidemic patients whose diseases are resistant to diet and drug therapy may benefit from plasmapheresis, due to efficient removal of offending total cholesterol, low-density lipoprotein (LDL) and other apoB-containing lipoproteins.[11] Serum lipoproteins serve as carriers for excessive phytanic acid in patients with phytanic acid storage disease (Refsum's disease), and plasmapheresis is a useful adjunct to dietary treatment.[11] Hyperviscosity syndrome, resulting from the accumulation of clonal immunoglobulins in Waldenstrom's macroglobulinemia or multiple myeloma, is also alleviated with plasmapheresis.[12] Circulating cytokines, such as tumor necrosis factor and interleukin-1, mediate some of the septic complications of severe protozoal infections, and plasmapheresis has been used to reduce their concentration as well as clear debris from hemolyzed red cells in severely infected patients.[19,21] Plasmapheresis has been used as adjunctive therapy to prevent recurrent focal segmental glomerulosclerosis following renal transplantation, and may remove a circulating factor that alters glomerular permeability.[46,47]

These plasmapheresis procedures utilize 5% albumin or a combination of albumin and physiologic saline as replacement fluids. Fresh frozen plasma may be added to the replacement regimen for patients with coagulopathy or risk of bleeding. Plasmapheresis has been used to treat DIC and clotting factor inhibitors, requiring extensive replacement of the patient's plasma with fresh frozen plasma and/or cryoprecipitate to prevent dilutional coagulopathy and to restore hemostasis. Fresh frozen plasma is also the primary replacement fluid for cases of thrombotic thrombocytopenic purpura (TTP), for reasons explained below.

Thrombotic Thrombocytopenic Purpura/Atypical Hemolytic Uremic Syndrome

Hemolytic uremic syndrome (HUS) is not a single disease entity but rather a heterogeneous group of disorders with different causes, clinical courses, and prognoses, characterized by thrombocytopenia, microangiopathic hemolytic anemia, and renal dysfunction. Principal categories of the disease have emerged, including classic (typical, epidemic, diarrhea-associated) HUS, atypical (sporadic, non-diarrhea-associated) HUS, and secondary HUS. Classic HUS accounts for approximately 90% of childhood cases, and is usually associated with infection with enterotoxigenic bacteria, such as *Escherichia coli* O157:H7.[11] The disorder demonstrates age and seasonal predilection, occurring most often in children under 3 to 5 years old during late spring, summer, and early fall. Onset of hemolysis and renal abnormalities is abrupt, usually occurring within a week of the hemorrhagic colitis or diarrheal illness. The vast majority of children with classic HUS recover fully with supportive treatment and dialysis and do not experience relapses or recurrences.

The remaining 10% of cases of childhood HUS are referred to as atypical, non-diarrhea-associated, or sporadic disease. A proportion of these cases are likely due to invasive pneumococcal infection[48,49]; while other cases have no clear etiology or disease association. Children with atypical HUS do not have diarrhea in the course of the disease, and there is no seasonal prevalence. The disorder is rare in children less than 2 years of age, may demonstrate a familial association, and may be recurrent. In contrast to the abrupt onset of classic HUS, atypical HUS has an insidious onset of anemia and thrombocytopenia. The clinical course and outcome in childhood atypical HUS varies greatly, likely reflecting the heterogeneity of diseases included in the group without diarrhea. With notable exceptions,[49,50] most case series have reported a less favorable prognosis for atypical HUS compared with classic HUS in pediatric populations.[51-54]

In addition to microangiopathic hemolytic anemia, thrombocytopenia, and renal function abnormalities, neurologic signs and symptoms may be prominent in atypical HUS. This clinical picture also describes TTP in adults, and the diseases have been described as a spectrum with TTP occurring primarily in adults with predominant neurologic symptoms and atypical HUS occurring mainly in children with predominant renal symptoms. However, TTP may occur with fulminant renal failure and HUS may demonstrate impressive neurologic symptoms. Use of the term TTP/HUS reflects this clinical overlap, and the condition is treated aggressively with plasmapheresis due to the severity of the disease and poor prognosis without prompt treatment.[55] TTP/HUS may be secondary to drugs, malignancy, marrow transplantation or systemic infections. Chronic relapsing TTP in children is a rare form of idiopathic TTP manifesting in childhood.[56]

Recent evidence regarding the pathogenesis of idiopathic TTP and HUS suggests a definitive means of discriminating between the two diseases. The vascular lesions in TTP and HUS are composed predominantly of aggregated platelets. Contributing to the tendency for platelet aggregation are unusually large von Willebrand factor (vWF) multimers circulating in the plasma and adhering to the platelets.[57] Defects in processing these unusually large forms of vWF to smaller, less platelet-adherent forms have been described in patients with TTP, but not in patients with HUS.[58,59] An absolute deficiency in the enzyme, vWF metalloprotease, has been described in children with chronic relapsing TTP, and enzymatic activity was reduced or absent in patients with idiopathic TTP but normal in patients with HUS.[58] An inhibitor of vWF metalloprotease was detected in adults with TTP during active periods of disease but not during remission.[59]

Role of Therapeutic Apheresis

Classic HUS in children is effectively treated with supportive care and dialysis in the vast majority of cases; consequently, plasmapheresis or plasma infusion is not recommended.[11] Because of the difficulty in distinguishing HUS and TTP in adult populations and the grave consequences of delayed treatment of TTP, plasma exchange with fresh frozen plasma replacement is recommended for the TTP/HUS syndrome in adults.[55] The use of plasma exchange dramatically converted TTP from a fatal disease with a mortality exceeding 90% to a curable one with a mortality of approximately 10% to 20% among adults.[55] The underlying rationale for the effectiveness of plasma exchange is likely the efficient removal of offending inhibitors of vWF metalloprotease activity and replacement with functional enzyme to process unusually large von Willebrand factor in affected patients.[56-58] Chronic relapsing TTP in children may respond to simple plasma infusions, because these enzyme-deficient patients require only periodic repletion of enzyme not removal of inhibitors.[59] Determination of vWF metalloprotease activity may be a useful way to discriminate between TTP and HUS or predict which patients will respond to therapeutic plasma exchange.

The role of plasma exchange in treating atypical, non-diarrhea-associated HUS in children is not clear. Pneumococcus-associated HUS is treated with supportive care and dialysis, and some authors caution against transfusing plasma-containing blood products to these patients because of the possibility of red cell T-activation and hemolysis.[60] In contrast, case reports of clinical response in patients with atypical HUS have been reported,[52,61] and some authors have recommended plasma exchange in the treatment of severe forms of HUS.[62,63] Similarly, plasmapheresis may be used to treat transplant-associated and other secondary forms of TTP/HUS, based on anecdotal experience with single case reports and small series of patients.[64]

Technical Aspects

If plasma exchange is used for atypical HUS or secondary forms of TTP/HUS, a strategy similar to that used for adult idiopathic

TTP is employed. Daily plasma exchange should be performed, replacing 1 to 1.5 plasma volumes with fresh frozen plasma or plasma depleted of cryoprecipitate (cryosupernatant or cryo-poor plasma),[65] until LDH normalizes and platelet counts increase to greater than 100 to 150 × 10^6/mL for 2 to 3 consecutive days.[55,66] Following this recovery, plasmapheresis is either discontinued completely or gradually tapered by prolonging the interval between treatments or reducing the volume of plasma exchanged. In a survey of 20 apheresis centers in the United States, 40% reported use of a tapering strategy that involved performing additional procedures after documenting a response to daily exchanges; however, there was no statistically measurable advantage to tapering compared with discontinuing treatment with respect to relapse rates.[66] The duration of treatment necessary to effect a response is variable, averaging 10 days with a range of 2 to 34 days.[66] If a patient experiences an acute exacerbation of TTP following withdrawal of treatment or a recurrence of the disease several weeks after treatment, plasmapheresis must be emergently resumed. The relapse rate following successful treatment is estimated as 40%.[66]

PANDAS

Pediatric autoimmune neuropsychiatric disorders associated with streptococcus (PANDAS) describe a group of patients with childhood-onset obsessive-compulsive disorder (OCD) and tic disorders.[67] These patients experience symptom exacerbations following group A beta-hemolytic streptococcal infections (GABHS). As with Sydenham's chorea, the neurologic complication of rheumatic fever, antibodies against GABHS are thought to crossreact with neuronal cells to produce inflammation in the central nervous system, particularly within the basal ganglia, in patients with PANDAS. Because autoimmunity was implicated in the pathogenesis of the disease, a controlled trial of plasmapheresis and IVIG was investigated as treatment.[68] Perlmutter et al[68] studied 30 children with severe, infection-triggered exacerbations of OCD or tic disorders who were randomly chosen to receive active treatment with either plasma exchange or IVIG or placebo (saline infusion). The plasma exchange group received five single-volume exchanges over 2 weeks, with 5% albumin and saline replacement. Symptom severity was rated at baseline, and at 1 month and 12 months after treatment by use of standard assessment scales for OCD, tics, anxiety, depression, and global function. The authors concluded plasma exchange and IVIG were both effective in lessening the severity of symptoms in children with infection- triggered OCD and tic disorders. This improvement persisted in all measures for most children at the 1-year point with both therapies, with a trend toward greater relief of OCD symptoms with plasma exchange than with IVIG.

Leukapheresis and Plateletpheresis

Therapeutic leukapheresis and plateletpheresis are used to remove cells circulating in great excess, such as leukemic blasts or platelets, from patients with hematologic malignancies or myeloproliferative disorders. Leukocytosis causes symptoms related to increased viscosity or metabolic derangement; and markedly elevated leukocyte or platelet counts increase the risk of thrombosis or bleeding. Cellular depletion with therapeutic apheresis is expected to provide temporary clinical improvement and symptomatic relief, but is not definitive treatment for the underlying disease. Consequently, therapeutic apheresis is used in conjunction with chemotherapy or as a temporizing measure if chemotherapy is contraindicated.

Leukocytosis

Extreme increases in peripheral leukocyte concentration, often exceeding 100,000/μL, occur in leukemia and may result in serious complications due to increased viscosity of whole blood and/or metabolic disturbances.[10,69] Symptoms of leukostasis and hyperviscosity reflect multi-organ involvement and include tachypnea, dyspnea, pulmonary insufficiency, blurred vision, diplopia, dizziness, slurred speech, and coma. Dire pulmonary and neurologic complications such as intracranial and pulmonary hemorrhage may ensue. Metabolic derangement resulting from increased cellular proliferation, metabolism, and cell death may result in hyperuricemia, hyperphosphatemia, hyperkalemia, hypocalcemia, and renal failure. Biochemical imbalances may be aggravated by chemotherapy-induced blast cell lysis. Patients with myeloid malignancies are more likely to experience symptoms of thrombosis or hemorrhage than those with lymphoid malignancies, due to large, relatively nondeformable myeloblasts that are more likely to sludge in capillaries and damage vessels.[69,70] Consequently, complications of hyperleukocytosis are more common in acute myelogenous leukemia (AML) or chronic myelogenous leukemia (CML) in accelerated or blast crisis, less common in acute lymphocytic leukemia (ALL), and rare in chronic lymphocytic leukemia (CLL). Leukostasis remains a risk factor in chronic phase CML patients with hyperleukocytosis due to the associated increase in immature myelocytes. A higher incidence of hyperleukocytosis and leukostasis in childhood CML than in adult CML has been reported.[71]

Role of Therapeutic Apheresis

Rapid cytoreduction with leukapheresis is widely accepted as a means to alleviate symptoms and prevent complications due to hyperleukocytosis in children with leukemia.[10,70,72] The threshold for treatment is extremely variable, as the cellular concentration that poses risk to an individual patient depends on a number of factors including physical properties of the circulating leukocytes, the status of the microvasculature, and the underlying medical condition. As a general guideline, patients with peripheral white cell counts greater than 100,000/μL, with a high percentage of blasts and promyelocytes, and neurologic or pulmonary manifestations of leukostasis are candidates for leukocyte depletion. Leukapheresis has also been used as an adjunct to chemotherapy to prevent metabolic complications associated with blast cell lysis in ALL and as a means to control leukocytosis in CML when cytotoxic therapy is contraindicated, as in early pregnancy.[73,74]

Technical Aspects

Leukapheresis may be repeated daily until clinical manifestations of leukostasis and hyperviscosity resolve or leukocyte count is substantially reduced. A general therapeutic endpoint with respect to the postprocedure leukocyte count cannot be specified; therapy must be tailored to the individual. Although some degree of cytoreduction is usually accomplished, the efficacy of the procedure is variable and reflects the total body tumor burden, cellular proliferative rate, physical properties of tumor cells, and response to concomitant chemotherapy. The procedure usually involves processing two or more volumes of the patient's blood, and the total volume removed varies depending on the patient's size and white cell count. Calculation of appropriate replacement fluids with leukocyte depletion procedures is extremely important to avoid hypovolemia, dehydration, and acid-base imbalance, especially in small children. In addition, clinical and laboratory monitoring of citrate toxicity is important during leukapheresis procedures, because large volumes of blood are processed and virtually all of the administered citrate is returned to the patient. Heparin may be used in conjunction with citrate anticoagulation, to decrease the amount of citrate administered to the patient, in the absence of specific contraindications such as coagulopathy or hemorrhage.

Thrombocythemia

Thrombocythemia occurs in myeloproliferative disorders, such as essential thrombocythemia, polycythemia vera, or chronic myelogenous leukemia. Thrombocytosis is frequently seen in conjunction with reactive or secondary megakaryocytic proliferation, as occurs following splenectomy or with underlying malignancy or inflammatory disease. Both malignant thrombocythemia and reactive thrombocytosis may result in platelet counts exceeding 1,000,000/μL; however, reactive thrombocytosis following splenectomy or other causes in children is transient and rarely requires treatment. In contrast, thrombocythemia associated with myeloproliferative disorders is persistent and may require treatment to prevent bleeding or thrombosis. Primary treatment requires myelosuppressive therapy to lower the platelet count. Such therapy usually alleviates symptoms, but takes up to 2 weeks to lower platelet concentrations. Consequently, plateletpheresis may be performed to lower the platelet count more rapidly. There is poor correlation between the platelet count and the risk of significant clinical problems. Plateletpheresis is generally recommended as an adjunct to chemotherapy for patients with platelet counts greater than 1,000,000/µL and for patients with markedly elevated platelet counts and manifestations of thrombosis or bleeding, irrespective of the exact platelet concentration.[10]

Modified Therapeutic Apheresis Methods

Modification of apheresis techniques permits more selective removal of pathogenic plasma components or manipulation of collected immune cells for cellular therapeutic applications. Selective plasma component removal is exemplified by staphylococcal protein A immunoadsorption and LDL apheresis.[75] With protein A immunoadsorption, plasma is separated by plasmapheresis and perfused through a column containing covalently bound protein A. Immune complexes and IgG bind to the column and the processed plasma is returned to the patient. The therapeutic effect of the procedure is more likely due to immunomodulatory effects rather than the direct removal of pathogenic IgG and circulating immune complexes. Protein A immunoadsorption may be effective adjunctive therapy for chronic, refractory idiopathic thrombocytopenic purpura (ITP) or other autoimmune conditions in children.[9]

LDL apheresis uses dextran sulfate columns to selectively remove apoB-containing lipoproteins from patients with familial hypercholesterolemia and other dyslipidemias refractory to diet and drug treatment. Treatment thresholds for heterozygous familial hypercholesterolemia patients already receiving maximal doses of lipid-lowering drugs depend on underlying cardiac status: LDL cholesterol levels >300 mg/dL for patients without evidence of coronary artery disease, or LDL cholesterol levels >200 mg/dL for patients with established coronary artery disease. LDL apheresis has been used successfully for children 5 years or older with homozygous familial hypercholesterolemia.[76,77] This therapeutic approach is limited in smaller children primarily by the large extracorporeal volume of the devices.

Photopheresis or extracorporeal photochemotherapy is a modified apheresis procedure to activate the host immune response against autoreactive or malignant lymphocytes.[78] Leukapheresis is performed to collect mononuclear cells, which are then treated with 8-methoxypsoralen and exposed to ultraviolet light. These chemically modified cells are reinfused to the patients and stimulate the host's immune system against pathogenic lymphocyte populations by mechanisms that have not been fully elucidated. Photopheresis has been used to treat cutaneous T-cell lymphoma, as well as other T-cell disorders, such as graft-vs-host disease.[78]

Conclusion

The use of therapeutic apheresis techniques is increasing in the pediatric setting. With careful attention to intravascular fluid volume and circulating red cell mass, as well as prompt recognition of adverse effects, therapeutic apheresis can be performed safely, even in small infants and critically ill children. The available published data supports the use of therapeutic apheresis in selected immunologic, hematologic, and metabolic diseases. Further clinical research is necessary to define the role of therapeutic apheresis in the management of other diseases and to derive optimal treatment schedules. Because therapeutic apheresis is often used for life-threatening medical emergencies or for rare diseases, a coordinated effort and multi-institutional approach to clinical research will be necessary.

References

1. Kim HC. Therapeutic pediatric apheresis. J Clin Apheresis 2000;15: 129-57.
2. Gorlin JB. Therapeutic plasma exchange and cytapheresis in pediatric patients. Transfusion Sci 1999;21:21-39.

3. Jeter EK, Rogers RL. Pediatric apheresis. In: McLeod BC, Price TH, Drew MJ, eds. Apheresis: Principles and practice. Bethesda, MD: AABB Press, 1997:409-21.
4. Kevy SV, Fosburg M. Therapeutic apheresis in childhood. J Clin Apheresis 1990;5:87-90.
5. Kasprisin DO. Techniques, indications and toxicity of therapeutic hemapheresis in children. J Clin Apheresis 1989;5:21-4.
6. Vamvakas EC. Evaluation of clinical studies of the efficacy of therapeutic apheresis. J Clin Apheresis 2000;15:6-17.
7. Strauss RG, Ciavarella D, Gilcher RO, et al. An overview of current management. J Clin Apheresis 1993;8:189-94.
8. McCleod BC. Introduction to the third special issue: Clinical applications of therapeutic apheresis. J Clin Apheresis 2000;15:1-5.
9. Koo AP. Therapeutic apheresis in autoimmune and rheumatic diseases. J Clin Apheresis 2000;15:18-27.
10. Grima KM. Therapeutic apheresis in hematological and oncological diseases. J Clin Apheresis 2000;15:28-52.
11. Winters JL, Pineda AA, McLeod BC, Grima KM. Therapeutic apheresis in renal and metabolic diseases. J Clin Apheresis 2000;15:53-73.
12. Weinstein R. Therapeutic apheresis in neurological diseases. J Clin Apheresis 2000;15:74-128.
13. Leitman SF, Kucera E, McLeod BC, et al. Guidelines for therapeutic hemapheresis. Bethesda, MD: American Association of Blood Banks, 1992.
14. Stockman JA. Red cell transfusions in pediatrics. In: Rossi EC, Simon TL, Moss GS, Gould SA, eds. Principles of transfusion medicine. Baltimore, MD: Williams & Wilkins, 1996:167-76.
15. Clough L, Dugan N, Hulitt C, et al. Improved method to estimate total blood volume for erythrocytapheresis using the COBE Spectra in pediatric sickle cell patients. J Clin Apheresis 1998;13:81.
16. McCleod BC, Sniecinski I, Ciavarella D, et al. Frequency of immediate adverse effects associated with therapeutic apheresis. Transfusion 1999; 39:282-8.
17. Francina A, Chassard D, Baklouti F, et al. Open heart surgery in a patient with a high oxygen affinity haemoglobin variant. Anesthesia 1989; 44:31-3.
18. Larson PJ, Friedman D, Reilly MP, et al. The presurgical management of a patient with a high oxygen affinity, unstable hemoglobin variant (Hb Bryn Mawr) with erythrocytapheresis. Transfusion 1997;37:703-7.
19. Golden PJ, Weinstein R. Treatment of high-risk, refractory acquired methemoglobinemia with automated red blood cell exchange. J Clin Apheresis 1998;13:28-31.
20. Phillips P, Nantel S, Benny WB. Exchange transfusion as an adjunct to the treatment of severe falciparum malaria: case report and review. Rev Infect Dis 1990;12:1100-8.

21. Weir EG, King KE, Ness PM, Eshleman SH. Automated RBC exchange transfusion: Treatment for cerebral malaria. Transfusion 2000;40:702-7.
22. Evenson DA, Perry E, Kloster B, et al. Therapeutic apheresis for babesiosis. J Clin Apheresis 1998;13:32-6.
23. Werch J, Todd C. Resolution by erythrocytapheresis of the exposure of an Rh-negative person to Rh-positive cells: An alternative treatment. Transfusion 1993;33:530-2.
24. Adams RJ, McKie VC, Hsu L, et al. Prevention of a first stroke by transfusions in children with sickle cell anemia and abnormal results on transcranial doppler ultrasonography. N Engl J Med 1998;339:5-11.
25. Cohen AR, Norris CF, Smith-Whitley K. Transfusion therapy for sickle cell disease. In: Capon SM, Chambers LA, eds. New directions in pediatric hematology. Bethesda, MD: American Association of Blood Banks, 1996: 39-88.
26. Cohen AR, Martin MB, Silber JH, et al. A modified transfusion program for prevention of stroke in sickle cell disease. Blood 1992;79:1657-61.
27. Miller ST, Jensen D, Rao SP. Less intensive long-term transfusion therapy for sickle cell anemia and cerebrovascular accident. J Pediatr 1992; 120:54-7.
28. Vichinsky EP, Neumayr LD, Earles AN, et al. Causes and outcomes of the acute chest syndrome in sickle cell disease. N Engl J Med 2000;342: 1855-65.
29. Hassell KL, Eckman JR, Lane PA. Acute multiorgan failure syndrome: A potentially catastrophic complication of severe sickle cell pain episodes. Am J Med 1994;96:155-62.
30. Siegel JF, Rich MA, Brock WA. Association of sickle cell disease, priapism, exchange transfusion and neurological events: ASPEN syndrome. J Urology 1993;150:1480-2.
31. Koshy M, Chisum D, Burd L, et al. Management of sickle cell anemia and pregnancy. J Clin Apheresis 1991;6:230-3.
32. Vichinsky EP, Haberkern CM, Neumayr L, et al. A comparison of conservative and aggressive transfusion regimens in the perioperative management of sickle cell disease. N Engl J Med 1995;333:206-13.
33. Kim HC, Dugan NP, Silber JH, et al. Erythrocytapheresis therapy to reduce iron overload in chronically transfused patients with sickle cell disease. Blood 1994;83:1136-42.
34. Adams DM, Schultz WH, Ware RE, Kinney TR. Erythrocytapheresis can reduce iron overload and prevent the need for chelation therapy in chronically transfused pediatric patients. J Pediatr Hematol Oncol 1996;18: 46-50.
35. Singer ST, Quirolo K, Niski K, et al. Erythrocytapheresis for chronically transfused children with sickle cell disease: An effective method for maintaining a low hemoglobin S level and reducing iron overload. J Clin Apheresis 1999;14:122-5.

36. Hilliard LM, Williams BF, Lounsbury AE, Howard TH. Erythrocytapheresis limits iron accumulation in chronically transfused sickle cell patients. Am J Hematol 1998;59:28-35.
37. Stramer SL, Caglioti S, Strong DM. NAT of the United States and Canadian blood supply. Transfusion 2000;40:1165-8.
38. Dodd RK. Germs, gels, and genomes: A personal recollection of 30 years in blood safety testing. In: Stramer SL, ed. Blood safety in the new millennium. Bethesda, MD: American Association of Blood Banks, 2000: 97-122.
39. Sosler SD, Jilly BJ, Saporito C, Koshy M. A simple, practical model for reducing alloimmunization in patients with sickle cell disease. Am J Hematol 1993;43:103-6.
40. Tahhan HR, Holbrook CT, Braddy LR, et al. Antigen-matched donor blood in the transfusion management of patients with sickle cell disease. Transfusion 1994;34:558-60.
41. Schmalzer EZ, Lee JO, Brown AK, et al. Viscosity of mixtures of sickle and normal red cells at varying hematocrit levels: Implications for transfusion. Transfusion 1987;27:228-33.
42. Kim HC, Dugan N, Clough L, et al. Comparison of erythrocytapheresis performed by intermittent-flow centrifugation (Haemonetics V50) and continuous-flow centrifugation (COBE Spectra) (abstract). In: ASFA 16th annual meeting final program. Tuscon, AZ: American Society for Apheresis, 1995:68.
43. Berdoukas VA, Kwan YL, Sansotta ML. A study on the value of red cell exchange transfusion in transfusion dependent anaemias. Clin Lab Haematol 1986;8:209-20.
44. Cohen AR, Friedman DF, Larson PJ, et al. Erythrocytapheresis to reduce iron loading in thalassemia (abstract). Blood 1998;92(Suppl 1):532a.
45. Plasma Exchange/Sandoglobulin Guillain-Barré Syndrome Trial Group. Randomised trial of plasma exchange, intravenous immunoglobulin and combined treatments in Guillain-Barré syndrome. Lancet 1997;349: 225-30.
46. Savin VJ, Sharma R, Sharma M, et al. Circulating factor associated with increased glomerular permeability to albumin in recurrent focal segmental glomerulosclerosis. N Engl J Med 1996;334:878-83.
47. Sharma M, Sharma R, McCarthy ET, Savin VJ. "The FSGS factor:" Enrichment and in vivo effect of activity from focal segmental glomerulosclerosis plasma. J Am Soc Nephrol 1999;10:552-61.
48. Cabrera GR, Fortenberry J, Warshaw BL, et al. Hemolytic uremic syndrome associated with invasive *Streptococcus pneumoniae* infection. Pediatrics 1998;101:699-703.
49. Mizusawa Y, Pitcher LA, Burke JR, et al. Survey of haemolytic-uraemic syndrome in Queensland 1979-1995. Med J Aust 1996;165:188-91.

50. Siegler RL, Pavia AT, Hansen FL, et al. Atypical hemolytic-uremic syndrome: A comparison with postdiarrheal disease. J Pediatr 1996;128: 505-11.
51. Fitzpatrick MM, Walters MDS, Trompeter RS, et al. Atypical (non-diarrhea-associated) hemolytic uremic syndrome in childhood. J Pediatr 1993;122:532-7.
52. Loirat C, Baudouin V, Sonsino E, et al. Hemolytic-uremic syndrome in the child. Adv Nephrol 1993;22:141-68.
53. Tonshoff B, Sammet A, Sanden I, et al. Outcome and prognostic determinants in the hemolytic uremic syndrome of children. Nephron 1994; 68:63-70.
54. Renaud C, Niaudet P, Gagnadoux MF, et al. Haemolytic uraemic syndrome: Prognostic factors in children over 3 years of age. Pediatr Nephrol 1995;9:24-9.
55. George JN, Gilcher RO, Smith JW, et al. Thrombotic thrombocytopenic purpura-hemolytic uremic syndrome: Diagnosis and management. J Clin Apheresis 1998;13:120-5.
56. Moake JL. Studies on the pathophysiology of thrombotic thrombocytopenic purpura. Semin Hematol 1997;34:83-9.
57. Furlan M, Robles R, Galbusera M, et al. Von Willebrand factor-cleaving protease in thrombotic thrombocytopenic purpura and the hemolytic-uremic syndrome. N Engl J Med 1998;339:1578-84.
58. Tsai HM, Lian ECY. Antibodies to von Willebrand factor-cleaving protease in acute thrombotic thrombocytopenic purpura. N Engl J Med 1998;339: 1585-94.
59. Chintagumpala MM, Hurwitz RL, Moake JL, et al. Chronic relapsing thrombotic thrombocytopenic purpura in infants with large von Willebrand factor multimers during remission. J Pediatr 1992;120:49-53.
60. Crookston KP, Reiner AP, Cooper LJN, et al. RBC T activation and hemolysis: Implications for pediatric transfusion management. Transfusion 2000;40:801-12.
61. Robson WLM, Leung AKC. The successful treatment of atypical HUS with plasmapheresis. Clin Nephrol 1991;35:119-22.
62. Slavicek J, Puretic Z, Novak M, et al. The role of plasma exchange in the treatment of severe forms of HUS in childhood. Int J Artif Organs 1995;19:506-10.
63. Gianviti A, Perna A, Caringella A, et al. Plasma exchange in children with hemolytic-uremic syndrome at risk of poor outcome. Am J Kidney Dis 1993;22:264-6.
64. Schriber JR, Herzig GP. Transplantation-associated thrombotic thrombocytopenic purpura and hemolytic uremic syndrome. Semin Hematol 1997;34:126-33.
65. Rock G, Shumak KH, Sutton DMC, et al. Cryosupernatant as replacement fluid for plasma exchange in thrombotic thrombocytopenic purpura. Br J Haematol 1996;94:383-6.

66. Bandarenko N, Brecher ME, and Members of the US TTP Apheresis Study Group. United States thrombotic thrombocytopenic purpura apheresis study group (US TTP ASG): Multicenter survey and retrospective analysis of current efficacy of therapeutic plasma exchange. J Clin Apheresis 1998;13:133-41.
67. Swedo SE, Leonard HL, Garvey M, et al. Pediatric autoimmune neuropsychiatric disorders associated with streptococcal infections: Clinical description of the first 50 cases. Am J Psychiatry 1998:155:264-71.
68. Perlmutter SJ, Leitman SF, Garvey MA, et al. Therapeutic plasma exchange and intravenous immunoglobulin for obsessive-compulsive disorder and tic disorders in childhood. Lancet 1999;354:1153-8.
69. Lichtman MA, Rowe JM. Hyperleukocytic leukemias: Rheological, clinical and therapeutic considerations. Blood 1982;60:279-83.
70. Bunin NJ, Pui CH. Differing complications of hyperleukocytosis in children with acute lymphoblastic or acute nonlymphoblastic leukemia. J Clin Oncol 1985;3:1590-5.
71. Rowe J, Lichtman M. Hyperleukocytosis and leukostasis: Common features of childhood chronic myelogenous leukemia. Blood 1984;63: 1230-4.
72. Lane TA. Continuous-flow leukapheresis for rapid cytoreduction in leukemia. Transfusion 1980;20:455-7.
73. Caplan SN, Coco FV, Berkman EM. Management of chronic myelocytic leukemia in pregnancy by cell pheresis. Transfusion 1978;18:120-4.
74. Strobl FJ, Voelkerding KV, Smith EP. Management of chronic myeloid leukemia during pregnancy with leukapheresis. J Clin Apheresis 1999;14: 42-4.
75. Vamvakas EC, Pineda AA. Selective extraction of plasma constituents. In: McLeod BC, Price TH, Drew MJ, eds. Apheresis: Principles and practice. Bethesda, MD: AABB Press, 1997:375-407.
76. Zwiener JR, Uauy R, Petruska ML, Huet BA. Low-density lipoprotein apheresis as long-term treatment for children with homozygous familial hypercholesterolemia. J Pediatr 1995;126:728-35.
77. Gordon BR, Kelsey SF, Dau PC, et al. Long-term effects of low-density lipoprotein apheresis using an automated dextran sulfate cellulose adsorption system. Am J Cardiol 1998;81:407-11.
78. Sniecinski I. Photopheresis. In: McLeod BC, Price TH, Drew MJ, eds. Apheresis: Principles and practice. Bethesda, MD: AABB Press, 1997: 521-35.

In: Herman JH, Manno CS, eds.
Pediatric Transfusion Therapy
Bethesda, MD: AABB Press, 2002

21

Adverse Reactions in Pediatric Transfusion

CATHY LITTY, MD

GENERALLY, THE TRANSFUSION of blood components is a safe and life-saving procedure. However, there are instances when transfusion may lead to an adverse outcome. Acute transfusion reactions in pediatric patients, especially the youngest patients, may differ from those seen in adults. This chapter discusses febrile reactions, allergic and anaphylactic reactions, bacterial contamination, acute lung injury, volume overload, and neonatal hypoglycemia. Hemolysis, transfusion-associated graft-vs-host disease, and cytomegalovirus transmission are covered in other chapters.

Cathy Litty, MD, Director of Transfusion Medicine, St. Christopher's Hospital for Children, Philadelphia, Pennsylvania

Febrile Nonhemolytic Transfusion Reactions and Leukocyte Reduction

Febrile nonhemolytic transfusion reactions (FNHTRs) are the most frequent complication of red cell and platelet therapy in adults. They also occur in children, but not as often. In infants, it is quite unusual to see a febrile reaction. These reactions consist of an increase in temperature of at least 1 C in association with transfusion, without any other cause. One cause of this reaction in multitransfused adults or multiparous women is antibodies previously formed to white cells. Transfusion in the neonatal period is different. The neonatal immune system is immature and cannot produce antibodies beyond IgM. Infants born prematurely are most likely to receive transfusion(s) during the neonatal period. A study of premature infants showed that, when transfusions begin in the neonatal period, antibodies to white cell antigens did not form.[1] Children whose transfusions begin at a young age are also less likely to form these antibodies.

Not all patients who have this type of reaction will have it after subsequent transfusions, and the reaction may be prevented by the use of antipyretics as pretreatment. Transfusing leukocyte-reduced components will reduce but not eliminate the occurrence of FNHTRs and is more likely to be of benefit with the transfusion of red cells than platelets.[2] The reason for the persistence of these reactions, even after leukocyte reduction, is the presence of cytokines in the blood component. Cytokines are soluble glycoproteins that regulate intercellular communication. Those seen in blood components are from the proinflammatory subset. For the important effects of these specific cytokines, see Table 21-1. The cytokines are produced by donor leukocytes in the product, rather than by the recipient at the time of transfusion, and therefore their presence does not differ whether the recipient is a child or an adult.

Heddle et al[3] first demonstrated that the age of platelet components, as well as the leukocyte count, correlated with the likelihood of a febrile reaction. A subsequent study showed that the supernatant portion of platelet concentrates was more likely to cause a reaction than the cellular portion, and, when a reaction

Table 21-1. Cytokines Produced by Monocytes in Blood Components

Cytokine	Actions in FNHTRs
Interleukin-1β	Pyrogen, causes hypotension
Interleukin-6	Pyrogen
Interleukin-8	Neutrophil chemotaxis and activation
Tumor necrosis factor	Pyrogen, causes hypotension

occurred, there was a positive correlation with high concentrations of interleukin (IL)-1β and IL-6.[4] Others also showed increasing levels of tumor necrosis factor (TNF), IL-1β, IL-6,[5] and IL-8[6] in platelets with greater lengths of storage and a greater risk of FNHTR with higher concentrations.[5] Prestorage filtration was shown to prevent the production of cytokines in the components during storage.[6,7] Cytokines increase in the supernatant portion of RBC units during storage, although not reaching the levels observed in platelet concentrates.[8] The reason for this is that monocytes, a large percentage of the white cells in platelet concentrates, remain active at room temperature, which is how platelets are stored. Red cells are stored at 1-6 C. However, red cells also are less likely to produce FNHTRs if white cell levels are reduced before storage rather than after storage.[9]

In a pediatric patient receiving platelets, when the clinician feels that avoiding transfusion reactions is key, platelets obtained by apheresis with modern machinery will be collected as leukocyte-reduced. Whole-blood-derived platelets are more difficult to obtain with prestorage leukocyte reduction. Leukocyte reduction in the hospital blood bank or at the bedside will remove only the white cells, not the cytokines that are already present. In a small child, however, an entire apheresis unit may be too large a dose.

When FNHTRs do occur, they are not serious, and antipyretics are an effective treatment. Because fever is the initial sign of a hemolytic reaction, however, it is necessary to stop the transfusion and proceed with a transfusion reaction evaluation. Other, more serious causes of the temperature elevation, such as hemolysis or bacterial contamination, will then be ruled out. FNHTRs are actually diagnosed by the exclusion of other causes of fever.

HLA Alloimmunization

HLA antibodies may form after exposure to HLA Class II antigens on white cells, and these antibodies may subsequently react with HLA Class I antigens on platelets. In adults, these antibodies cause patients to be refractory to platelet transfusions, which can lead to serious difficulty in achieving adequate post-transfusion platelet levels. The antibodies will not form if the recipient is exposed only to Class I antibodies, such as those seen on platelets. It has been shown that leukocyte reduction of blood components helps to prevent the formation of the antibodies, thus reducing the occurrence of antibody-mediated refractoriness to platelet transfusions.[10]

A study of preterm infants showed that 7 of 19 neonates who received nonleukocyte-reduced red cell transfusions were able to form HLA antibodies, while those receiving leukocyte-reduced red cells did not.[11] This finding for HLA antibodies differs from the study above, which evaluated antibodies to white cells,[1] but the authors state that the HLA antibodies may be transient. In addition, these infants were receiving red cells, not platelets. There is no evidence that platelet refractoriness would have resulted.

Both of the above studies evaluate premature infants. Studies of the capacity of the immune system in older children have not been performed. It is believed that starting red cell transfusions before age 10 in sickle cell patients leads to a tolerance, and fewer red cell alloantibodies are formed, but the same knowledge is not available for HLA and white cell antibodies.

On rare occasions, children do receive HLA-matched platelet transfusions, because they are exhibiting refractoriness to platelet transfusions. In many of these cases, however, when testing is performed to identify lymphocytotoxic HLA antibodies, none are identified. This is the case in teenagers as well, who may be thought to have immune systems more like those of adults.

Leukocyte Reduction for All Components

The question of whether leukocyte reduction of all components for pediatric transfusion would provide enough benefits in preventing febrile reactions and refractoriness to platelet transfusion to be justified is a difficult one. Leukocyte reduction has clear benefits in preventing cytomegalovirus infection, and this additional use may cause children's hospitals to use it for all three reasons. Although the neonate's immune system is immature, the system in older children may behave more like that in adults from an immunologic standpoint. It is unknown at what age this maturity is likely to be reached, and pediatric patients may survive their illness to go on and develop adult illnesses. Keeping them free of HLA antibody at a young age may have more benefits later on. All of this is subject to great debate at the current time, as the decision to leukocyte reduce all components for adults is still controversial.

There is wide difference of opinion as to whether transfusion-related immunomodulation in adults is a real phenomenon. This is defined as an immune alteration due to allogeneic white cells that makes the recipient more susceptible to postoperative wound infections and other septic events. There is an abundance of adult literature, not all reaching the same conclusion, but there is only one prospective study of the same phenomenon in low birth weight infants. Preterm infants were randomly assigned to receive standard or leukocyte-reduced red cell transfusions. It suggested that red cell transfusions induce selective lymphocyte alterations that are less pronounced in leukocyte-reduced blood. Because of small sample size, no trends reached statistical significance. There was also a trend toward more serious infections in those infants who received standard red cells.[12] A larger study should be performed, as should similar studies in older children.

Anaphylactic and Cutaneous Hypersensitivity Reactions

Life-threatening anaphylactic reactions may occur within minutes after the infusion of only a few milliliters of blood. The patient may exhibit coughing, bronchospasm, and respiratory distress, followed by vascular collapse and shock. Fever is absent, but flushing of the skin and gastrointestinal symptoms such as nausea, vomiting, or diarrhea may occur. The absence of IgA, which occurs in approximately 1 in 700 persons, is often a factor, but the recipient must also have anti-IgA present, so the actual occurrence is substantially lower than 1 in 700 transfusions. Previous transfusion might account for the presence of anti-IgA, but, in most people with the absence of IgA who have anti-IgA, the immunizing event is not clear. The antibodies may be class-specific, directed against the alpha heavy chain, or type-specific, directed against the heavy chain subclass. People with normal or deficient levels of IgA may make antibody to the heavy chain subclass that they do not possess (two antigenically distinct subclasses exist). Severe reactions are most often class-specific. The anti-IgA, which causes these reactions, is almost always a potent IgG or IgM antibody, not IgE. Other antibodies can occasionally be the cause, directed at soluble plasma proteins or even drugs, such as penicillin.[13] This reaction is rare in all age groups, but it occurs in the pediatric age group.

Anaphylactic reactions can have a severe and rapid onset even with only 10-15 mL of the blood component. Transfusion must be stopped immediately and the hypotension vigorously treated. Epinephrine given subcutaneously early in the course of treatment is vital. Known IgA-deficient patients with anti-IgA should receive blood from an IgA-negative donor. Deglycerolized or extensively washed RBC units will suffice. It is also possible to wash platelets if an IgA-negative donor cannot be identified, although not all blood centers are prepared to do this. If plasma components are needed, there is no other alternative: IgA-negative components from an IgA-deficient donor must be provided.

Cutaneous hypersensitivity or allergic reactions commonly cause urticaria and local erythema in the absence of fever. The allergies may be to plasma proteins. These reactions are mild and are most common in patients undergoing therapeutic plasmapheresis with plasma as the replacement fluid. The reactions may worsen with repeated exposure. Possibly because this type of plasmapheresis as well as diagnoses requiring large amounts of plasma are more common in adults, this reaction is seen more often in adults. It is, however, one of the more common reactions seen in children.

It is sensible to conserve the blood component, rather than increase donor exposure by discarding the component and transfusing another one. The transfusion may be paused while an antihistamine is administered and then restarted when the symptoms subside. If a patient has a history of these reactions, pretreatment with antihistamines is helpful.

Transfusion-Related Acute Lung Injury

Transfusion-related acute lung injury (TRALI) is a rare, but potentially life-threatening complication. Passive transfer of donor white cell antibodies reacting with the recipient's white cells is the usual cause of TRALI. Any blood component containing plasma can be implicated. RBCs in additive solutions have such a small residual volume of plasma that they are the component least likely to cause this. This reaction has been described in all age groups, and thus the same risk exists in children as in adults. Respiratory distress develops with severe hypoxemia, and the chest x-ray shows pulmonary edema, while the patient is not experiencing volume overload or cardiac failure. Fever, chills, and hypotension are often present. The mechanism for the injury and the reason it occurs in the lungs are unclear, but it is believed that complement is activated and that C5a, a granulocyte chemotaxin, recruits leukocytes to the lungs. An animal model has suggested a requirement for complement in the presence of an antigen-antibody reaction.[14] Damage from neutrophil lysosomal enzymes is sustained in the endothelial wall, and this is followed by the entrance of fluid into the alveolar space.

In a review of 36 cases, Popovsky and Moore[15] found that all reactions began within 4 hours of transfusion. All patients required oxygen support, with most needing mechanical ventilation, but 81% made a complete recovery within 4 days. Two patients died, and it was believed that the episode of respiratory distress was a contributing factor. In 89% of the cases, granulocyte antibody or granulocyte and HLA antibodies were found in the donors.

In another series, Popovsky et al[16] discuss five patients from the Mayo Clinic, where leukoagglutinating antibodies were found in the serum of one donor for each patient. Four of the donors had HLA-specific antibodies, and, in three cases, one antibody corresponded to an HLA antigen in the recipient. Three granulocyte-specific antibodies corresponding to recipient granulocyte antigens have been documented in cases of TRALI.[17-19] In one case,[17] investigation showed the donor to be a 44-year-old woman who had had three pregnancies. She had donated 21 prior times, and TRALI had never occurred, even though the frequency of her antibody (NB2) is 32%. There are many women with multiple prior pregnancies in the donor pool, but this type of transfusion reaction is rare. In the above reports, most patients had undergone general anesthesia. The patient who received plasma from the 44-year-old woman discussed above had thrombotic thrombocytopenic purpura and was undergoing plasmapheresis.

The authors in the above study suggest that hypoxic tissue damage makes the patients more susceptible.[17] This theory is important, because it implies that only the sickest patients are susceptible. In these persons, it is likely that respiratory distress would be thought to be part of the underlying illness. Yet, with aggressive support, sometimes including steroids, TRALI is reversible, and lung function can be expected to return completely. Thus, recognition is imperative for successful treatment of this reaction. The above theory is not proven. It is important to think of TRALI in any patient who develops the described symptoms, no matter what the underlying illness is. Once a donor has been found to have an antibody that causes this complication, most blood centers will defer the person as a donor of components containing plasma.

Bacterial Sepsis

Bacterial sepsis is an underestimated cause of transfusion-related morbidity and mortality. The reaction is often attributed to other causes of infection, and, because of the concentration of organisms present or the patient's underlying condition, the reaction may not even be apparent. Normal skin flora such as *Staphylococcus epidermidis,* diphtheroids, and *Micrococcus* and *Sarcina* species[20] are more likely to grow in platelets because they are stored at room temperature. These organisms are gram-positive. Psychrophilic organisms are those that can proliferate at cold temperatures and that when present are a hazard of red cell transfusion, as red cells are kept in refrigerated storage. Examples are *Yersinia enterocolitica* and *Pseudomonas* and *Serratia* species, which are gram-negative. Red cells are a rich energy source for most organisms, and a bag of blood is a well-suited environment for these organisms that can grow in the cold. *Y. enterocolitica* in particular grows better with increasing concentrations of iron. Psychrophilic organisms do not necessarily grow only in the cold; *Pseudomonas* and *Serratia* species can also grow in platelet concentrates. There has even been one case of *Y. enterocolitica* traced to a platelet transfusion.[21]

Bacteria may enter the blood component at any time during its life span from collection to transfusion. The possible sources include incomplete cleansing of the phlebotomy site, contamination of equipment used for collection, asymptomatic infection of the donor, or introduction into the unit during preparation for transfusion. This reaction, like TRALI reactions, can occur in transfusion recipients of any age, including infants and children, because the contamination is specific to the blood component transfused.

The clinical symptoms seen after the transfusion of bacterially contaminated platelets and red cells differ as a result of the type of organisms present in each component. After platelet transfusion, symptoms can vary from none to frank sepsis. There may be a delay of up to 6 hours in onset. Skin organisms can also be implicated in catheter infection, and patients who are receiving platelet transfusions are often neutropenic as well, and thus there may be other potential sites of infection to complicate the diagnosis. Symptoms associated with contaminated red cells are more severe and rapid in onset than those associated with platelet transfusion, because gram-negative organisms produce significant amounts of endotoxin. Fevers greater than 105 F, chills, and rigors are likely. Hypotension may also occur and the patients often rapidly progress to endotoxin-mediated shock.

To confirm a septic reaction, cultures of the blood component and the patient's blood must grow the same organism. A gram-stained smear of the transfused component may be positive, but, if not, sepsis is not ruled out. In febrile reactions, it is important that the remainder of the component be sent to the blood bank, so it can be forwarded for culture, as the original segments from the unit are not adequate for this. During storage, the organism may not have grown to the same concentration as that in the unit, because of the small volume in the segment. It might not always be clear which blood component was responsible if the transfusion was of more than 1 unit, and thus all units would have to be investigated. Treatment includes intravenous antibiotics and appropriate care for endotoxic shock (fluids, vasopressors, etc).

Morrow et al[22] described a series of seven septic reactions, one fatal, that were caused by platelet concentrates. The temperature elevations in the patients were higher than those of FNHTRs, but they took as long as 4 hours to peak. Five of these infections were due to skin flora, and four of the platelet concentrates had been stored for 5 days. Thus, these organisms may need to grow to high concentrations before being able to cause infection. In many situations, the bags have already been discarded by the time this reaction becomes apparent. This contributes to the difficulty of describing these reactions.

Y. enterocolitica can be present in persons with a gastrointestinal illness. Unfortunately, it also can be present in asymptomatic donors. The Centers for Disease Control and Prevention investigated seven patients who developed transfusion- associated *Y. enterocolitica* between 1987 and 1989.[23] All seven had received RBC units, and five died. After an investigation identified the implicated donors, testing for antibody against the specific strain found in each case was performed, and six of the donors had the appropriate serologic findings. Four reported a gastrointestinal illness in the month before donation, and one developed symptoms the day he donated. Two donors denied any illness, but one stated that household members had had a gastrointestinal illness. This organism is a gram-negative endotoxin-producing organism that begins to exhibit logarithmic growth after a lag phase of up to 20 days in RBCs stored at 4 C.[24]

Three cases of *Serratia marcescens* were found in Denmark in 1991, all resulting from RBCs transfused after collection into contaminated blood bags.[25] This organism is a gram-negative bacillus that occurs ubiquitously in soil and water and on plant surfaces. *Serratia liquefaciens*, another gram-negative bacillus, has become increasingly recognized as a cause of transfusion-transmitted sepsis. A recent report of five fatal cases highlights the seriousness of this contaminant. In addition, despite investigation, the source was not found in any of these cases.[26]

Circulatory Overload

Increases in blood volume, which are possible with transfusion of any blood component, may result in circulatory overload, manifesting as dyspnea, a rapid increase in systolic blood pressure, and pulmonary edema. Premature infants and children with pre-existing cardiac disease are the most susceptible of pediatric patients. In premature infants, hypervolemia is linked to the development of systemic patent ductus arteriosus, congestive heart failure,[27] and intraventricular hemorrhage.[28] Neonates are likely to receive small-volume transfusions to replace iatrogenic blood loss. When red cells in additive solutions are used, the advisable transfusion amount is 15 mL per kg of body weight. Transfusions should proceed at a slow rate. Some patients in this age group receive large-volume transfusions, including those undergoing exchange transfusions, extracorporeal membrane oxygenation, or cardiothoracic surgery with cardiac bypass. Careful attention to volume status is essential.

Chronic anemia is often compensated with an increased plasma volume. Chronically anemic patients may experience volume overload if RBCs are transfused too rapidly. Any pediatric patient can experience hypervolemia or polycythemia if the physician ordering the transfusion is not mindful of the size of the patient. Transfusions for small children should be ordered in milliliters rather than units. A range of 10 to 15 mL/kg is appropriate, and the blood bank will make aliquots from complete units.

The concern for volume overload in neonates in the 1980s led to the routine centrifugation of platelet concentrates by many hospitals. This is not necessary for the neonate who receives platelets. Because of improvements in the plastics used for the manufacture of blood bags to allow more oxygen permeability, whole-blood-derived platelets have become more concentrated over the last decade. Most centers produce this component with concentrations of 8 to 9 × 10^{10} platelets in 40 to 50 mL of plasma. Transfusions of 5 to 10 mL/kg will increase the neonate's platelet count by 50,000 to 100,000/μL, which will adequately treat the thrombocytopenia with acceptably small transfusion volumes.[29] In addition, there are risks to further volume-reduction of this component. The platelets may sustain some degree of damage because of the excess manipulation of this fragile component. The procedure delays transfusions because it takes about 2 hours to perform, and, because of the small remaining volume, clinicians may inadvertently increase the number of units requested and actually overtransfuse.

Hypoglycemia in Neonates

Hypoglycemia was described in 1985 as a consequence of transfusion in the neonate.[30] It was recognized that this may occur as a result of the decrease in glucose infusion rate when the dextrose infusion was discontinued to use the existing intravenous line for transfusion. It was also noted that the smallest and most unstable neonates were at greater risk, probably because they are less likely to have a second intravenous site and more likely to be on fluid restrictions. However, hypoglycemia may complicate any neonatal transfusion. This was occasionally seen with fresh frozen plasma, but it more commonly occurred with red cells drawn into the anticoagulant used at that time, CPDA-1.

Today it has become widely accepted that neonatal transfusions can be performed with red cells stored in additive solutions. An additional benefit is that, when these solutions are used, there is a greater final concentration of dextrose in the component. This is described in detail with AS-1.[31] Other additive solutions also will have greater concentrations than CPDA-1 RBCs, but in varying degrees.

Three additive solutions are available: AS-1 (Adsol, Baxter Healthcare Corporation, Deerfield, IL), AS-3 (Nutricel, MedSep Corporation, Covina, CA), and AS-5 (Optisol, Terumo Medical Corporation, Somerset, NJ). They all contain dextrose, and, in addition, some of the dextrose from the primary anticoagulant will end up in the RBC component. For the amount of dextrose in the entire container and the amount of dextrose in a 15-mL aliquot, see Table 21-2. A 15-mL aliquot is the standard dose per kg of body weight. The dextrose concentration in an aliquot will vary depending on the amount of cells in the original unit. In contrast, when CPDA-1 RBCs are used, a 10 mL per kg aliquot would be the standard dose, because the hematocrit is higher. The average concentration of dextrose is 24 mg.

Table 21-2. Dextrose in Red Cells Stored with Additive Solutions

Additive Solution	Dextrose in Fresh Product*	Dextrose in 15-mL Aliquot
AS-1	2361 mg	101-118 mg
AS-3	1422 mg	61-71 mg
AS-5	1061 mg	45-53 mg

*Final product consists of cells, residual primary anticoagulant, and additive solution.

Regardless of the type of red cell component, glucose should be monitored at 30-minute to 1-hour intervals during transfusions. Point-of-care glucose testing is optimal. Glucometers or glucose-measuring strips may be used.

ABO Compatibility and Washing of Components

ABO compatibility in pediatric platelet transfusion can be a source of difficulty. Because of shortages, sometimes the patient's type or a type that is plasma compatible to the patient is not available. In adults, it is common to transfuse a type that is not compatible and have a good clinical result. Infrequently, a single-donor platelet collected from a group O donor with high ABO system antibody titers will cause acute intravascular hemolysis of the patient's red cells when the recipient is group A.[32] Because this is so rare, screening for high anti-A and anti-B titers is not performed before group O single-donor platelets are transfused out of group, and in older children this is usually adequate.

In infants and small children, however, it is possible to see a positive direct antiglobulin test or even hemolysis due to an antibody incompatible with the patient's red cells. The difference is due to the smaller blood volume, which makes the transfused amounts of antibody more significant, even in a donor without high ABO system antibody titers.

If compatible platelets cannot be obtained, it may be necessary to volume-reduce the platelet concentrate by centrifugation, as discussed in the above section on circulatory overload. The reason does not have to do with volume, but the plasma contains the incompatible antibodies, and this is a method to remove them. The time issue and concerns for manipulation of the platelets still exist. The actual patient size and/or age at which incompatible plasma and hemolysis are no longer a major concern has not been identified.

Washing red cells was common to remove white cells before leukocyte reduction filters were available. Because of the switch to additive solutions, when transfusing compatible but not identical red cells, there is not enough plasma present to make it necessary to wash away incompatible antibodies. Washing red cells is rarely performed anymore. It may still be necessary in unusual circumstances, however, such as the case of a large-volume transfusion when only older red cells are available and high levels of potassium may be an issue because of rapid transfusion rates. In exchange transfusion, cardiac procedures, or priming of an extracorporeal membrane oxygenation circuit, if RBCs less than 7 days old are not available, washing to remove potassium is advisable. For a complete discussion of additive solutions and product age in small-volume transfusions, see Chapter 6.

Conclusion

Whereas some adverse reactions to transfusion are similar in character to those seen in adult transfusion medicine, others are less common. It should never be assumed, however, that a specific reaction cannot occur. The transfusionist should always be alert for signs of reaction. Because of the smaller patient size, there may well be a shorter time frame for limiting the adverse effects after transfusion is halted.

It is also important to keep in mind that the literature is not complete for patients of all age groups and for each type of reaction. We still do not have complete knowledge of all of the possible factors that put patients in the different age groups at risk for specific reactions.

References

1. Floss AM, Strauss RG, Goeken N, Knox L. Multiple transfusions fail to provoke antibodies against blood cell antigens in human infants. Transfusion 1986;26:419-22.
2. Mangano MM, Chambers LA, Kruskall MS. Limited efficacy of leukopoor platelets for prevention of febrile transfusion reactions. Am J Clin Pathol 1991;95:733-8.
3. Heddle NM, Klama LN, Griffith L, et al. A prospective study to identify the risk factors associated with acute reactions to platelet and red cell transfusions. Transfusion 1993:33:794-7.
4. Heddle NM, Klama L, Singer J, et al. The role of the plasma from platelet concentrates in transfusion reactions. N Engl J Med 1994;331:625-8.
5. Muylle L, Joos M, Wouters E, et al. Increased tumor necrosis factor α (TNFα), interleukin 1 and interleukin 6 (IL-6) levels in the plasma of

stored platelet concentrates: Relationship between TNFα and IL-6 levels and febrile transfusion reactions. Transfusion 1993;33:195-9.
6. Stack G, Snyder EL. Cytokine generation in stored platelet concentrates. Transfusion 1994;34:20-5.
7. Aye MT, Palmer DS, Giulivi A, Hashemi S. Effect of filtration of platelet concentrates on the accumulation of cytokines and platelet release factors during storage. Transfusion 1995;35:117-24.
8. Stack G, Baril L, Napychank P, Snyder EL. Cytokine generation in stored, white cell-reduced, and bacterially contaminated units of red cells. Transfusion 1995;35:199-203.
9. Federowicz I, Barrett BB, Andersen JW, et al. Characterization of reactions after transfusion of cellular blood components that are white cell reduced before storage. Transfusion 1996;36:21-8.
10. The Trial to Reduce Alloimmunization to Platelets Study Group. Leukocyte reduction and ultraviolet B irradiation of platelets to prevent alloimmunization and refractoriness to platelet transfusions. N Engl J Med 1997;337:1861-9.
11. Russel ARB, Rivers RPA, Davey N. The development of anti-HLA antibodies in multiply transfused preterm infants. Arch Dis Child 1993;68:49-51.
12. Wang-Rodriguez J, Fry E, Fiebig E, et al. Immune response to blood transfusion in very-low-birthweight infants. Transfusion 2000;40:25-34.
13. Mollison PL, Engelfriet CP, Contreras M. Blood transfusion in clinical medicine. 9th ed. London: Blackwell Scientific Publications, 1993: 690-6.
14. Seeger W, Schneider U, Kreusler B, et al. Reproduction of transfusion-related acute lung injury in an ex vivo lung model. Blood 1990;76: 1438-44.
15. Popovsky MA, Moore SB. Diagnostic and pathogenic considerations in transfusion-related acute lung injury. Transfusion 1985;25:573-7.
16. Popovsky MA, Abel MD, Moore SB. Transfusion-related acute lung injury associated with passive transfer of antileukocyte antibodies. Am Rev Respir Dis 1983;128:185-9.
17. Van Buren NL, Stroncek DF, Clay ME, et al. Transfusion-related acute lung injury caused by an NB2 granulocyte-specific antibody in a patient with thrombotic thrombocytopenic purpura. Transfusion 1990;30:42-5.
18. Yomtovian R, Kline W, Press C, et al. Severe pulmonary hypersensitivity associated with passive transfusion of a neutrophil-specific antibody. Lancet 1984;1:244-6.
19. Nordhagen R, Conradi M, Dromtorp S. Pulmonary reaction associated with transfusion of plasma containing anti-5b. Vox Sang 1986;51:102-7.
20. Goldman M, Blajchman MA. Blood product-associated bacterial sepsis. Transfus Med Rev 1991;5:73-83.
21. Kuehnert MJ, Jarvis WR, Schaffer DA, Chaffin DJ. Platelet transfusion reaction due to *Yersinia enterocolitica* (letter). JAMA 1997;278:550.

22. Morrow JF, Braine HG, Kickler TS, et al. Septic reactions to platelet transfusions. JAMA 1991;266:555-8.
23. Tipple MA, Bland LA, Murphy JJ, et al. Sepsis associated with transfusion of red cells contaminated with *Yersinia enterocolitica*. Transfusion 1990;30:207-13.
24. Franzin L, Gioannini P. Growth of *Yersinia* species in artificially contaminated blood bags. Transfusion 1992;32:673-6.
25. Heltberg O, Skov F, Gerner-Smidt P, et al. Nosocomial epidemic of *Serratia marcescens* septicemia ascribed to contaminated blood transfusion bags. Transfusion 1993;33:221-7.
26. Roth VR, Arduino MJ, Nobiletti J, et al. Transfusion-related sepsis due to *Serratia liquefaciens* in the United States. Transfusion 2000;40:931-5.
27. Bell EF, Warburton D, Stonestreet BS, Oh W. Effect of fluid administration on the development of symptomatic patent ductus arteriosus and congestive heart failure in premature infants. N Engl J Med 1980;302: 598-604.
28. Goldberg RN, Chung D, Goldman SL, Bancalari E. The association of rapid volume expansion and intraventricular hemorrhage in the preterm infant. J Pediatr 1980;96:1060-3.
29. Strauss RG, Levy GJ, Sotelo-Avila C, et al. National Survey of Neonatal transfusion practices: II. Blood component therapy. Pediatrics 1993;91: 530-6.
30. MacMahon P, Jones ST, Kovar IZ. Hypoglycemia and blood transfusions in the newborn (letter). Lancet 1985;2:388.
31. Goodstein MH, Locke RG, Wlodarczyk D, et al. Comparison of two preservation solutions for erythrocyte transfusions in newborn infants. J Pediatr 1993;123:7833-8.
32. Larsson LG, Welsh VJ, Ladd DJ. Acute intravascular hemolysis secondary to out-of-group platelet transfusion. Transfusion 2000;40:902-6.

Index

Page references in italics refer to figures or tables

B

C

I

J-K

L

M

N

O

Q-R

S

X-Y